1980   *Sister M. Rozar...*

HUMANIZING HEALTH CARE

HEALTH, MEDICINE, AND SOCIETY:
A WILEY-INTERSCIENCE SERIES

DAVID MECHANIC, Editor

JAN HOWARD, Ph.D.

ANSELM STRAUSS, Ph.D.

VOLUME EDITORS

HUMANIZING

HEALTH CARE

A WILEY-INTERSCIENCE PUBLICATION

JOHN WILEY & SONS

NEW YORK · LONDON · SYDNEY · TORONTO

Library of Congress Cataloging in Publication Data:

Main entry under title:

Humanizing health care.

   (Health, medicine, and society)

   "A Wiley-Interscience publication."

   "Early drafts of most of the papers were presented
at the National Symposium on Humanizing Health
Care, held December 1-2, 1972, in San Francisco."

   Includes bibliographical references and index.

   1. Social medicine—Congresses. 2. Medical
personnel and patient—Congresses. 3. Social
interaction—Congresses. 4. Sick—Psychology—
Congresses. 5. Medical care—United States—Congresses.
I. Howard, Jan. II. Strauss, Anselm L.
III. National Symposium on Humanizing Health Care,
San Francisco, 1972. [DNLM: 1. Health Services—Congresses.
2. Quality health care—Congresses. W84 H918 1972]

RA418.H86   362.1'04'25   75-12874

ISBN 0-471-41658-4

Printed in the United States of America

10 9 8 7 6 5 4 3 2

NOTES ON THE EDITORS

Jan Howard is a research sociologist and lecturer in the School of Medicine at the University of California in San Francisco. She serves on the faculty of the Health Policy Program, the Division of Ambulatory and Community Medicine, and the Hooper Foundation. In addition to studies in humanization of health care, she is engaged in research concerning the epidemiology of breast cancer.

Dr. Howard received her Ph.D. in sociology from Stanford University in 1961. Before joining the faculty at UCSF, she taught and conducted research at Stanford and participated in the Law and Society Center at the University of California in Berkeley, where she explored inequities in civil justice. She is well known for her research and articles on hypertension among blacks, needle sharing among drug shooters of the Haight-Ashbury district, access of the poor to legal representation and justice, and dehumanization in social institutions.

In 1967 Dr. Howard coauthored (with Jerome Carlin and Sheldon Messinger) *Civil Justice and the Poor* for the Russell Sage Foundation. In 1971 she set forth a theoretical model for resisting dehumanization in bureaucratic organizations. Her article "Resisting Institutional Evil from Within" appeared in *Sanctions for Evil*, published by Jossey-Bass. Currently Dr. Howard is completing a series of articles on social-psychological correlates of breast cancer severity at diagnosis. During her "off-hours" Dr. Howard enjoys the beauty and relaxed pace of Los Altos Hills where she lives with her eight-year-old son.

Anselm Strauss is widely known for his research in medical sociology. He helped initiate and chaired the Graduate Program in Sociology at the University of California Medical Center in San Francisco, where he currently teaches both in this program and the School of Nursing. After receiving his Ph.D. from the University of Chicago in 1945 he taught sociology at Indiana University and later at the University of Chicago. From 1958 to 1960 he headed the social science laboratory at the Institute for Psychosomatic Medicine and Psychiatry, Michael Reese Hospital, Chicago.

Professor Strauss has written many books and articles in the field of health and illness. They include *Psychiatric Ideologies and Institutions* (coauthored with others); *Awareness of Dying* and *Time for Dying* (coauthored with Barney Glaser); and *Where Medicine Fails* (which he edited). In press are *Nurses at Work* (which he coedited) and a volume on chronic disease.

At present Dr. Strauss is especially interested in studies of chronic illness and organizational and interactional aspects of pain management in hospitals. A city dweller by birth and temperament, he lives in the heart of San Francisco.

PREFACE

This book is the intellectual product of a large number of practicing health professionals and behavioral scientists representing more than a dozen disciplines. Early drafts of most of the papers were presented at the national symposium on Humanizing Health Care, held December 1–2, 1972, in San Francisco. Approximately 40 persons participated in the symposium. When the papers were being revised for publication in this volume, several additional articles pertaining to research issues were solicited by the editors.

David Mechanic's introduction underscores the importance of the central theme, places it appropriately in the larger social context, and sets the stage for chapters to follow. We begin with Jack Geiger's perceptive discussion of "The Causes of Dehumanization in Health Care and Prospects for Humanization." Dr. Geiger, a physician by training, is especially known for his vanguard contributions to community medicine. The two commentators on his paper are Rashi Fein, an economist, and Price Cobbs, a psychiatrist.

Part II, which focuses on Jan Howard's article, "Humanization and Dehumanization of Health Care: A Conceptual View," is more theoretically oriented. In a review and analysis of relevant literature, Dr. Howard considers the state of the art and provides her own conceptual scheme from a sociologist's perspective. Robert Cooke, a pediatrician, and Eugene Feingold, a political scientist, offer comments.

Part III is more empirically grounded. Howard Leventhal, a social psychologist, presents an information-processing model of the causes and consequences of self-depersonalization and dehumanization during illness and treatment. His model is discussed by Irving Janis, also a social psychologist, and Jeanne Benoliel, a researcher and administrator in nursing.

Part IV focuses on possibilities for cultural and subcultural change toward greater humanism in health services. The major paper, "Adaptation to More Humanizing Forms of Health Care," is the work of Donald Kennedy, an anthropologist. The commentaries are by a social-work researcher, Elliot Studt, and a sociologist, Eliot Freidson.

Part V summarizes pertinent remarks of participants at the symposium. Following each major presentation and critiques by the two discussants, members of the audience gave their views on the subject at hand. Jan Howard and Carole Tyler organized the material around a number of issues and questions that cross-cut comments regardless of the topic being considered.

Part VI consists of five research perspectives concerning the admittedly complex problems of humanization and dehumanization of care. The authors are Charles Lewis, a research-oriented physician; Clifford Barnett, an anthropologist; Anselm Strauss, a sociologist; Sol Levine, a sociologist; and Roslyn Lindheim, an architect-planner. Their differing research priorities reflect the varied experimental and professional bases of the authors.

In his epilogue, Philip Lee, director of the Health Policy Program at the University of California, San Francisco, looks to the future and weighs the potential implications of national health insurance for humanization and dehumanization of care.

We particularly thank the National Center for Health Services Research and Development for sponsoring the symposium. Sherman Williams, Dennis Webb, and Jere Wysong of the Social Analysis Division provided essential organizational support. We also thank the Carnegie Foundation for subsidizing research efforts of the subcommittee on Humanizing Health Care of the American Sociological Association. This committee was chaired by Jan Howard and helped formulate the task of the conference. The able, generous assistance of Nancy Hill and Patricia Lund, our administrative associates, made it possible for us to coordinate the cooperative endeavor that resulted in this book.

Finally, we express our gratitude to Professor Robert Crede, chairman of the Division of Ambulatory and Community Medicine at UCSF, and

Professor Philip Lee, former Chancellor of UCSF. Doctors Crede and Lee contributed helpful suggestions and preliminary funding until the National Center undertook sponsorship of the symposium. Since the conference, the Division of Ambulatory and Community Medicine and the Health Policy Program have funded Dr. Howard's work on this publication through grants from the Robert Wood Johnson Foundation and the Henry J. Kaiser Family Foundation.

We greatly appreciate the enthusiastic cooperation of all participants in the conference, especially those whose ideas are expressed here. They were willing to tackle a fundamental issue without clear cognitive or empirical guidelines. By so doing they have broken the ground for others. The editors and authors of this book were motivated by more than intellectual curiosity. They combine a deep concern for human dignity with a firm conviction that scientific knowledge enlarges man's capacity to help his fellow man.

JAN HOWARD
ANSELM STRAUSS

*University of California
at San Francisco, April 1975*

CONTENTS

PART VI   RESEARCH ISSUES

HUMANIZING HEALTH CARE

INTRODUCTION

DAVID MECHANIC, PH.D.

With the expansion of medical technology, the accelerated increase in the costs of medical care, and the growing expectation of expanded access to health-care services, the concepts most frequently advocated are efficiency and improved management. More and more we are told that medicine, as a major sector of our economy, must be subjected to the same incentives, controls, and administrative devices that allegedly bring order and efficiency to other sectors. There is no reason to quarrel with improved efficiency and management; we all wish to use our resources wisely and to achieve as much for a given level of expenditure as is humanly possible. But as the terms of reference change to efficiency and management, there has been more than a noticeable lack of concern with medicine as a humane institution and with the motivations and ethics that govern its endeavors.

The working conference on which this book is based attempted to develop carefully the assumptions and ethical bases of medicine as a humane social institution and to consider the implications of these assumptions and perspectives for policy as this nation looks toward national health insurance. The project began jointly between the Medi-

David Mechanic is the John Bascom Professor of Sociology at the University of Wisconsin in Madison.

cal Sociology Section of the American Sociological Association, supported
by the Carnegie Foundation, and the University of California Medical
Center at San Francisco. It was through the encouragement and support
of the Carnegie Foundation—and particularly Margaret Mahoney—that
the effort at the University of California Medical Center was stimulated;
and with the assistance of the Carnegie grant and a grant from the
National Center for Health Services Research and Development, a
diverse and interdisciplinary group was brought together to thrash out
the issues and problems. Sociologists and physicians, administrators and
activists, government officials and theologians all came with different
concerns, diverse views of the world, and varying ideas as to what was
humanizing and dehumanizing about modern medicine.

Although there is a vast literature on the humanization of medical
care, it soon became obvious that the area is in a state of conceptual
chaos. Everyone seems to know what is dehumanizing about health care,
but as one considers various points of view, contradictory and inconsistent
formulations are apparent. The reader can sense the tension as the
participants, trained in different disciplines and committed to different
types of professional activities, came to terms with one another and with
the mandate of the conference to move toward greater clarification of
concepts, further specification of theory, and the formulation of appropriate research questions. There was a general awareness that any fool
can ask a question; the trick is to ask one in a way that allows a useful
answer.

Throughout the conference there was considerable attention to larger
issues and perspectives that have vast influence on how the problem of
humanization is formulated. Is dehumanization of medical care simply
a reflection of the larger culture and utilitarian perspectives of the society
and, if it is, is it possible to intervene effectively? To what extent is dehumanization a product of the perceptual process of being ill, focusing
on one's own symptoms and fears, and lacking consensual validation for
one's feelings and thoughts? Is the supremacy of medical technology—
and the forms of social organization required to support it—inherently
dehumanizing, or can the technology be structured to facilitate compassion and the optimization of human choice? Is humane care and
respect for the dignity of individuals possible as social organizations
strive for efficiency and maximal use of social resources?

The confusion generated about the definition and significance of the concept of humanization makes it abundantly clear that we require a more sophisticated conceptual and theoretical basis from which to attack the issue. We must have a clearer sense of the biological and psychological needs of the sick person and of the roles and functions of medical institutions within the larger social and cultural system. We must also have a clearer view of the motivations and perspectives of both patients and health personnel and the cultural and personal incentives that affect their behavior.

A historical or anthropological view of medicine would make apparent the complexity of the systems of belief and behavior that surround illness. Why, indeed, do human beings seek to assist those who are afflicted, and from what ethical and cultural roots have helping institutions developed? It is evident that medicine as a social institution existed well before it had an effective technology for intervention, and that the mandate for its existence reflected a certain concept of humanity and of ethical and social norms. For most of the history of medicine, *caring* and not cure was the issue, and practitioners mainly functioned to sustain persons in distress, to alleviate pain if they could, and to provide hope. It is essential that we focus on the fact that medicine has important humane as well as technical functions; and despite impressive technical achievements and the elaboration of medical knowledge and technology, caring and the ethical context of medicine are perhaps more important than ever before.

In recent decades, medicine has undergone enormous change. Not only has the scientific basis and technology of medicine developed remarkably; the institutional forms for providing care are in the process of revolution as well. Within the traditional medical model, the contract was between the patient and the practitioner, and the ethical responsibility of the physician was clear even if the reality departed from the norm. But, increasingly, the technology of medicine requires new forms of organization, and the physician's primary responsibility to the patient may come into conflict with the physician's responsibility to the institution, the medical group, the community, and even the future development of medical science and medical education. Medicine now consumes a larger proportion of the gross national product and greater government expenditures than in the past, and government—as well as a variety of other third parties—has greatly elaborated the complexity of the relationship between the patient and helping institutions and has a stake in the way medicine is practiced. Greater complexity of medicine is inevitable, but this makes it even more important that we give special attention to the ethical and humane basis of medical practice and that we develop mechanisms to preserve individual dignity and choice.

The technology of medicine itself confronts society with a variety or new and awesome dilemmas. We have developed the capacity to keep persons alive well beyond the time that their social identities are intact; we have enabled persons with genetic disabilities to survive and have offspring; we have developed techniques, such as amniocentesis, that make possible choices that were inconceivable several decades ago. With a growing proportion of older persons in the population and a changing pattern of morbidity, an increasing proportion of medical resources is used to stave off the consequences of one chronic illness among the aged only to confront another. The point is not that such efforts are unworthy of the investment, as some have argued, since human beings are to reach for whatever possibilities offer some reasonable chance to reduce likely discomfort and to increase functional vitality. It is, rather, that medicine as an activity must consider the human consequences of its activities. Medicine must be more than technically successful; it must have the capacity to provide sustenance, to preserve dignity, and to relieve psychological as well as physical distress.

Many of the dilemmas of medical care are inherent in its emerging organization. As we strive to bring medicine to more people at less cost, we inevitably increase the work load of health personnel and develop organizational forms to expedite their tasks. But the process of meeting some problems brings on others, since it is the harassed and busy health worker who is most likely to attend to the specific task and not to the person. As we seek to reap the benefits from increased knowledge, we have created a highly specialized and elaborate division of labor in carrying out medical efforts. But as specialists attend to their particular roles, continuity and coordination of care frequently suffer. As we look toward the future, we must seek models of care that allow us to take advantage of what we know and what is possible, but we must also develop means to better control the consequences of specialization, fragmentation, routinization, and dehumanization.

Dehumanization is more than a product of individual thoughtlessness or failure of supervision. Its antecedents are inherent in the process of sickness and the organization of medical work itself. Moreover, it is not simply an issue of not caring to do better; instead the problem is that if we choose to do better on some problems we face difficulties in dealing with others. No doubt medicine is more humane when physicians provide patients more time, and feel themselves less hurried and harassed. But what may be humane for the individual who receives care may result in excluding others who need care from opportunities to receive it.

The purpose of this conference was not to lament those instances of dehumanization in medical care and in other life endeavors with which we are all too familiar. The goal was to develop some coherence out of the vagueness that now prevails, to better define what we mean by humanization, and to locate its roots and consequences. It would be naive to anticipate that such a conference could lay to rest competing definitions and formulations, or come to substantial agreement as to the issues of greatest importance. But reading these papers and comments, which encompass various disciplines and contrasting points of view, will stir up in the active reader's mind innumerable research issues and policy questions that, however difficult they may be to appraise and investigate, are too important to the future of medicine and society to be left outside the arenas of policy debate and social research.

PART ONE

CAUSES

David Mechanic's introduction gives us an overview of the problem of dehumanization and identifies some of the causes of this phenomenon. In Chapter 1, Jack Geiger looks more deeply into the question of causes and, through a series of vignettes, tells us what humanization and dehumanization of health care mean to him. In training and experience Dr. Geiger is ideally suited to address the central theme of this section. An M.D., he holds a master's degree in public health, and trained as a postdoctoral research fellow in the Harvard Department of Social Relations. Before he became involved with the health problems of impoverished populations in the United States, he studied and worked in developing nations in Africa and Latin America.

While serving as professor of preventive medicine at Tufts Medical School, Geiger focused his attention on community aspects of health and disease. He was director of two nationally known Office of Economic Opportunity health projects: the Delta-Mississippi Health Center and the Columbia-Point Boston Health Center. More recently Dr. Geiger has been chairman of the Department of Community Medicine at the

State University of New York at Stony Brook. During the academic year 1972-73 he was a visiting professor of medicine at Harvard Medical School. He is now a Professor of Community Medicine at Stony Brook. In 1974 he was the recipient of the first annual Rosenhaus Award of the American Public Health Association for "outstanding contributions to the health of the American people."

Among Dr. Geiger's research interests, the following areas are most relevant: problems of health and poverty, community organization among urban and rural low-income populations, and health and social change. Almost all of Professor Geiger's writings bear on the topic he discusses here. Several recent articles are especially cogent: "Hidden Professional Roles: The Physician as Reactionary, Reformer, Revolutionary," *Soc Policy,* vol. 1, March-April 1971, pp. 24-33; (with S. Bellin) "The Impact of a Neighborhood Health Center on Patients' Behavior and Attitudes Relating to Health Care," *Med Care,* vol. 10, May-June 1972, pp. 224-239; "The New Physician," in *The New Professionals,* edited by R. Gross and P. Osterman, New York: Simon & Schuster, 1972, pp. 95-116; "Health Services in the Concentration Camp: Prospects for the Inner City in the 1970's," in *The Urban Theme in the Seventies,* edited by J. F. Blumstein and E. J. Martin, Nashville: Vanderbilt University Press, 1974, pp. 145-174.

The two commentators on Jack Geiger's paper have diverse academic backgrounds. Rashi Fein is a world renowned medical economist. He is presently professor of the economics of medicine at Harvard University, serving on the faculty in the Department of Preventive and Social Medicine and the Center for Community Health and Medical Care. He is also a member of the faculty of Public Administration in the John Fitzgerald Kennedy School of Government, Harvard University. Dr. Fein is anything but a provincial dollars-and-cents economist. He keeps abreast of developments in the whole field of behavioral science and displays a keen appreciation for the importance of political, sociological, and psychological parameters governing man's actions. His major books and articles include: *Economics of Mental Illness,* New York: Basic Books, 1958; *The Doctor Shortage: An Economic Diagnosis,* Washington, D.C.: Brookings Institution, 1967; (with G. Weber) *Financing Medical Education: An Analysis of Alternative Policies and Mechanisms,* New York: McGraw-Hill, 1971; and "On Measuring Economic Benefits of Health Programmes," in *Medical History and Medical Care,* edited by G.

McLachlan and T. McKeown, London: Oxford University Press, 1971, pp. 179-218.

Price Cobbs is a psychiatrist focusing on the interface between individuals and society. As a black therapist and academician he is particularly interested in the impact of social norms, values, and constraints on the self-definitions and behavior of black patients. His concerns are not parochial, however. Dr. Cobbs is a student of power, victims, and victimizers whatever their social and personal attributes. Although he recognizes and condemns the effects of persecution, he adopts a positive approach to change. As a member of the clinical faculty of the University of California at San Francisco he has been instrumental in organizing black-white groups to improve communication and reduce racial tension among employees from different ranks and ethnic backgrounds.

Dr. Cobbs practices psychiatry in San Francisco and conducts ethnotherapy training sessions throughout the United States. His major publications include: (with W. Grier) *Black Rage*, New York: Basic Books, 1968; (with W. Grier) *The Jesus Bag*, New York: McGraw-Hill, 1971; "White Mis-Education of the Black Experience," *The Counseling Psychologist*, vol. 2, February 1970, pp. 23-27; and "Ethnotherapy in Groups," in *New Perspectives on Encounter Groups*, edited by L. N. Solomon and B. Berzon, San Francisco: Jossey-Bass, 1972.

CHAPTER ONE

THE CAUSES OF DEHUMANIZATION IN HEALTH CARE AND PROSPECTS FOR HUMANIZATION

H. JACK GEIGER, M.D.

The practice of medicine, and in a larger sense the social provision of mechanisms for the protection of the healthy and the care of the sick, is an intrinsically human enterprise. It exists in one form or another in every human society and culture, everywhere on earth. It is, simultaneously, an increasingly dehumanized process.

The recognition of this paradox, this uncomfortable conflict, is what gives us concern: we are simply less willing to accept dehumanization in health care than in public transportation, for example. All of the contributors to this book presumably share this discomfort, and all of us presumably favor humanization and oppose dehumanization, however we define these terms.

To ask a physician to discuss the causes of humanization and dehumanization, however, is certainly to risk some biases and perhaps to express some. Physicians almost inevitably talk from their own particular platform of "professional" experience, beginning with their own social class background, going on to their medical education and training—their socialization into the tacit rules and values of the profession as well as its manifest technical content and skills—and continuing in their experience with patients, with the health-care system, and with the rest of the society. Every step of the process is a biasing one. To that extent, since I am a physician, my view of humanization and dehumanization in health care is unlikely to be the same as the social scientist's, the nurse's, or the orderly's. It is even less likely to resemble the view of the patient or the sick person who cannot even obtain health care and become a patient. The decision to ask a physician to discuss dehumanization therefore may express biases I can only guess at: the belief that doctors are the major cause of dehumanization, for example, or the idea that they are the best instruments for change.

In any case, in addition to specific professional experiences, I have particular political views and social values, as well as some personal experiences that helped me to resist my socialization as a professional. To help identify and articulate these biases, I think it is important to drop the pretense of value-free objectivity. Therefore, I shall postpone a more formal attempt at analysis, and begin with some personal comments.

When I began the reading, reflecting, and remembering involved in the preparation of this paper, I defined the subject almost entirely as "the causes of dehumanization," omitting the question of humanization. Even now, I am more comfortable defining the task as identifying dehumanization and fighting it, rather than identifying humanization and supporting it. This says something either about my training as a physician, with its massive emphasis on identifying and treating pathology, or about my personal emotional bent toward finding pathology and fighting it, or both. Perhaps it suggests one of the moral and psychological reasons for my eventual decision, and those of many like me, to become a physician and to work in social medicine.

I think it also suggests that many of us in our professional roles would rather objectify our own dehumanizing impulses toward other people and deal with them as an external evil called dehumanization than struggle with the uncomfortable task of fully defining humanization and accepting our own humanity. One recalls, for example, how many northern white liberals found it easier to go freedom fighting in the "evil" South than to deal with their own racism. Indeed, I believe this preference for externalizing threatening impulses may be an important part of self-selection for the helping professions and of the very process of professionalization.

The second comment is that my views and feelings about dehumanization in health care were shaped not only by formal study and experience but also by some personal, even intensely emotional events—precisely the kind of material that is avoided in most academic presentations. They seem to me, in retrospect, to be crucial experiences in this regard, and so I begin with them.

The first of these crucial experiences occurred when I was an intern on the Harvard medical service at Boston City Hospital. In the eighth month of my internship, I had the good fortune, as I now see it, to become seriously ill. I had to be hospitalized, suddenly and urgently, *on my own ward*. In the space of only an hour or two, I went from apparent health and well-being to pain, disability, and fear, and from staff to inmate in a total institution. At one moment I was a physician: elite, technically skilled, vested with authority, wielding power over others, affectively neutral. The next moment I was a patient: dependent, anxious, sanctioned in illness only if I was cooperative. A protected dependency and the promise of effective technical help were mine—if I accepted a considerable degree of psychological and social servitude.

Like the subjects of Goffman's observations,[1] I underwent some of what he calls "mortification procedures," and they were particularly acute: from civilian clothes to hospital johnny is bad enough, but from hospital whites to hospital johnny is worse. I also experienced the medical equivalent of Goffman's moral career of the mental patient, for my diagnosis proved difficult. It started as a suspected coronary insufficiency, and my reaction was real fear. When the necessary organic and biochemical indicators did not appear, I worried that I would be classified as a "crock,"* and I felt outraged indignation and defensiveness. At last it was confirmed that I had viral pericarditis. My reaction was vast relief. To survive with minimal dehumanization in a teaching hospital, there is nothing better than a moderately serious, reasonably benign, incontrovertibly organic illness with a good prognosis and just enough rarity to interest the physician.

---

* "Crock" is a derogatory term used by some physicians to describe patients who do not present clear-cut symptoms of an organic disease, who are suspected of having only neurotic anxiety—and who do not gratify the physician.

Of course, my transition was not complete. Everyone was aware of my special status. I even got the only private room on the ward, a symbolic gesture that I have long suspected was not so much for my benefit (after all, I *knew* that it was the isolation room, most recently inhabited by a patient suspected of tuberculosis, since I had put him there) as for the unconscious benefit of the rest of the staff. Had I been put among the other patients, the permeability of role and status barriers might have been too clear, and they might have perceived too directly the message that members of the physician caste were mortal, after all.

Nonetheless, I was there long enough to learn something of life on the other side. I experienced some of the humility enforced by pain and illness, some of the humility required by the system, and some of the distinctions between them. I learned the daily feeding, cleaning, watering, and medicating routines on the ward. I learned the meaning of sounds: the ebb and flow of the shifts, new admissions, crises, deaths. I suffered the patient's eye view of full-scale ward rounds.

Despite my friendships and collegial relationships with other interns and residents, I learned that the most personal care, and the attention most related to my physical comfort and my emotional needs, came from the ward aides and orderlies. My room was opposite the ward kitchen, their main work place, and so I had a chance to watch and listen. Gradually it became clear to me that their experience of the ward, and their perceptions of it, differed enormously not only from my own as a patient, but also from what mine had been as an intern. The aides were excluded from the professional work team and the central curative work of the ward. By and large, they were denied the opportunity either to contribute to it their knowledge of the patients or to learn from it in any structured way.

In a sense, they dealt with two kinds of patient "scut work" whose juxtaposition could not be accidental: with a selected set of physiological processes (eating, vomiting, urinating, and defecating) and with interpersonal and emotional needs. I am not contrasting their work with the manifest attitudes of other workers such as nurses and doctors; some of the latter were genuinely concerned about the personal and emotional needs of patients, but even they spent far less time than the aides at this aspect of patient care. Neither do I mean to sentimentalize or glorify the aides' functions. If I *had* to choose between having my illness accurately diagnosed and competently treated or having my emotional needs as a patient filled, I would choose the former every time. Perhaps no choice was demanded; clearly, there was a division of labor for these functions, but this major aspect of work performance by the aides was neither recognized nor given dignity.

I was back working on that ward as a physician in six weeks, but it never looked quite the same to me as it had before my illness. What else emerged from this experience? Although I tried, I found that it was really impossible to maintain affective neutrality or detached concern about myself as a patient, and somewhere in that realization was the glimmering of the idea that the detached concern I manifested as a physician about my patients might not be as detached as I had thought.

Finally, I learned what I believe is the real reason why physicians make notoriously terrible patients. It is not primarily that their technical knowledge enables them to imagine the worst, mistrust the encouraging, hypothesize all dangerous alternatives, and criticize all decisions and techniques, although we do all of that. It is because surrendering the professional, controlling, and elite role is so painful, so damaging to the sense of self into which the professional role has been deeply incorporated, and so ego-damaging. And that means that some of the changes we discuss in this book may be particularly difficult to accomplish, for many physicians will see them—however irrationally—as deeply threatening, for reasons they may be unwilling or even unable to articulate.

The second crucial experience, really two experiences, occurred when I had the opportunity as a medical student to live and work in a non-Western culture for a considerable period. The first was one full day I spent with a Zulu nyanga (a kind of diagnostician) and her patients in the company of a gifted Western physician who understood and respected what she did. I had the chance to see that healing—attempting to deal with both physical and emotional problems—could be approached in ways radically different from the one I had been learning back in Cleveland, Ohio. There were other ways to be a healer, and there were other kinds of relationships between healer and client than the one into which I was being socialized. A few weeks later I learned that there were other ways to be a patient.

I was standing at sunset in the courtyard of a place called McCord's

Zulu Hospital, an institution of about 200 beds in Durban, South Africa. The wards and balconies opened onto a courtyard filled with flowering trees and warm subtropical air. Suddenly a single soprano voice soared from one of the wards, wavered, was joined and sustained by a chorus of women's voices, and rose again. After a moment, a great deep harmonic counterpart swelled; the men's wards had joined in. And for the next 10 minutes, the whole hospital sang. Someone translated for me. The Zulu song was about the pain of being ill, the loneliness and fear of being in the hospital, and the goodness of being with the people—other patients —for sharing and support. Every day at twilight, I learned, the whole hospital sang—all the patients and some of the staff. It was a profoundly moving experience.

At intervals since, I have tried to imagine patients so sustaining themselves in a hospital in Boston. I cannot. The problem is not just that our culture does not provide the resources for this feeling of being together and sharing a painful experience. If it did happen—if there were this spontaneous, unsupervised collective patient action, not controlled or directed by staff—I wonder: would the professionals panic?

Finally, I remember one day in 1965 in Selma, Alabama, just after a mob of white "sheriff's deputies" had savagely beaten black civil rights protesters on the Edmund Pettus Bridge. Although few of us there that day knew it, that was the start of two weeks of confrontation between the Alabama white power structure and blacks and civil rights workers led by Martin Luther King—a confrontation that became a kind of existential crisis for many white Americans who came by the thousands from across the nation to join the protest. (Many of the same whites would be on the other side of the fence less than five years later when the battleground had shifted to their own cities in the north and blacks had taken militant control of the movement.)

On that day in Selma, an 11-year-old black girl was brought to our improvised first-aid station for help. She was not sure whether she had been hit by a horse's hoof or by a deputy's club, and it hardly mattered; she had a hot, swollen, and painful knee. Training and routine carried me through the processes of history and examination, treatment, and bandaging, but as I worked I was seized with the most intense feeling that these technical skills were deeply irrelevant to the real damage. Furthermore, I had a sense that all the affective support I might offer, all the concern, kindness, or respect I might express within the confines of the "physician-patient relationship" were equally irrelevant or, even worse, further damaging. I was white and a professional; she was black and a patient. Another dose of dependence and status inequality, and across racial lines to boot, did not seem to be the right prescription for Selma, no matter how worthy my motives.

There was little in my professional medical training, or within the usual *professional* behaviors, that pointed the way toward being human in this situation, that is, toward giving full recognition to the girl's humanity. (The black power movement, as a way of saying that such recognition is not to be "given" but must be asserted and won, had not yet flowered.) Both the girl and her knee needed care. My training to deal with the knee was excellent; my training to deal with the inter-personal dynamics was fair. But my preparation for understanding the social, racial, and political context—which were not context but the very core of the pathology afflicting this girl—had to come entirely from sources outside my professional training.

Later, planning a health center in Mississippi, I had to be reminded by people that what they saw as most relevant to their health was not medical care but food, jobs, cash income, basic housing, shoes and clothing, clean water, and the right to vote. Once again it seemed clear that profes-sional training had blinded some of us to all except the most abstract recognition of human needs if those needs were not precisely congruent with the specific technical skills we had to offer and could not be met in ways consonant with our usual modes of self-gratification.

In addition to clarifying the platform of experiences and personal values on which "formal" discussion really stands, I feel that these ex-periences point the way toward any reasonable analysis of the sources of humanization and dehumanization. They all deal, in one way or another, with what I consider are the four major origins of humanizing and dehumanizing phenomena in health care:

1. Sources in the social order—the general society with its culture, values, and institutions.

2. Sources in our Western rational science, our consequent view of man, our technology, and our consequent development of large and complex systems.

3. Sources in the subculture, values, institutions, and organizations of the health professions, particularly of physicians.

4. Sources in political movements and organizations attempting to defend—or change—the health care system.

Before turning to these categories, there are problems of definition and quantification. Howard[2] suggests eight components of humanization, of which six seem to me to be relevant here: recognition of inherent worth, the uniqueness of the individual, the wholeness of person, freedom of action, equality of status, and shared decision-making between patient and practitioner. In place of her categories of relationships (1-1 and 1-n versus n-1 and n-n) I substitute what I believe to be most patients' perception of duality: those instances of humanization (or more likely dehumanization) that they perceive as directed toward them personally and those that they perceive as aspects of the system, impersonally directed toward everyone although, of course, affecting them as patients.

Quantification is an even more difficult problem. I know of no specific data to support my opening statement that there is greater dehumanization in health care now than in the past. Innumerable survey research and interview studies, from Koos[3] to Freidson,[4] have dealt with one or several of the components mentioned above, or with broader rubrics like "patient satisfaction." Fewer have dealt with humanization and dehumanization as such. Furthermore, concepts like "uniqueness of the individual" or "equality of status" may have very different meanings to different cultural, racial, or social class groups, or in different medical care settings. A black patient who is required to wait an hour to see a physician may view the experience quite differently if the physician is black or white, or if it occurs in a private office or an outpatient department.

It is not clear, therefore, to what extent questions like "Do you think the doctors at ——— care about you as a person?" denote humanization or dehumanization. Similarly, one cannot be certain of the humanization or dehumanization content of categories like "patient satisfaction," which may reflect satisfaction with costs, treatment outcomes, technical procedures, or other less personal factors. Despite the work of Cartwright,[5] Field,[6] Paul,[7] Saunders,[8] and others, it is even more difficult to interpret data that might reflect on humanization or dehumanization in other societies or systems of medical care organization, where the terms may have somewhat different meaning.

It would be a desirable undertaking to organize a systematic review of the literature on components or aspects of humanization/dehumanization as both independent and dependent variables in different health care settings, kinds of illness, types of health-worker contact, by social class, race, and so on. Lacking such a review, we can only examine the four broad areas I have mentioned as humanization/dehumanization sources in more general, descriptive, and even speculative ways.

SOURCES IN THE SOCIAL ORDER.   Few societies have made more explicit, central, and prolonged professions of commitment than has the United States to the ideas of inherent human worth, uniqueness of the individual, freedom of action, equality of status, and shared decision-making. Only the "wholeness of person" concept remains vague, perhaps because it is a less political value than the others. These ideas are the central set of our formally espoused values, the dogma of our claim to be a democratic society. They are overtly affirmed over and over again in the use of symbolic documents—the Declaration of Independence, the Constitution and the Bill of Rights, and so on—and they are embodied in our figures of speech, our political mythology, our folktales, and our public rituals. They are part of our earliest socialization, and they are rapidly internalized. Almost all children believe in them, at least for a while, and most adults persist in using them as a formal political reference standard.

Most of us, in fact, do believe that these are our rights as human beings and as citizens—rights to be acknowledged in interpersonal relationships, by government, and by its mediating institutions, including the health-care system. As such, these political concepts are the source of the idea that health care should be egalitarian and humane in the first place, as a matter of right rather than of compassion, and it is these concepts that fuel most attempts to humanize (as well as equalize) health care.

These ideas are only variably embodied in specific law, however, and the interpretation, enforcement, and implementation of law is a social matter—that is, it is skewed and biased to conform to the realities of the existing social order.

That social order is, of course, something else. It is racist, nonegalitarian, characterized by gross maldistributions of power (and therefore of income and opportunity) and, in most respects, exploitative of the many, including the weaker and the deviant, for the benefit of the few. Furthermore, the formal adherence of this social order to the rights of man did not for several centuries seriously interfere with the genocide of native Americans, the enslavement of blacks, the subjugation of women, the enforced labor of children, the disfranchisement of the poor, the exploitation of the immigrant, the capitalist coalescence of economic with political power at home, or the imperialist conquest (whether economic or military) of other peoples abroad. The gap between professed values and the reality of the social order has been maintained by a long tradition of social Darwinism in American popular thought (a process currently summarized by Ryan[9] as "blaming the victim"), and by a long tradition of violence.

These are hardly novel observations—the spectrum from American Dream to American Dilemma to American Myth has been described countless times. The obvious point is that the health-care system, like every other major system or set of institutions, expresses and reflects the general social order. Just as the general social order is, in its formal value statements, one major source of humanizing trends in health care, so it is in its day-to-day functioning and latent values one major source of dehumanization in health care.

And so where everyone is human, but some are less human than others, it is hardly surprising that there is a finely graded hierarchy of dehumanization in health care that operates along racial, social class, and economic lines. The latter are made more intense by the fact that—although everyone has the right to life—the basic human services and necessities essential to support life are treated over most of the spectrum as commodities to be purchased, and therefore to be distributed unequally in accord with the unequal distribution of political power and economic resources. Of course much more is involved than money; there is also access to the health-care marketplace, and the right to unbiased diagnosis and treatment. Studies in every setting—physician's office, group practice, outpatient department, emergency room, general hospital and mental hospital, drug treatment center—have repeatedly shown that race and social class powerfully and irrationally bias diagnosis, rapidity and type of response to the patient's needs, type of treatment, length of treatment, and so on.

As anyone who has worked for long in an emergency room knows, there are even race- and class-determined differences in the response to those who are dead on arrival and in the choice of patients for resuscitation. The purest examples were provided by Hollingshead and Redlich:[10] the lower classes tend to be diagnosed as psychotic, are electroshocked, and are sent to essentially custodial institutions; the middle and upper classes tend to be diagnosed as neurotic, talked to and mildly drugged, and given intensive care. But the counterparts in physical illness are just as real. Since these biases have nothing to do with individual human beings —their real natures or the real nature of their illnesses—they are the very essence of dehumanization.

There is no need, I think, to belabor the point that inherent worth, uniqueness as an individual, wholeness of person, freedom of action, equality of status, and shared decision making are accorded differentially to patients by health workers and the health-care system in accordance with the biases of the rest of the social order. Since extremes can be illustrative, I suggest that:

1. The most humanized health care in the nation is that offered to a white, independently wealthy, U.S. Senator of upper-class family origin, hospitalized for minor surgery at the U.S. Naval Hospital in Bethesda, Maryland, at a time when he is chairman of the Senate committee controlling appropriations for the armed forces.

2. The most dehumanized health care in the nation is that offered to a black, lower social class convicted criminal, perceived as politically "radical" or "militant," with a diagnosis of mental illness, in a so-called hospital for the so-called criminally insane.

3. The health care the rest of us get has a humanization/dehumanization content, quite apart from its technical quality or physical amenities, that falls between these two poles. Where it falls on this scale depends on the clarity with which our race, social class, economic status, and degree of deviance can be determined.

It is important to note that these kinds of dehumanization are not limited to care of the individual patient. They powerfully influence other activities of health workers involving whole populations. Leaving aside other implications of the professional epidemiological phrase, "captive populations," it is no accident that most populations chosen for experimentation and study are lower social class, nonwhite, seen as deviant (e.g., the mentally retarded), institutionalized, or all of the above. It is no accident that the subjects (victims is the more accurate word) of the Tuskegee Study were black Southern sharecroppers.[11]

The treatment of the Tuskegee subjects, in fact, raises an additional point of importance. It is reported that the physicians and nurses conducting the study (after penicillin was available and even long after the value of the arsenicals had been definitively established) attempted to keep their black subjects from seeking treatment at venereal disease clinics by threatening to withdraw the food and cash supplements used as inducements in the experimental program, supplements that, in the Southern cotton plantation economy, represented the only available margin over sheer survival levels. (They also offered free burials in return for permission to conduct autopsies on the untreated syphilitic patients when they died.)[12] Their attempt suggests how far health workers, and the health-care system, not only reflect and express aspects of the general social order, but *work actively to maintain it*. A more recent example is the cooperative involvement of law enforcement and health-care systems in using drug-related diagnoses and treatments to control political and social deviance, and as instruments of intergenerational and racial conflict.

These biases in the social order are not the only causes of dehumanization in health care, and their removal would not totally end dehumanization. Nor of course is the health-care system unique among other major systems or institutions in reflecting them. Most of what has been said here could be said about the school system or about housing. There is one respect, however, in which the health-care system may be particularly vulnerable to a recognition of the gap between our professed humane and egalitarian values and our performance, and therefore more vulnerable to efforts at change. It is widely perceived as working for the sustenance and protection of human life—somehow as being even more involved with the maintenance of life than are food or the money to buy food, on which our record is just as bad—in a society that says, more insistently than many others, that life is priceless.

Yet here we come to some curious paradoxes, contradictions within the general culture. Life is priceless, but health services that may protect, prolong, or save life are treated essentially as commodities for individual purchase rather then as a general social investment, despite the fact that this policy is demonstrably costly both to the individual and to the society. We do, of course, make a wide variety of provisions—some mere tokenism, others more effective—for medical care for the poor and indigent. We maintain the fiction that even those totally without resources can get medical care, and we offer a profusion of school health services, and so on, under government and voluntary auspices. More often, for substantial segments of the population, we force choices between medical care and other essentials of life: food, housing, job income, and so on. And I know that it is still possible, in many rural Southern areas, for indigent blacks *and* poor whites not covered by federal or private third-party mechanisms to be turned away from emergency rooms and physicians' offices, with obvious and urgent life-threatening problems, because they have no money, and to die.

But the economists have shown us that the demand for health services does not behave like other commodity demands. Even if we decided that health services were a social investment, not just a commodity in the individual's economy, we would still be faced—in the presence of massive demands—with this problem: how much health service shall we provide? Which leads to the next paradox. Life may be priceless, but the resources of any society are finite. What is the upper limit, whether expressed as percentage of gross national product or by other indicators, that any Western society can rationally allocate to health care? There is no way to distribute and allocate finite resources to protect against *all* needless death, avoidable disability, or preventable illness; at any given level, what we devote to catastrophic illness reduces what we devote to primary care, and vice versa. And I think it is likely that, at any given level, some dehumanization will persist. Humanized care, responding to such factors as individual uniqueness, may in fact cost more, although I doubt that has been demonstrated.

We tend to deal with this paradox in health and in other fields by making intermittent, nonroutine, expensive symbolic statements as if to reassure ourselves. Periodically, enormous expenditures of money, manpower, and other resources will be made to save a single miner trapped in a shaft, a child trapped in a well, a burn victim, or a hemophiliac. If we cannot meet all legitimate health care demands, and if we cannot eliminate all dehumanization—if, in short, those are not rational or achievable goals—then we can still set as our goal the elimination of *inequality of risk* of inadequate care or dehumanized care.

Even this much will require vast changes in the priorities of our society, although not nearly so much as the task in health care we have most studiously avoided working at and thinking about—to eliminate, or at least equalize the risks of, the causes in the social order of so much ill health: inadequate food, bad housing, sudden crowding, and toxic environments in the work place and the neighborhood. As long as we ignore these, our best efforts at improving medical care, even for those who are now most denied it, will be reminiscent of bringing a few Vietnamese children to the United States for extensive plastic surgery, bone and skin grafts, prostheses, and physical therapy, while continuing to drop bombs and napalm on Vietnam. Aside from the question of our willingness, I believe we know very little (other than what common sense tells us about things like the economies of providing safe water instead of treating cholera) about the economics of investment in health. For example, under any given set of circumstances, does a dollar invested in housing, for example, have a higher yield than a dollar invested in medical care?

There is one other major source of dehumanization in the general social order that powerfully influences health care. This is the problem of maintaining human identity in the urban and particularly in the megalopolitan environment. In 1850, there were 4 cities of the world with more than one million people. In 1950, there were about 100 cities with a million or more population. By 2000—less than a quarter-century away—there will be more than 1,000 cities of this magnitude.[13]

How can a megalopolitan population retain or reorganize values inherent in independent small communities? How can inhabitants create islands of identifiable wholeness in a sea of spreading, anonymous bigness? Is the megalopolitan scale, and the complex systems needed to maintain it, consistent with the dignity of the individual? Or, more specifically for our purposes, with the components of humanization? The intermediaries between nuclear family and the huge, impersonal systems of a megalopolis grow steadily fewer. The great majority of the inhabitants of a megalopolis step straight from their front door into the impersonal, faceless city with no human intermediary. As stress on the nuclear family increases, the basic need for continuity of human relationships with a diversity of others becomes more and more difficult to meet. Ethological studies of sudden crowding and enforced high densities, both in rats and primates, show consequences—to individuals and to social groups—that are strikingly like those in the inner-city slums.[14] In *The Pursuit of Loneliness*, Slater[15] suggested that the attempted middle-class solution of suburban flight leads to a different kind of isolation in which most relationships are discontinuous and abrasive and the sense of community is submerged.

This change in scale is accompanied by centralization, systematization, and computerization. These are processes that usually respond not to the uniqueness of the individual but to some characteristic shared with large numbers of others; not to wholeness of person but to some fragment that is operationally useful for a particular purpose. They offer equality of status only in the sense of a shared anonymity. They limit freedom of action and shared decision making by being inaccessible to communication, and the communication that does exist tends to be unidirectional and stereotyped. And they are, at best, indifferent to the idea of inherent worth. In other words, these processes are (at least in their present forms) intrinsically dehumanizing. Yet they are necessary, and urban (let alone megalopolitan) life could not exist without them.

There is, consequently, a wide and growing urban sense of the increasing dehumanization of everything, not just health care. The remaining urban villagers—East Boston, an Italian community in the city of Boston, is a good example—may have their solo-practice family doctors, but there are only 12 left (most over age 60) for 35,000 people. Residents of the community are more and more likely to end up in the outpatient clinics or wards of Massachusetts General Hospital or Boston City Hospital. The care may be technically better, the treatment outcomes better, the records better, but there is no one who knows you very well or has known you very long. We must also wonder how much real humanized content there is in a 6-minute visit with an exhausted local general practitioner who sees 60 or 80 patients a day, even if the doctor has known you since birth, treated your father and, as is rarely the case, except in television serials, knows what is now going on in your family.

SOURCES IN WESTERN SCIENCE AND TECHNOLOGY.   A second major category of the sources of dehumanization in health care is the view of man provided by Western science, particularly by the advances in the biological sciences over the last hundred years. Although biology has made enormous progress in integration and in understanding the links between seemingly disparate but complexly related phenomena, it has been become increasingly reductionist. We tend to think more about (and know more about) the molecular biology of Hemoglobin C or the impact and mode of action of serum potassium on cardiac contraction than we do about the problem of the relationships between mood and affect, the cerebral cortex, the autonomic nervous system, and cardiovascular events—let alone the relationship of all of these to phenomena outside the skin and the skull, such as the sociopolitical system.

Put another way, biologists and physicians have learned, and learned to use, much more information about the biological substrate—the processes we share with other primates, other mammals, or other forms of life—than about what is uniquely human or related to groups of humans. The result, as we all know, is an overwhelming tendency toward fragmentation and against wholeness of person. In the following quotation, a surgical intern summarizes his observations on evening ward rounds:

> Everybody on ward service was under control. Both hernias were in good condition, already walking; the gastrectomy had taken a full meal; the veins were ready to go home in the morning; one of the hemorrhoids had had a bowel movement.[16]*

Even in his eyes, however, the ward is not entirely populated by this grisly collection of anthropomorphized bits and pieces, remnants and organs. The intern does acknowledge that there are human beings there, although they are still identified not by their humanity but only by their organic pathology:

> My abscess patient, not unreasonably, wanted to know why I had squeezed his fingers, and the edema man asked again about his pills . . .[17]†

Patients, of course, have long known about this attitude. We are all indebted to Erik Erikson for the following excerpt from a commencement address at Harvard Medical School:

> Let me ask first, what is a patient, and answer by telling you one of my favorite stories, undoubtedly known to most of you. An old patient comes to the office and says, "Doctor, my feet hurt, I have headaches, my bowels

---

* Robin Cook, from *The Year of the Intern*. Copyright © 1972 by Robin Cook and reprinted by permission of Harcourt Brace Jovanovich, Inc.
† Robin Cook, from *The Year of the Intern*. Copyright © 1972 by Robin Cook and reprinted by permission of Harcourt Brace Jovanovich, Inc.

are sluggish, my heart pounds. And you know, Doctor, I myself don't feel so good either." As always, there is a Jewish version which throws additional light on the matter. Here the patient says, "das Ganze von mir"—"the whole of me" doesn't feel so good either. In both versions, the patient complains that he has lost the connection between the various parts of him. Tell me, he seems to plead, what is wrong with all of my parts—but tell me in such a way that I myself, the whole of me, the middle of me, can feel "Yes, I understand, and I will help you help me to handle it." This, in fact, is the true meaning of the term "ego": it is the middle that holds us together.[18]*

As both these quotations suggest, reductionist science and technology can be abused to fragment the whole person, deny equality of status, block shared decision making based on intelligible information, and thus limit freedom of action. One has only to examine the processes involved in many efforts to obtain "informed consent" to find examples of all three.

Medical schools, medical sociologists, and humanist physicians have, for decades, attempted to restore the balance without great success. There is nothing automatically dehumanizing about physiology, biochemistry, or pathology, only about some of the ways in which they are used clinically. But teaching about "the whole man" or "comprehensive care" has tended to have much less scientific content, and therefore to be much more exhortative than substantive. For a long time, such teaching seemed to consist of normative prescriptions for tender loving care. It was operationally almost useless—that is, it did little for the student faced with the pragmatic problem of a particular patient with a particular set of symptoms—and, lacking data, it was inconsistent with the general scientific, technological milieu of the teaching hospital.

Furthermore, as I mention in the next section, the curriculum of professional medical education makes it clear that this approach, and this kind of information, is not important. Only recently, with the coalescence of contributions from medical care research, psychiatry, social epidemiology, ecology and environmental concerns, and, most centrally, political interests drawn from outside the usual requirements and content of professional preparation, have some health workers begun to recognize that their humanizing desire to do the patient good may require social and political intervention as well as technical biological intervention.

Another dehumanizing aspect of science and technology has less to do

---

* Erik Erikson, "On Protest and Affirmation." Copyright © 1972 and reprinted from *Harvard Medical Alumni Bulletin*, July-August, 1972.

with the specific content of biological science than with the professional and public attitudes toward science in general. I mean the acceptance of what might be called a "tyranny of technology," the idea that every scientific or technological advance is synonomous with "progress" and must be applied. In medicine, the push for ever-newer clinical technologies may be initiated as much by public demand as by professional interest or by commercial exploitation by pharmaceutical manufacturers or the producers of complex electronic medical equipment.

Often it occurs without adequate prior testing and with little knowledge of cost-benefit ratios. For example, it is not at all clear that massive expenditures on renal dialysis (with an average dialysis patient survival time of about three years) would be as useful as the same expenditure on primary care and primary prevention of renal disease; that expenditures on heart transplantation have the same impact on the health of the population as an equivalent expenditure on other, earlier forms of diagnosis and treatment; or that intensive coronary care units materially affect the survival time of several categories of coronary patients.

In the past decade, resistance to this "tyranny" has increased, along with awareness of environmental concerns and tragedies of the thalidomide type. Our sophistication about unanticipated effects of innovation has also increased. These are, in my view, humanizing trends. They are statements that the tests of technological application must be human and social as well as narrowly "scientific," and that reasonable measurements of effectiveness must be made along several parameters. The substitution of ethical and social concern for half-conscious ideas about the "autonomy" of biological technology can be seen most clearly in the discussions of new biological potentialities such as genetic engineering, human cloning, or *in vitro* fertilization, as well as in the continuing examination of older issues like abortion and euthanasia.

The technological contribution to the development of large, impersonal systems—particularly computerization—has already been mentioned, though again this is not a problem unique to health care. The human experience with such systems often defines them as sharing what Goffman called "the key fact of total institutions": the handling of many human needs by the bureaucratic organization of large blocks of people, regardless of whether this is a necessary or effective means of social organization. The problem in health care, obviously, is not whether or not to have computer systems. Their value is enormous, whether they are simultaneously monitoring and analyzing complex respiratory and cardiac functions during anesthesia, facilitating the transfer of medical histories from one center to another, or making possible third-party payment and billing schemes on a large scale. Instead, the problem is to identify the ways in which, directly or as a side effect, they contribute to dehumanization, and then to provide alternatives for those aspects of their use.

SOURCES IN THE SUBCULTURE AND ORGANIZATION OF THE HEALTH PROFESSION. Health professionals and the institutions and organizations that comprise the health-care system incorporate, as central aspects of structure and performance, both humanizing and dehumanizing elements from the general social order and from the orientations of science and technology. In many ways the physician and the hospital are the embodiment of dominant cultural values. But they also have evolved special characteristics of their own, a discrete subculture and unique methods of organizing and controlling their work and their relationship with clients and with the larger society, which are major sources of humanization/dehumanization.

The first of these is the definition of professionalism itself. Freidson[19] has identified the professions as occupations whose practitioners uniquely define and control their own work. While this may serve (or be invoked to serve) a multiplicity of other purposes—control of professional deviance, quality control, and so on—we are beginning to see the extent to which it can be self-serving for the professional, rather than socially serving. (For example, effective quality control simply does not exist in most of the settings in which medicine is practiced, and its avoidance is a matter of powerful, if tacit, policy.) This aspect of the "professional" is, by definition, a denial of status equality.

In more social terms, it means *nonaccountability*, relative immunity both to patient control and to societal regulation. Erikson has pointed out that there are whole categories of roles, usually dealing with ultimate matters of life and death—priests, doctors, and even the military—to which society gives this relative immunity, extracting in return certain oaths for superior sanction and social loyalty.[20] But if this is not effective, if there is no professional accountability—if not to the individual patient as a status equal, then to extraprofessional societal groupings representing patients as a class—then dehumanization is almost inevitable.

In narrower focus, other aspects of dehumanization may be seen in microcosm in the physician-patient relationship, the patterned content of interaction between two role players that nonetheless exists in and expresses a sociocultural matrix. In Parsons's view,[21] the role relationships are designed to serve the social good. Illness is social deviance, since patients are, by definition, thwarted by their incapacity and unable to perform their normal social roles. Patients legitimate this incapacity by seeking and cooperating with the practitioner, trading dependency for technical intervention, and "trying to get well." Professionals, as agents of social control, require that patients transfer some of their allegiance from the society—the performance of their normal social roles—to them. The deference is usually expressed in the phrase, "Well, you're the doctor!" In return, practitioners offer expertise, technical proficiency, pragmatic efficacy, affective neutrality, universalism—a uniform orientation toward all patients—and functional specificity, or adherence to those things that are strictly "medical."

This model is intrinsically a denial of status equality. Wilson[22] wrote of the patient's role that "to be a patient is to be a man but not quite a man, to be human without the full responsibilities and privileges of humanity." That is beyond status inequality; it is the Patient as Nigger. The status inequality limits shared decision-making, as does the technical orientation of the model. The technical orientation and the universalism militate against wholeness of person and individual uniqueness, respectively, and the whole model at least limits inherent worth by implying that it is greater in health than in illness—that is, that worth is not inherent but achieved. And as Freidson argued at length, the model does not accurately describe what the professional really does, anyway.[23]

This does not mean, I think, that the Parsonian model of the physician-patient relationship reflects an exclusively professional conspiracy of self-interest. Much of the impetus comes from patients, who have been socialized to it from early childhood. For a variety of reasons, they may insist on associating expertise with elitism; and they insist vigorously on a technical orientation. A friend of mine has cleverly turned this shared technical impulse of patient and physician inside out. The one sure way, she insists, to get an absolutely thorough examination from an internist is to present a symptom, and argue heatedly at the outset that the whole thing is psychosomatic, thus at once preempting his diagnostic function and downgrading the relevance of his technical skill. It is then certain, she says, that the internist, jaw clenched and teeth gritted, will leave no stone unturned, no instrument unused, and no organ unpalpated in the effort to find an organic explanation.

We may gain further insight into this, I think, by asking this fascinating question: Why are some occupations professions and others not? I puzzle over this most often in relation to airline pilots. Certainly they make thousands of life-and-death decisions (far more than the physician), they must have a high degree of technical knowledge, they are schooled by experts and must undergo a long process of training and licensing; they are highly paid, better than many physicians, although more as a result of union than of guild actions. On the other hand, they are not ordinarily in a personal relationship with their clients. Their services are only one part of the commodity purchased directly by the consumer. Their relationship with passengers is discontinuous, if indeed a "relationship" exists at all, and although pilots are recognized as an elite there is not necessarily a status inequality (although the pilot, as "captain," has certain controlling and paramilitary powers.)

In short, being an airline pilot is not a profession. The most important difference is in occupational regulation and quality control. It must be done by other pilots. But it is not done by pilots acting as a professional association (like a medical society). It is done by a public agency with at least nominal public (i.e., nonpilot) representation, and by pilots employed by the airline company, whose loyalties presumably are to the company rather than to their pilot-peers. The pilot is not an independent entrepreneur, but neither are many physicians; perhaps the crucial difference is that the institutions and systems of air travel are not organized and dominated by pilots. In any case, there is regular sampling of performance, regular reexamination, and mandatory relicensing, and some pilots are grounded. (The effectiveness of even this kind of quality regulation in achieving airline safety is uncertain. Perhaps the most powerful factor leading to quality control is that the pilot, unlike the physician, is at simultaneous risk.)

Another source of dehumanization is outside the physician-patient relationship itself: the hierarchical ordering of health workers and health-care institutions, and the barriers to upward mobility, which are barriers to communication as well. I have already noted the functional division of labor on the ward, with the assignment of technical functions to professionals and human or personal functions to aides and orderlies.

Information of both types is necessary to humanized care, yet it has been observed repeatedly that where staff stratification is high, communication to and about the patient is decreased, and vice versa.

Finally, I discuss the last major source of dehumanization in health care, which is the training of health professionals. Humanizing impulses are extraordinarily high in medical students just beginning their training. Six or eight years later, at the other end of the training funnel, such impulses are much harder to find. It is not surprising that professional training should be, in part, socialization into these aspects of professional behavior. The curriculum of medical school and teaching hospital makes very clear the primacy of technical orientations, appropriately elitist behavior, and professional control.

The process is facilitated by the sharply skewed selection for professional training. The great majority of medical students are white, male, middle class and upper class in origin, with high family incomes and a high frequency of professional and executive family backgrounds. About 13 percent are the sons or daughters of physicians.[24] Some of the necessary social/professional "learning" thus long precedes formal professional training and, of course, almost every medical student has been a patient, has experienced the physician-patient relationship, and has one or more professional role models. What does not ordinarily get as much attention is the professional and emotional consequence of the dehumanization most professionals-in-training themselves must suffer. The same surgical intern who (not coincidentally) saw his patients as dehumanized organs and diagnoses describes it well:

> Perhaps this is a natural effect of the system, the final result of too much intensity and repression through too many years of training. I had begun to see it in myself. If he wants to get ahead, an intern learns to keep his mouth shut. Later, as a resident, he learns the lesson so well that it becomes internalized. Underneath, however, he is angry much of the time. No matter how cleansing it might have been to tell some guy to stuff it, I never did, and neither did anybody else. Being at the bottom of the totem pole, we naturally aspired to rise higher, and that meant playing the game.
>
> In this game, fear was symbiotic with anger. If anything, the fear portion of it was more complicated. As an intern, you were scared most of the time; at least, I was. At first, like any good little humanist, you were afraid to make a mistake, because it might harm a patient, even take his life. About six months along, however, the patient began to recede, becoming less important as your career went forward. You had by then come to believe that

no intern was likely to suffer a setback because of official disapproval of his practice of medicine, however sloppy or incompetent. What would not be tolerated was criticism of the system. No matter that you were exhausted, or were learning at a snail's pace, if at all, and being exploited in the meantime. If you wanted a good residency—and I wanted one desperately—you just took it without a murmur . . .

Most of us didn't believe in the devil theory of history, or in an extreme notion of original sin, and so we knew that these older men we hated so much must have once been like us. At first idealistic, then angry, and then resigned, they had finally come to be mean as hell. At last the anger and frustration, held in so long, were gushing out in a gorgeous display of self-indulgence. And at whose expense? Who else? The sins of the fathers and grandfathers were visited on us, the sons of the system . . . the wonder of it to me was that any doctors at all came out as whole human beings. Apparently, few did.[25]*

This man is in the fifth year of professional training. His eye is accurate and his description eloquent, but you will notice that his concern for the consequences is selective. For the most part, he sees himself—not the patient—as the most important victim. To that extent he is already, in the worst rather than the best sense of the word, a professional.

SOURCES OF HUMANIZATION IN LIBERAL AND RADICAL HEALTH MOVEMENTS. Others in this book suggest ways to reduce dehumanization in health care. What follows in these remaining comments, then, is not intended as a prescription, although I am sure my own biases will be evident. I believe the intensifying drives, over the past decade, for liberal reform and/or radical change in health care have important consequences for issues of humanization/dehumanization, and I briefly note some of them. They include:

1. The change from dyadic to group relationships, from the patient's relationship with a solo practitioner (or a small group or partnership functionally indistinguishable from solo practice) to a relationship with a group. This is particularly important if the cost is met not by fee-for-service or by health insurance as an actuarial mechanism for funding essentially fee-for-service relationships, but rather by prepayment and

capitation as the expression of a contractual, continuing relationship between patients and a professional group that will be concerned with both their illnesses and their healthy life course. Groups, of course, can be even less personal and more dehumanizing; but they also offer the opportunity for a wider choice of relationships, and they can be held accountable far more easily than can the individual practitioner.

2. The development of a variety of new health careers, including physician surrogates and physician substitutes for some functions, particularly if there is upward mobility within the career ladder. The important *process* here is demystification of professionals and their skills. The important *problem* is to distinguish between expertise and elitism, and to keep the former.

3. The rejection, by a growing number of health professionals, of the concept of illness (particularly mental illness) as social deviance, and the use of professionals, their technical knowledge and skills, and their therapies as agents of social control.

4. The attempt by some health professionals to form alliances with organized groups of health-care consumers—that is, patients and potential patients united by some geographic, racial, class, or political sense of identity—rather than merely with other professionals.

5. The introduction by some health workers of social and political issues as proper matters for their explicit professional concern, particularly where these issues relate not merely to patients but to the inequalities of risk of illness (or possibility of health) in the social order, and the attempt to develop social and political ethics, rather than traditional medical ethics, as one underpinning for professional work.

6. The definition of health care as a right, rather than a marketplace commodity, and the application to health care of ideas of self-determination on the part of traditionally dehumanized groups: nonwhites, the poor, women, prisoners, and homosexuals, among others.

7. Finally, and most importantly, the change that I believe has the greatest potential for humanization of health care: consumer participation, the organization of people to share with (or control) professional activities in the design, regulation, and management of basic human services. This movement accepts some of the enforced dependence of the sick patient on the skilled professional in the physician-patient relationship and the health-care institution; but it helps to *restore the balance* by requiring the professionals also to interact with, and have some

accountability to, organized groups of currently healthy persons whose interest is determined both by their knowledge that they will someday be patients and by their concern for the quality of their own lives. Consumer participation—directly, rather than by mediation through the upper-class groups that control most health-care institutions or the public agencies that turn out to be under effective professional control—can be a way of making the most powerful statements about shared decision making, equality of status, freedom of action, wholeness of person, inherent worth, and even individual uniqueness.

Like all changes, these pose not only new benefits but new dangers. The abandonment of expertise is one. The "humanizing" content of substituting an overriding social ethic for a true professional ethic is another. It depends on the nature of the society; in China the barefoot doctor serving the people is attractive, but in Nazi Germany the physician performing concentration-camp experiments is not. The conflict between human and political priorities is another danger that professionals (and the public) must face more and more as professionals abandon their pretense of nonpolitical objectivity, and such conflicts are inevitable.

Even what is most desirable—the broadening of the professional's public accountability—has its dangers in excess. The physician whose reference group is exclusively the consumer (as it now is almost exclusively their peers) may become a W. C. Fields pitchman, selling extract of ipecac to cure hoarseness. The internal politics of consumer groups could conceivably make political conformity a part of the price of access to health care, just as money, social class, and race are now; and the leadership of such groups is as vulnerable to the distortions of personal self-interest as are professionals.

But all these risks and more, in my view, are clearly justified by the potential gains. These gains, in the last analysis, must be won by forces outside the health professions, for we are unlikely to have more humane health care until we have a reordered society with more humane priorities.

NOTES

1. E. Goffman. "The Characteristics of Total Institutions." In *Symposium on Preventive and Social Psychiatry*, Walter Reed Army Medical Center—National Research Council. Washington, D.C.: U.S. Government Printing Office, 1958, pp. 43-85.

2. See Jan Howard. "Humanization and Dehumanization of Health Care: A Conceptual View," Chapter 2 in this book.

3. E. L. Koos. *The Health of Regionville*. New York: Columbia University Press, 1954.

4. E. Freidson. *Patients' Views of Medical Practice*. New York: Russell Sage Foundation, 1961.

5. A. Cartwright. *Human Relations and Hospital Care*. London: Routledge and Kegan Paul, 1964.

6. M. Field. *Doctor and Patient in Soviet Russia*. Cambridge: Harvard University Press, 1957.

7. B. D. Paul. *Health, Culture and Community*. New York: Russell Sage Foundation, 1955, pp. 460-471.

8. L. Saunders. *Cultural Difference and Medical Care*. New York: Russell Sage Foundation, 1954.

9. W. Ryan. *Blaming the Victim*. New York: Pantheon Books, 1971.

10. A. B. Hollingshead and F. C. Redlich. *Social Class and Mental Illness*. New York: John Wiley & Sons, 1955.

11. *Hospital Tribune*, vol. 6, no. 18, September 18, 1972, p. 1.

12. E. Rivers et al. "Twenty Years of Followup Experience in a Long Range Medical Study." *Public Health Rep*, vol. 68, April 1953, p. 393.

13. G. Bell and J. Tyrwhitt, eds. *Human Identity in the Urban Environment*. Middlesex, England: Penguin Books, 1972, p. 15.

14. J. B. Calhoun. "Population Density and Social Pathology." *Sci. Am*, vol. 206, February 1962, pp. 139-148. J. J. Christian. "The Potential Role of the Adrenal Cortex as Affected by Social Rank and Population Density on Experimental Epidemics." *Am J Epidemiol*, vol. 87, March 1968, pp. 255-264.

15. P. Slater. *The Pursuit of Loneliness*. Boston: Beacon Press, 1970.

16. R. Cook. *The Year of the Intern*. New York: Harcourt Brace Jovanovich, 1972, pp. 191-192.

17. Ibid. p. 192.

18. E. Erickson. "On Protest and Affirmation" *Harv Med Alumni Bull*, vol 46, July-August 1972, pp. 30-32.

19. E. Freidson. *Profession of Medicine*. New York: Dodd, Mead & Company, 1972.

20. E. Erikson. *Op. cit.*, p. 31.

21. T. Parsons. *The Social System*. Glencoe, Ill.: The Free Press, 1951, pp. 428-479.

22. R. N. Wilson. "Patient-Practitioner Relationships." In *Handbook of Medical Sociology*, edited by H. E. Freeman, S. Levine, and L. G. Reeder. Englewood Cliffs, N.J.: Prentice-Hall, 1963, p. 276.

23. E. Freidson. *Op. cit.*, p. 140.

24. A. R. Crocker and L. C. R. Smith. "How Medical Students Finance Their Education: Results of a Survey of Medical and Osteopathic Students, 1967-1968." In *Financing Medical Education*, edited by R. Fein and G. Weber. New York: McGraw-Hill, 1971, p. 103.

25. R. Cook. *Op. cit.*, pp. 189-190.

CHAPTER TWO

A REQUEST FOR PRECISION:

Commentary on Jack Geiger's Causal Analysis

RASHI FEIN, PH.D.

Jack Geiger's beguiling paper was obviously composed by one who truly cares about humanization. Professor Geiger is to be commended for his willingness to tackle a very difficult area, for there are few landmarks in this new and unfamiliar terrain. His contribution represents an attempt to open a subject for discussion.

As I read the paper, I felt that Geiger had sketched a vast mural into which he had inserted a number of asides and highly personal observations. At times I wondered whether the asides added to or detracted from the richness of the mural's argument and central thesis. Because the asides are interesting we may focus on them and miss the central points. It is even possible that this happened to the author and that, as a result, the rigor of the argument is not as highly developed as it might be. Yet perhaps at this stage Geiger had no choice. Perhaps only after future scholars continue to define and refine the subject will we be certain what is essence, what is illustration, and what is interesting but irrelevant.

There are three paths I might take. I will not choose the usual alternative: to present the paper I might have written instead of commenting on the one I have been asked to review. Nor will I go through Geiger's paper section by section, noting areas of agreement and disagreement.

I have done that for myself, and I have a marked-up copy with a number of questions in the margin, a number of exclamation points, a number of X's, and, in the British tradition, an occasional "Here, Here!" In reviewing these marginal notes I find that they fall into categories, that there are some general themes to my line-by-line commentary. I therefore adopt a third alternative and attempt to generalize my comments and reactions. It seems to me that our objectives will be better served by attempting to understand a few general themes than by picking at specific phrases.

Geiger begins with a complex model to explain the variables that cause (or are associated with) dehumanization. He rejects a much simpler model, one with considerable appeal in some Washington circles. He does not say that Americans (or patients) are like children; that if you pamper them you are going to make them soft, spoiled, and, eventually, very weak individuals. Had he said that, life would be much simpler, and we would know what to do: presumably, ask them—tell them?—to stand on their own two feet (which may be as bad medical advice as it is social policy).

In Geiger's view, however, the problem does not derive from the patient. It is the fault of society, the system, the physician, or other health providers. This makes the list of causes much longer, the analysis more complex, and the remedial actions to be taken not quite so clear. That, however, is in the nature of the problem, and Geiger cannot be faulted for finding complexity where it exists. If we live in a complex world, it is all the more important that we attempt to understand each of the interrelated elements.

The major difficulty I had with the paper concerns the lack of definition of dehumanization. We need very badly a more precise idea of the central concept, one that would make possible a more precise description of the problem and thus provide a base of agreement upon which an analytical structure could be erected.

Geiger fails to define the term "dehumanization" sufficiently. As a result, we are not clear as to the "pathology" we face. At times the problem seems to be the system of medical care, a system that provides unequal services to various groups. At times it seems to be the lack of knowledge on the part of consumers, an ignorance that makes them fearful. At times it is the fact that the physician does not know the patient and there is no personal relationship. On other occasions, dehumanization seems to mean the lack of a smile on the face of a health worker or the absence of meaningful contact because the physician is too busy. Further still, we seem to be discussing the quality of medical care or constraints on the total quantity of care that can be delivered. Perhaps it can be argued that dehumanization encompasses all of these elements. But if it does, we cannot speak about the concept in general but instead must speak about a specific component of dehumanization in a particular context.

There are a number of components to the dehumanization process, each of which must be examined separately since each may stem from a different cause. We may, therefore, require a set of different remedies (or, if it exists, such a very general remedy—such "radical" treatment— that it affects all parts, all components). If we do not succeed in isolating the particular characteristic and the particular cause, we will fail to find the needed remedy. We will be at sea and will be tempted to rely on anecdote rather than analysis.

For example, Geiger suggests the need for personalization. Yet he makes clear that he would still feel that the *system* is dehumanized if poor people received poor-quality treatment in distressing surroundings, even though from nurses who provided highly personalized, tender loving care. The converse is also true: high-quality care from dour-faced physicians and irritable nurses is, in Geiger's terms, dehumanizing. But the solution to each of these different problems is likely to be different. Precision—not looseness—of definition is needed.

This vagueness leads to one important contribution, however. It permits Geiger, even at this early stage, to explore problems that come out of the culture and values of society. If the various definitions of dehumanization were made as precise as will ultimately be necessary, Geiger might well be constrained to focus on each one separately and to lose sight of the overall systemic problem. I cannot refrain, however, from noting two places where the broad-brush approach contributes, in my view, to an easy acceptance of language and ideas that may not be helpful.

The first such case involves Geiger's discussion of the "investment" in health and the investment rationale for the provision of health services. If words do mold ideas and, ultimately, actions, the word "investment" may turn out to be incompatible with humanization. The second occasion on which I am troubled occurs when Geiger places significant emphasis on the usefulness of a cost-benefit approach. It should be pointed out that the typical cost-benefit calculation fails to include any empirical estimates of the cost of dehumanization or of the advantages of humanization. Reliance on cost-benefit analysis may be misplaced.

The difficulty that is created when we use the same word—"dehumanization"—to mean many widely different things has unfortunate implications. It leads to further confusion in drawing inferences and conclusions. Thus, for example, Geiger complains, in his recounting of Selma, that "there was little in my professional medical training, or within the usual *professional* behaviors, that pointed the way toward being human in this situation, that is, toward giving full recognition to the girl's humanity." I have some difficulty with the account in general for Geiger does not, in my view, sufficiently answer the question of his role and the issue of the child as an *individual* as contrasted with a *member of a group*.

Given the "hot, swollen, and painful knee" is it really true that—at *that* moment—the "social, racial, and political context . . . were not context but the very core of the pathology"? This is the child seen as group member, a perspective that is important and vital. Yet, I rather think that at the time of the swollen knee the child needed Geiger, not Gunnar Myrdal. Surely, a sensitive Geiger could be, and was, even more helpful than a theorist, and it is in this context that he complains about his *professional* medical training. But should it, does it, require professional training to be human? I doubt it. I hope that is not the case.

Medicine, after all, is not the only dehumanized sector, and in an economy that is more and more service-oriented, one likes to think that humanization can be achieved without having to give every provider of services professional training in being human and fully recognizing the next person's humanity. I do not want to be misunderstood on this point. I am not saying that the issues are not important and that there is no problem. I do note, however, that Geiger found that he behaved "correctly" and that this came from sources outside his professional training. Before concluding that we all need special training, I would prefer to examine the sources that influenced Geiger—and the factors that inhibit others from being human. The solution to the problem may not lie in professional training at all.

Given a precise definition of dehumanization and its various components and an analysis of its origins, I believe we would find it possible to conceive of mechanisms that would cause the system and the people in it to behave "decently." Here we come to an important question. Are we talking about behavior or about attitudes? Is it the process that counts or the motivation? These distinctions are important in the determination of what it is we seek. Are we interested in having physicians love their patients or do we want them to behave as if they loved their patients? Many of us, I suspect, would be satisfied with the latter—and it may be much easier to achieve. We would not really care whether the health workers loved us so long as they behaved as if they loved us, as if they cared. Such behavior can be induced by structuring environments and situations. It is worth noting, too, that there is growing evidence that, in time, behavior can affect attitudes. Thus, we may reap even wider benefits than we now realize from the implementation of mechanisms to change behavior.

We must remember that there is no single or simple solution to the multidimensional problem of dehumanization. Just as dehumanization exists at various levels, so it has various sources. Surely, the sources at "system" level are different from those at "tender loving care" level. It is, therefore useful to ask whether there already exist sectors of the medical-care system that are more humane or more humanized than others, and if that is the case, why is it so? It is worth asking whether there is a relationship between dehumanized behavior and the size (or nature) of the institution in which care is rendered; between dehumanization and the amount of competition and the nature of the market forces in a particular care sector; between dehumanization and a wide variety of other variables of an institutional, structural, economic, and sociological kind. All of these, and more, are research questions. The answers would help illuminate the nature of what Geiger calls the "pathology" and the possible cure. The research agenda is long and the issues important, but this is all the more reason to get on with the job.

My request for precision in definition and for research could, I fear, be interpreted as a delaying tactic. Too often these days the call for more research seems to be motivated by a desire for less action. I do not mean to delay. The problems we are discussing are pressing. They lie at the core of what a good deal of medical care is really all about. My desire for precision and analysis derives from the fact that in its absence we are likely to thrash about, dissipate a good deal of energy, and accomplish relatively little.

I confess that I do have a bias—a belief that we can create situations, environments, and structures that will cause providers of care to behave in certain desirable ways. The answer lies in instituting appropriate rewards for humanistic behavior. I recognize how difficult that may be since health-care systems reflect the values and attitudes of the larger society. But I see more hope here than in trying to change the tacit curriculum of medical schools (desirable as that might be) and teaching people how to be decent and expecting them to remember that when they graduate.

I also have faith in consumers, particularly when they are members of groups and at moments when they are not actually seeking care. They do more to create a humanized health system than all the professionals in all the medical schools given all the time to teach all the right values. Consumers rather than providers will bring change to medical systems. Indeed, they are the ones who will and should define the dehumanization we are examining.

Thus, even in arriving at a definition we have to be extremely careful not to impose on others—the consumers of medical care—the definition that we think they should have. Physicians and even some of us who are not physicians begin at a different starting point—at least in terms of knowledge about the health-care system—and this colors our perspective. In spite of the experiences that Geiger relates, including his experience as a patient, he is not and never will be the typical patient. He has a special characteristic: an M.D. As a result of the knowledge he possesses, he does not have the same fears so many patients have. I doubt that, sensitive as he may be, he can really understand what it is to be a frightened patient. The same comment might apply to a number of us who are social scientists. We may not know medicine, but we know "the system" and, to some degree, how to cope with it. As a result, I doubt that those involved in operating or studying the health system are well qualified to judge what patients want, perhaps not even what patients ought to want.

It is possible—perhaps likely—that we would find a trade off between humanization, with its by-product of patient satisfaction, and satisfaction derived from the quantity or quality of medical care that can be delivered. Let consumers decide these trade-off questions. It is their definition and desires that we must take into account. These may be very different from those that we, as professionals, may hold. Introspection is NOT a sufficiently powerful research methodology.

But definitions and solutions lie in the future and, having called for research, it ill behooves me to speculate instead of analyze. It is, nevertheless, to Geiger's credit that he causes us to speculate. He has many ideas worth grappling with and his enthusiasm carries us along. I hope that we can put this stimulation to good use.

CHAPTER THREE

THE VICTIM'S PERSPECTIVE:

Commentary on Jack Geiger's Causal Analysis

PRICE M. COBBS, M.D.

Jack Geiger has written a stimulating paper that I have read with great interest. Its broad scope and scholarly nature crystallize many thoughts and provoke new questions and concerns. By graciously allowing us to share some of the thinking and feeling processes involved in the preparation of his paper, Dr. Geiger gives us an opportunity to learn more fully the origins of his ideas and concepts. These origins, unfortunately omitted from most presentations in the name of scientific objectivity, are important for understanding another's life work.

In the opening paragraph Jack insightfully states the central historical paradox in the delivery of health care; that is, the practice of medicine is at once an intrinsically human concern and an increasingly dehumanized process. We who contribute to this volume, and our colleagues at large who are responsible for the delivery of health care, return again and again to this paradox.

Without labeling it as such, we confront it daily as we decry our inability to get closer to the motivations, perceptions, and reactions of certain patients. In attempting to protect the healthy and care for the sick we sense a gap, a seemingly unbridgeable chasm and, try as we might, a helplessness envelopes us as we try to close it. In our work most of us seek to be more humane and empathic; yet, the dehumanizing process has been historically relentless and irreversible, and we have few clues as to why.

Perhaps a clue can be found if we focus on several stages or landmarks in the making of a physician. Dr. Geiger's comments prompt me to speculate that doctors may be major causes of dehumanization, or could be forceful instruments for change. If this speculation is accurate, and most of us would probably agree that it is, then at what stage in the making of a physician should we attempt to shape the human product? In my view a crucial landmark occurs somewhere in what has been called "the process of professionalization."

After appropriate initiation rites, students are granted the privilege of wearing a short white coat and are turned loose (under rigorous supervision, of course) to play doctor. They are entreated to auscultate properly and accurately, to know what lab test to order, and how to read an EKG correctly. In bewildering succession there are countless diseases to study, symptoms to remember, and correct diagnoses to make. In all of this hectic activity, wise forbearers and department chairmen feel confident that students will be exposed to most of what they need to know in order to function in a humane fashion.

Any study of the delivery of health care, however, quickly dispels this confidence. Even after acquiring a mountain of useful knowledge and applying it in clinically approved ways, most students lack the personal tools and comprehension of skills that favor humanization. In fact, they may have unlearned humane approaches they once knew. In this important regard we must conclude that the process of professionalization has failed.

However, we should scrutinize this conclusion further. As a psychiatrist I am unwilling to suggest that people who choose medicine as a career have greater potential than others for impersonal and inhuman conduct. Most medical students make the choice at least partially as a result of strivings, perhaps deep and hidden, toward serving and relieving the suffering of fellow human beings. Nevertheless, I do agree with Dr. Geiger about certain biasing factors and how they influence a particular view of the world. In broadening this view we may find the greatest prospects for developing humanization in health care.

Before proceeding with that discussion, there is another important and frequently overlooked dimension to be recognized. As medical curricula and services have become more and more technologically-oriented, medical care has become less and less intrinsically human. To be sure, technological advances have generated exciting breakthroughs, yielding knowledge about the cause and prevention of disease. Even when some advances have been oversold and overpublicized, there remains, on balance, solid evidence of great progress in humanity's fight against disease. But biasing factors have limited our creative thought as to how technology should be used to make medical practice a more intrinsically human concern.

Geiger points this out vividly in relating his dilemma when defining the task of his paper. He found it much easier and more natural to identify and fight dehumanization than to identify and give support to humanization. Without question there is built into our training and experience as deliverers of health care a focus on the identification and treatment of pathology. Equally without question, most of us have a personal bent toward finding and fighting pathology. No doubt this bent plays an important part in the decision to become either a physician or some other worker in the health-care field.

In our search for clues as to the causes of dehumanization, let us now look deeper into this personal bent and, hence, the view of the world of those who deliver health care; those who, for the most part, share many important cultural characteristics, such as social class background, the Puritan ethic, a white skin, scientific reasoning, and the attainment of economic security. These attributes need not be viewed as intrinsically negative. This society, we are constantly reminded, has grown and flourished by adhering to a particular way of life and shared view of the world.

However, according to a central theme in Geiger's paper, our way of life is rapidly changing and our view of the world is frighteningly distorted. Many of the cultural characteristics thought to serve us well in earlier days now seem just so much excess baggage. Where previously those who delivered health care were regarded, by themselves and others, as selfless servants of mankind, the contemporary view of them is, to say the least, less lofty.

Individual patients and organized groups who do not share the cultural characteristics mentioned above have become more vocal, and are demanding changes favoring humanization. Too few professionals, however, understand them and heed their words. Even where those working in health care want to respond, up to now, most changes have been idio-syncratic and haphazard.

Indeed, the gap between the perceptions of the servers and those of the served is ever-widening. What is considered humane to one is con-sidered inhumane by the other. Policies and practices carried out by individuals and institutions and long thought to be beneficial or at least benign to patients now are questioned, challenged, ridiculed, and ig-nored. Even when, as is often true, all concerned are dissatisfied with many of the same issues, such gaps between professionals and patients can result in volatile clashes.

The new approaches and altered mind-sets that might allow for solid change continue to elude us. Too often, what purports to be new and creative only serves in practice to perpetuate dissatisfaction, and what previously worked no longer seems useful. Our dominant cultural char-acteristics have become cultural biases.

When aware and thoughtful practitioners wish fervently to close a gap, their most trusted method in doing so will probably be to retreat into the confines of their experience. Regardless of the breadth of that experience, something would be missed, biases would be perpetuated, and the gap might only widen.

What then, we ask? If our personal experiences and good intentions no longer serve us well, where do we go next? If our curricula, the process of professionalization, and advanced technology all contribute to dehumanization, what then? Given our dissatisfaction with things as they are now, how do we discover and actualize the prospects for humanization?

A logical and illuminating pathway to help us ease this uncomfortable conflict and in the process, better accept our own humanity is readily available. Up to the present, our view of the world and our shared per-sonal and emotional bents have prevented us from either seeing or using this pathway. Very simply we must journey beyond the confines of our own experience. We must break the bonds of cultural bias, chiefly by seeking guidance from people whom we are sworn to serve—people who are, in many ways, quite different from us.

For health professionals to follow this pathway is to accept a moral and psychological imperative, one that dictates the acceptance and utilization of experiences and perceptions of the perennial victims of medical de-humanization. By perennial victims I refer to people of color, the poor, and those deemed social and psychological misfits in this society. In short, those who are and have been fundamentally and unchangeably different from America's norm or, more specifically, America's ideal of what the norm should be.

An analysis of our existing practices in health care might be helpful at this point. Basically, most assumptions and judgments, methodologies, and programs utilized in effecting change and progress in the delivery of care have derived from the "haves," who think up and structure something for the "have-nots." The frame of reference of the "haves" has naturally and inevitably shaped how health-care services should be delivered and how the recipients of such services should receive them.

Even where efforts have been well intentioned, and to be honest, many have, the opinions of those served have rarely been sought; even more rarely have their opinions been regarded. Unfortunately and tragically, the bias inherent in such a frame of reference has served as a major cause of medical dehumanization. Also, the perspective builds failure into much of the research and many of the policies designed to solve problems in delivery systems. Those individuals and groups who are victimized in health care can contribute something of great value in helping us rectify our failure by tilting our cultural bias in a positive direction. We have not seen this because we have not looked.

When groups historically have been victims in other spheres of this society, they have remained victims of the health-care system. They have remained in a state of being acted upon, spoken for, and, in general, disregarded. And when so often these victims have been black, this has provoked a rage directed at the medical establishment no less than at other institutions in our society.

In studying the rage of blacks and their heroic struggle to undo the crippling effects of American racism, I note strivings and stirrings that compel a march to a different drummer. The crucible of history has forced redefinitions of self and group. In their relentless search for an American identity, black people are turning their backs and refusing to be defined by others (whites). Black is now beautiful. Inherent in this powerful reversal is a bias toward humanization. Concepts of health rather than disease are expressed. The frame of reference, indeed the group mind-set, has moved away from feelings of deficiency and formerly accepted labels of cultural deprivation. My hunch is that other oppressed groups will find a similar reversal as they mobilize around common difficulties.

In its entirety and at its best, this trend represents thoughts, feelings, and ideas that, if tapped, will propel us toward new and more effective research, better-designed programs, and more purposively conceived and executed policies. In saying this, I am not advocating a romantic or condescending stance toward those who are different. What is needed is intense personal commitment and rigorous intellectual work by health-care workers that will compel us to use the experiences and incorporate the perceptions of the previously ignored.

And now, a final point about victimization. In defining the concept of ritual mortification, Erving Goffman was referring to persons of victim status who possessed little ability, even after leaving the hospital, to alter the content and quality of their lives. This distinction between long-term and temporary victimization should give us pause. Being thrust temporarily into victim status can certainly help us learn more about the victim's plight and lack of options. In a hospital setting, the change to such status is swift and dramatic and, to the perceptive patient-observer, important learning about its consequences can occur. But we have a special obligation not to confuse this transient state with a permanent one, and thereby fail to understand the powerlessness "no exit" victims feel about changing the conditions of their lives.

To learn about life on the other side—its enforced humiliations and personal outrages, its joys and pleasures—we as health workers must be continually motivated to do so. Only by continuing education will we challenge and change our usual frame of reference and automatically come to think of humanization and health instead of dehumanization and pathology.

Another clue as to how we can support humanization is contained in the poignant incident about the 11-year-old black girl from Selma. It points to something we all need to think deeply about. For all our vaunted technological advances, for all our skill in diagnosing and treating illness, most of us face far more situations than we are aware of where our professional skills are "deeply irrelevant to the real damage."

Therefore, if we are to treat the real damage in many of our patients, we must drop the pretense of clinical neutrality and move to a concept of advocacy. For those who deliver health-care services, a concept of advocacy should mean a commitment to the eradication of adverse influences in the lives of people, adversity beyond the pathology that is seen through a microscope or that responds to antibiotics. For too long, the social and economic system in which our patients live has been ignored. Health professionals have not viewed their obligation as including efforts to alter major inequities in the lives of patients.

Advocacy means that health workers must summon up the courage to challenge the injustices of America. There must be challenges to injustices in income distribution, slavelike conditions of the welfare system, inadequate education, and indecent housing. All of these conditions impinge on the lives of many patients as primary or secondary agents that create, exacerbate, and perpetuate pathology.

In conclusion, I found the excerpt from Erik Erikson's commencement address at the Harvard Medical School quite helpful. Dr. Erikson has provided a working definition of humanization. If dehumanization pertains to a person who has "lost the connection between the various parts of him," then humanization is making connection with parts of ourselves and subsequently with one another. This, above all else, will allow us to drop the barriers of race and class, cultural bias, and the isolation bred by modern technology. In dropping these barriers, we shall find and utilize the prospects for humanization.

PART TWO

CONCEPT

The reader has now been exposed to the idea of dehumanization in health care and has seen how various authors use the concept descriptively. Because humanizing behavior and its antithesis are critical variables in this book—whether the concern is causes, consequences, or modes of change—a systematic analysis of these focal concepts is called for. This is the task of Part II. Jan Howard, who opens the discussion, is a research sociologist and lecturer in the School of Medicine at the University of California, San Francisco. Over the last 10 years Dr. Howard has studied the issue of dehumanization in a number of contexts. Her investigations of hypertension among blacks convinced her that differential access to new forms of therapy resulted in a widening gap between black and white mortality from this disease.

Studies of legal representation and civil justice broadened Dr. Howard's knowledge of the problems that poor people encounter in dealing with our legal system. While conducting this research she also gained an understanding of the politics of confrontation and the impact of civil rights tactics on self-concepts of black participants. More recently Dr. Howard joined an interdisciplinary exploration of social and psychological factors in man's inhumanity to man. The Nazi experience served as a point of departure for analyses of dehumanization in other cultural and bureaucratic settings. As a result of this work Dr. Howard became interested in processes and techniques of resisting depersonalization from within institutions. She focused on selection, socialization, and social control within systems and possible means of countersocialization and countercontrol. Relevant, too, were her studies of the changing professional attitudes of law, medical, and nursing students.

Dr. Howard is currently expanding her research on dehumanization of patients and personnel. She is also engaged in a cooperative investigation of breast cancer among black and white women, exploring factors that affect etiology, morbidity, and survival.

The reader can gain a deeper understanding of Jan Howard's perspective from the following cogent publications: "Race Differences in Hypertension Mortality Trends: Differential Drug Exposure as a Theory," *Milbank Mem Fund Q*, vol. 43, April 1965, pp. 202-218; (with J. E. Carlin) "Legal Representation and Class Justice," *UCLA Law Rev*, vol. 12, January 1965, pp. 381-437; (with J. E. Carlin and S. L. Messinger) *Civil Justice and the Poor: Issues for Sociological Research*, New York: Russell Sage Foundation, 1967; "The Provocation of Violence: A Civil Rights Tactic?", *Dissent*, vol. 13, January-February 1966, pp. 94-99; and (with R. H. Somers) "Resisting Institutional Evil from Within," in *Sanctions for Evil*, edited by N. Sanford and C. Comstock, San Francisco: Jossey-Bass, 1971, pp. 264-289.

Professors Robert Cooke and Eugene Feingold comment on Dr. Howard's paper from divergent viewpoints. Dr. Cooke is a pediatrician well known for his research in biology, his chairmanship of the Department of Pediatrics at Johns Hopkins, and his academic and applied interest in mental retardation. In 1973 Dr. Cooke left Johns Hopkins to become Vice-Chancellor for Health Sciences at the University of Wisconsin in Madison, where he is also a professor of pediatrics. He continues to serve as a senior advisor to the Joseph P. Kennedy, Jr., Foundation (on mental retardation). During recent years Professor Cooke has focused his attention on moral and legal aspects of health, illness, and treatment. Thus, he spent his 1972-73 sabbatical year at Harvard University exploring questions in medical ethics. This interest is evident in his critique of Dr. Howard's paper.

Professor Cooke's most recent publications include: *The Biologic Basis*

CONCEPT 55

of Pediatric Practice, edited by R. Cooke, New York: McGraw-Hill, 1968; "The Child in the Hospital," *Ibid.*, pp. 1683-1685; *The Biosocial Basis of Mental Retardation*, edited by S. F. Osler and R. Cooke, Baltimore: Johns Hopkins University Press, 1965; and "Ethics and Law on Behalf of the Mentally Retarded," *Pediatr Clin North Am*, vol. 20, February 1973, p. 259.

Eugene Feingold received his doctoral degree in political science from Princeton and served as a research fellow in governmental studies at the Brookings Institution. In the mid-1960s he conducted a national study of the administration of antidiscrimination laws in the housing field. With this exception he has dedicated 10 years to health-care research. Dr. Feingold is currently chairman of the Department of Medical Care Organization and Director of the Bureau of Public Health Economics at the University of Michigan School of Public Health.

Professor Feingold's range of theoretical and action-research interests include government policy making, health planning, organization of delivery systems, and health services for the poor. He tempers intellectual speculation with a strong commitment to rigorous methodology. In his comments on Dr. Howard's paper he underscores the need for improving research techniques in studies of human interaction.

The following publications by Dr. Feingold are particularly relevant to the contents of this book: *Medicare: Politics and Policy*, San Francisco: Chandler Publishing Co., 1966; (with M. Taubenhaus) "Physician Response to a Governmental Health Plan: The Saskatchewan Experience," in *Health Services Administration: Policy Cases and the Case Method*, edited by R. Penchansky, Cambridge: Harvard University Press, 1968, pp. 45-81; "A Political Scientist's View of the Neighborhood Health Center as a New Social Institution," *Med Care*, vol. 8, March-April 1970, pp. 108-115; (with S. Bernard) "The Impact of Medicaid," *Wis Law Rev*, vol. 45, May 1970, pp. 726-755; and "Politics of National Health Insurance," in *The Social Welfare Forum 1972*, New York: Columbia University Press, 1972, pp. 48-67.

CHAPTER FOUR

HUMANIZATION AND DEHUMANIZATION OF HEALTH CARE

A Conceptual View

This paper attempts to define and operationalize humanization and dehumanization of health care. In it I discuss the necessity for clarification; describe the use of the terms by laymen and scholars; explore alternative frames of reference for defining the central concepts; and consider various contexts in which the terms apply and possible implications of environmental variation. Finally I suggest some essential ingredients of humanized care and how researchers might determine their presence or absence in particular situations.

THE IMPORTANCE OF PRECISION. The idea of "humanized" or "personalized" care and its antithesis is very familiar to patients, practitioners, administrators, and "impartial" observers. The terms or synonyms are

Carole C. Tyler helped compile the references for this paper.

widely used in professional and lay critiques. Yet those employing these concepts rarely specify their meaning or dimensions. They assume that the words trigger a clear and common frame of reference. They are partly correct. The idea of humanizing health care does call forth certain shared images.

But when one considers research, gut interpretations of depersonalization are inappropriate launching pads. Whether analysts treat humanization as a dependent or as an independent variable, they have to know whether that which they are predicting to or from exists. Further, they need a concept general enough to transcend the wide variety of health-care environments and possibly also sufficiently universal to apply to providers of care as well as to consumers.

If researchers have no clear conception of their focal variable, a myriad of problems will arise, some endemic to fuzzy research and others generated by the particular concept involved. Endemic problems include confounding related but different variables. For example, the time that practitioners spend with patients undoubtedly correlates with humanized treatment, in the sense at least that some minimum contact is necessary for personalized care.[1] But is time merely a catalyst allowing the professional to comprehend the whole patient, show warmth and empathy, and stimulate reciprocal communication, or does "sacrifice" of time itself index humanized interaction? Researchers must spell out the dimensions of personalized treatment so that factors such as time can be catalogued as predictors, end points, or intervening variables.

More specifically relevant to humanized and dehumanized care is the danger of globally equating them with good and evil.[2] If they are not operationally linked to definitive behaviors, cognitions, and feelings, they are likely to have such broad connotations as to be almost useless for research. A caveat is in order. Investigators might conclude that humanization and dehumanization do have global referents such as patient satisfaction,[3] excellence of care,[4] and dignity of man.[5] If this view stems from systematic research, investigators will have some understanding of the different manifestations of the central concept and how they relate to one another. This should help them disentangle causes and effects. If, however, they try to operate with an all-embracing concept without knowing how it is expressed in particular settings and situations, they are likely to be locked in tautologies. By circular reasoning they may conclude, for example, that if bad deeds are being done, bad people must be responsible.

CONCEPTUALIZATION IN THE LITERATURE. "Humanization" and "dehumanization" of care (or substitute terms) have a variety of meanings in the literature. Definitions are seldom set forth,[6] but inferences may be drawn from the larger analytic context. For heuristic purposes relevant materials can be divided into descriptive essays and more scholarly analyses of interactions and environments. The distinction is not clear-cut since case histories, loaded with insights, serve as points of departure for higher-level abstractions,[7] and many scholarly works rely for impact on illustrations.[8]

The descriptive essays are written by novelists, journalists, patients, or health professionals. They appear as books or in newspapers, magazines, and scholarly journals.[9] Occasionally authors wear two hats, for example, those of patient and doctor.[10] Writings in this category are generally critiques of health-care systems or specific situations having universal relevance. The concept of dehumanization or depersonalization symbolizes negative states that patients or professionals experience. Vulnerability and loss of identity in large faceless institutions are stressed: totally dependent patients at the mercy of those who must care for them or keep them out of mischief;[11] salaried professionals who fear punishment if they deviate from rules beyond their control.[12]

Some people are obviously painted as bad guys, running the gambit from money-hungry physicians to "crocks."[13] Who is labeled "bad" depends on the victim's vantage point, that of the medically indigent patient or the overworked practitioner. With rare exceptions[14] critics are reluctant to blame and identify particular culprits. They fault society in general or technological change or the rat race—some impersonal process or bureaucracy against which they feel powerless.[15] The meaning of humanization or dehumanization is often communicated by contrast and juxtaposition: life on the outside versus life on the inside, people who care versus people who couldn't care less, vulnerable victims versus invulnerable victimizers, what could or should be versus what is.[16]

In many essays or case histories the wrongness of the event speaks for itself. The authors try to reach their readers by shocking them and calling out an empathetic response based on identity of experience, sympathy, or fear that "there but for the grace of God go I." Implicit if not explicit is the notion that health-care systems should not replicate the impersonality of the larger culture but should set exemplary standards as humanitarian institutions. When reality suggests that humanism is being subverted by the same profit motives, bureaucratic red tape, and sterile relationships that typify economic and political institutions in our society, the writers express disillusionment or contempt and ask with defiance: must medicine go this route, too?[17]

In the scholarly studies of depersonalization, the theoretical and methodological approaches tend to be more rigorous, with definitive identification of the data base and research techniques. In both the scholarly and descriptive works, the concept of dehumanization appears to have a number of meanings, briefly summarized below.

People as Things ("Thinging"). A common referent of dehumanization is "thinging"—reducing a human to something reproducible like an IBM card. Individuals are transformed into ciphers, the better to administer them.[18] In the process of rationalization people are viewed as constellations of standardized needs and wants that are answerable by standardized units of service. They are quantified into elements the totality of which is no more than the sum of the parts.[19]

Things tend to be viewed as objects of action rather than as subjects. They are done to, not doers. An obvious implication is powerlessness and absence of reciprocity. If things cannot initiate action they cannot maintain themselves and must be directed, manipulated, and supported in life endeavors.[20]

Absence of feeling is another connotation. Humans sense pain, fear, anxiety, love, and hate; but things lack the capacity for subjective experience. The only emotional response associated with things is the affect called out in the initiator of action upon completion of an act toward a thing. Initiators essentially receive their own message. Thus, when people are defined as things, they are perceived as insensitive objects that psychologically, at least, do not exist at all. This obviously influences their treatment.

People as Machines: Dehumanization by Technology. Related to thinging is the idea of machines as substitutes for people and people as extensions of machines. Many types of hardware have replaced human beings in delivering health care. The "carer" may be totally absent while the patient "interacts" with technology and its products (computers, electronic monitors, X rays, etc.).[21]

Because of technological advances and consequent organizational change, patients with acute problems may be viewed as extensions of machines. In intensive care, coronary care, or neonatal units it may be questionable where the person leaves off and a mechanical apparatus begins. Since many of these patients are comatose, heavily sedated, asleep, or irrational, they are more easily perceived as extensions of tubes, respirators, and signaling devices. Professionals responsible for them may spend more time adjusting parts of machines than parts of people.[22]

Analogous to this conception of depersonalization is its use in referring to persons with artificial and transplanted organs. As vital parts of the body are replaced by foreign tissue or inorganic facsimiles, recipients allegedly lose some of their identity and humanness. The more vital the organ, the greater the loss[23]—for donors as well as for recipients.

People as Guinea Pigs: Dehumanization by Experimentation. Dehumanization concepts are frequently used in describing medical research on human beings. Obviously the "doctors of infamy" in concentration camps dehumanized prisoners, treating them as guinea pigs without considering longevity or pain, and totally disregarding humanitarian ethics.[24] However, the Nazi prototype is too extreme for most experimentation. The closest approximations in this country probably occur in involuntary institutions such as prisons and the military where traumatic experiments have been conducted.[25] The Tuskegee syphilis study is another illustration.[26]

Recently, dehumanization has been mentioned in connection with heart transplants,[27] referring to a constellation of attitudes and actions by health professionals: obsession with research and abstractions like "progress" that blind them to negative consequences for patients; use of success criteria contrary to those of the patient, for example, quantity of life versus quality; notions of ultimate good for mankind that supersede present realities; omnipotent behaviors that insulate the scientist from appraisal and reproach; and competition with other experimenters that works to the patient's detriment.[28]

Relevant to human experimentation is the question of informed consent.[29] Supposedly, subjects who are cognizant of all the ramifications of the experiment are more like partners than guinea pigs. The greater their understanding and freedom to opt out, the less probable the charge of dehumanization.

People as Problems.   Many who have studied professionalization have observed that over time health students become problem- rather than person-oriented.[30] In Parsonian language, trainees move toward specificity and away from a diffuse approach to patients,[31] gradually ignoring aspects of the case which they define as professionally irrelevant and sharing only those facets of themselves that bear on the patient's problem. Some investigators have described these changes as dehumanizing, with cynicism increasing and humanitarian idealism decreasing.[32]

The issues of fragmentation and specialization are obviously related. When patients are seen as summations of ad hoc disease entities rather than as whole persons with interrelated or conflicting problems and needs, the focus is narrow, compartmentalized, and disease- rather than person-oriented.[33] Terms like "dehumanizing" are often used to describe specialists, while general practitioners are portrayed as more human.[34]

Some have interpreted this problem versus people focus as a failure in communication between professionals and patients.[35] Health providers control the interactions, concentrating on factors they deem important instead of allowing patients to communicate their perspectives. The absence of reciprocity depersonalizes the patient because the relationship is frozen at the level prescribed by the provider.

People as Lesser People: Dehumanization by Degradation.   A widely used referent of dehumanization is the behavior of health professionals toward "nonpeople," and the actions of consumers toward providers they deem lesser professionals. "Nonpeople" are culturally defined and include ethnic groups; social deviants;[36] the physically, mentally, and economically disabled;[37] the aged;[38] and women.[39] For nationalists and reverse chauvinists, they include whites, gentiles, and men.[40] Professionals or semiprofessionals may also be perceived as lesser beings because of an ascribed characteristic such as sex or failure to achieve maximum training and prestige.[41]

When depersonalization is carried to extremes, the victim's self is "stripped, trimmed, mortified, defaced and otherwise disfigured,"[42] and treatment is laced with malice.[43] This frequently occurs in public "total institutions" for the mentally ill.[44] Under continuous degradation patients gradually become institutionalized, totally accepting the values of the system and merging into a faceless mass that can be easily controlled.

Indignities suffered by outpatients are conceptually related but tend not to destroy the whole self.

It is debatable whether providers of care ever undergo the degree of humiliation experienced by patients. Their position in the social structure may protect the last vestiges of their selves from complete destruction. They certainly become institutionalized and thereby controllable, but dehumanized professionals are not usually portrayed as being as degraded as many groups of patients, such as those confined to mental hospitals.

People as Isolates. The concept of depersonalization frequently signifies physical and psychological isolation or abandonment. Patients are pictured as alone and lonely, embedded among overworked personnel who have neither the time nor desire to speak to them.[45] Mental and geriatric patients are characteristic because of long confinements, involuntary and abrupt disruptions of normal living patterns, and hopeless prognoses.[46] Descriptions of waiting periods in outpatient clinics and private offices also connote abandonment.[47] Substitution of technology for human providers may exacerbate the consumer's sense of detachment. Where patients relate to each other, the milieu is less dehumanizing.

Health professionals themselves may feel isolated. Descriptions of personnel who deal with mental, geriatric, and terminal patients portray relationships devoid of two-way communication.[48] The provider may speak or reach out, but nobody reciprocates. The provider, too, is alone.

Akin to isolation is alienation, although the concept has many connotations besides detachment from other humans.[49]* According to Herbert Gintis, "the root meaning of the verb 'to alienate' is 'to render alien' or, more concretely, 'to separate from' . . . when the structure of society denies you access to life-giving and personally rewarding activities and relationships, you are alienated from your life. Alienation, on the subjective level, means that elements of personal and social life that should be meaningful and integral, become meaningless, fragmented, out of reach, and—if one has an existentialist bent—absurd."[51]†

* Other referents of alienation, such as fragmentation of productive effort (alienation from product),[50] are also relevant to dehumanization in health care and are covered in other sections of this paper.
† Herbert Gintis, "Alienation in Capitalist Society." Copyright © 1972 and reprinted by permission of Herbert Gintis.

Thus, alienated persons are not only isolated from others; they are estranged from themselves. This is perhaps the epitome of dehumanization and the essence of institutionalization.

People as Recipients of Substandard Care.   Dehumanization sometimes refers to substandard medical practice, a lower quality of care than could be provided, given available knowledge and technology. Usually some institution or group is accused of indifference or negligence toward particular patients, and the level of treatment is negatively compared with that enjoyed by others.[52] Specific situations may be described where care was far less than optimal; or the focus may be widespread mistreatment or nontreatment of special groups, with such dehumanizing consequences as higher rates of disabling morbidity, infant mortality, adult deaths, and subtle psychological impairments.[53]

People without Options.   The idea of options and degrees of freedom or its antithesis "powerlessness" is portrayed in many discussions of humanizing and dehumanizing actions toward patients and personnel.[54] Absence of control is also a significant ingredient of alienation. The literature stresses structural rather than psychological causes of helplessness in depersonalizing institutions. People appear to be crushed by hierarchies of power, often arbitrary in application, and rendered impotent by bureaucratic inertia that frustrates attempts to change "evil" norms, behaviors, and values.[55]

People "Interacting" with Icebergs.   A common connotation of depersonalization is coldness and absence of feeling. Related terms such as "dehumanization" may convey negative affect springing more from hate than from neutrality or indifference.

Objective detachment has been identified as a functional attribute of professional status, particularly in the healing arts.[56] Providers of care are admonished to maintain emotional distance commensurate with objective decision-making. And like icebergs, much of themselves remains a mystery to their clients, heightening the coldness of interaction. Emotional restraint may also apply to relations among health professionals, reflecting the social distance that accompanies differential power and prestige. However, detachment may not be applicable to consumers of care. Professionals are supposed to be reserved, but not necessarily their patients.

People in Static, Sterile Environments.   Health planners and architects view dehumanization as failure to respond to comprehensive and changing needs of human beings.[57] Depersonalizing milieus are those that deviate from natural ones and thereby constrict people's freedom, sense of growth, and completeness.

Some researchers stress particular conditions such as pregnancy and attempt to design environments for delivery that permit families to experience the event to its maximum.[58] The goal is to mold medical settings to the needs or assumed needs of the whole patient rather than to force consumer accommodation. A kind of romanticism permeates the literature; the home is portrayed as the ideal model for simulation regardless of its functional or dysfunctional qualities.[59]

Authors look backward in time for prototypes: when babies were born at home, the elderly died at home,[60] and physicians were decentralized in private practices.[61] They argue that today's static and sterile health factories should be scrapped or drastically revamped so providers as well as consumers can relate on a human-to-human level.[62] Where the clock cannot be turned back because the patient's life depends on technology in large-scale institutions, a humanized environment is seen as most approximating the natural world.[63]

A related approach stresses human variability and tries to match health environments with individual capabilities and desires, determined in part by physiological development.[64] If children walk, there should be walking areas; if adolescents need peers, areas should be allocated for peer-group interaction; if the aged want privacy, there should be ways for them to escape the multitude.

Neighborhood health centers have improvised on this theme, recognizing community needs and preferences. Facilities in black areas may stress African art while hippie clinics display psychodelic posters. Multipurpose health theaters may be designed to double as sites for education or recreation.[65]

People Denied Preservation of Life.   A number of scholars believe that
humanized or dehumanized care is a moral question in God's domain.[66]
The dividing line between decisions ordained by God and those in the
human province of debate is fuzzy, but a central dilemma concerns
death and responsibility for preserving life.[67] In the view of some theologians, laymen, and medical personnel, health professionals are obligated to keep people alive by any means possible and are morally forbidden to end the life of any organism defined as human.[68]

Dehumanization refers to acts that terminate life: abortion, euthanasia,
and detachment of respirators. Definitions of life and death vary greatly,
encompassing spiritual and legal as well as biological parameters.[69] Coun-
tergroups argue that it is more unethical to maintain "life" under certain conditions than to let death occur.[70] Their concept of dehumanization is commensurate with physiological pain, economic destruction, or
overwhelming psychological strain.

The moral conflicts associated with life and death may be so soul
shaking that what appears to be inaction substitutes for action. Health
professionals may not turn off the respirator; they may simply elect not
to treat an acute condition such as pneumonia. Their "nonresponse" is
defined by them as humanistic.

To summarize: depersonalized people are viewed as inanimate, un-
feeling objects or machines to be manipulated, experimented upon, fragmented into problems, and treated with detachment. In more extreme
cases they are isolated, alienated, stripped of dignity, and given few if
any opportunities to escape from the static, sterile, degrading environments in which they are enmeshed. Their care is often substandard in
accord with society's perception of their lesser worth.

The last connotation discussed (the taking of life or failure to preserve
it) has a somewhat different meaning, reflecting the theological and ethical approach of scholars concerned with these problems.

MODELS AND REFERENCE POINTS FOR CONCEPTUALIZATION.   In trying to
specify and operationalize the ingredients of humanized care, it is helpful
to have a theoretical frame of reference. Several alternatives are possible.

The first approach is based on the premise that human beings have
certain biological or physiological needs and that humanized behavior is
oriented toward fulfilling those needs, while dehumanizing behavior sub-

verts them. Institutions dedicated to the preservation of life and reduction of suffering are humanitarian from a biological perspective, and the quality of treatment received by patients is a relevant variable.

If one acknowledges that needs can be partly as well as totally filled, we can think of continuums and degrees of humanizing or dehumanizing behavior. In some nursing homes, diets are inadequate according to nutritional standards, or a patient's need for sleep may be continually frustrated by health professionals on rigid schedules, or by other patients. These recipients of care are unable to reach their full human potential because certain biological needs are not being met. Whether this results from actions of specific people or from the workings of systems that seem to be devoid of decision makers is immaterial. The end-product is dehumanization of patients.

Although an exact line between physiological and psychological needs probably does not exist, for heuristic purposes we can designate a second frame of reference based on psychological needs. These could include self-expression, self-respect, affection, sympathy, and social intercourse.[71] They may not be as important as needs for food, water, sleep, and elimination, but people can die psychologically as well as physiologically. The combination of physiological and psychological deprivation was the key to Nazi success in dehumanizing concentration-camp prisoners;[72] and a number of American studies suggest that patients in mental hospitals and custodial institutions undergo similar psychological regression.[73]

Where the scholar's reference system is based on psychological rather than physiological needs, it may be more difficult to measure the presence, absence, or magnitude of depersonalization in given situations because standards for assessing dehumanization in psychological terms are more relativistic, depending to a greater degree on individual or subgroup values than some universal or absolute constellation of needs. The researcher would have to ascertain how patients and health professionals define their situation with respect to depersonalization.[74] This might pose major problems because the investigator could not rely entirely on post facto perspectives since institutionalization (socialization to the norms of an institution) is a process of value change.[75] As individuals become dehumanized they also become desensitized to what is happening to them, and thereby become incapable of objectively evaluating their situation in before-and-after terms.[76]

In addition to models based on physiological and psychological needs, one might set forth a frame of reference based on social parameters, adopting a cultural perspective that defines humanizing and dehumanizing behavior in terms of relevant images of man and relationships among human beings.[77] Here, too, the researcher would be dealing with a relativistic model since humanistic values and views of the rights of man vary greatly over time and cultures.[78] Even in a short time span greater or lesser emphasis may be placed upon individualism versus conformity, equalitarianism versus differentiation, wholeness versus specificity, and rights versus privileges.[79] Scholars who attempt to define the ingredients of humanism at any particular moment will find it difficult if not impossible to free themselves from societal definitions, however independent they they may try to be.

Perhaps there is really no dilemma for students of humanism. Since values and ideologies are relative, they might well accept a sociology of knowledge perspective and not try to transcend the macrocosms and microcosms in which they are embedded. They must, however, acknowledge subgroup variations in social themes and not arbitrarily assume that a particular view is universal. Thus, they must identify their reference groups and randomly or systematically vary them to cover the relevant range.

Under some circumstances researchers may feel they can designate a set of social needs from a humanistic perspective without assessing opinions of particular patients or providers. These researchers might analyze goals of health institutions and attempt to determine what behaviors are functional and dysfunctional for their achievement. At some point, however, they will have to specify whether the goals are humanizing or dehumanizing; and biological and psychological models may not help them differentiate. Thus, they will be forced to rely on an implicit or explicit set of social definitions, which again makes them culture bound.

ENVIRONMENTAL CONTEXTS FOR ANALYSIS. Typically one thinks of human-to-human relationships in one-to-one terms. This perspective characterizes analyses of health-care settings as well as relations in other environments. The rationale is simple. At a minimum, human interaction necessitates two people; and at any given moment a particular person usually communicates with only one other. For health care, the historical prototype of the family doctor who performs a "laying on of hands" is still an idealistic model that influences scholarly as well as lay thinking about provider-consumer relationships.[80]

Much theorizing about professional behavior vis-à-vis clients and patients has been based on a one-to-one conceptual scheme.[81] Where others are deemed relevant to the interaction, they are usually portrayed as silent figures in a larger frame of reference. Thus, in his typology of professional-client relations, Parsons stresses the appropriateness of a specific rather than diffuse focus.[82]

I acknowledge that the 1:1 model can be useful in studying health-care relationships, but it has limitations. Even in the idealized days of the solo practitioner, official providers of care had their helpers (midwives, family members, etc.), and consumers were not always dealt with as single persons divorced from larger milieus in which they functioned. More important is the debatable relevance of the 1:1 model today, with group practice on the rise and aggregated care in the form of HMO's (health maintenance organizations) advocated as the prototype of the future.[83] On the consumer side, we see a proliferation of group therapy, not only for psychiatric patients but also for those with other disabilities in common, such as diabetics and paraplegics.[84]

Furthermore, modern health professionals stress comprehensive and primary care, which enlarges the scope of the *one* on the patient side of the interaction because the patient's whole environment is potentially relevant to the provider's diagnosis and recommendations. Thus, in setting forth the ingredients of humanization I recognize multiple providers and consumers as well as 1:1 relationships. To be parsimonious while still touching all theoretical bases, I take into account four models of interaction between professionals and patients: 1:1, 1:n, n:1, and n:n.

1. The 1:1 model essentially assumes one provider relating to one consumer. Patients as wholes are not necessarily ignored, but are viewed through their own eyes rather than through those of family, friends, or work associates.

2. The 1:n model assumes one provider relating to more than one patient or more than one person representing the patient's perspective. The n has a number of possible connotations: groups of patients with whom the provider interacts simultaneously (e.g., rap sessions and health

education);[85] anomic collectivities of patients who are examined sequentially in the presence of others (e.g., military sick call*); masses of patients to be screened or immunized in prevention programs; family units†
that are treated as gestalts by general or family practitioners;[86] consumer bargaining units represented by designated leaders or ombudsmen; and total populations of n patients (in waiting rooms, homes, and hospitals) for whom particular practitioners feel responsible, forcing them to balance gross patient needs against their own capacities to fulfill them.‡

Given finite time, energy, and skill, providers think in terms of seeing n numbers and types of patients over a given period of time.[87] This might be considered a "greatest good for the greatest number" approach or one that reduces existing and potential patients to common denominators; thus the relevance of n on the consumer side of interactions.

3. The $n:1$ model typifies relationships between at least two providers and one patient. A professional team may simultaneously deal with a patient or see the patient in consecutive or rotating order.[88] Two or more teams may be involved (such as dialysis and transplant groups for end-stage renal-failure patients) with or without integrated decision making between them.[89] Even if various professionals see the patient at the same time, not all may relate directly to the person being treated. In teaching hospitals with sharp status delineations, surgery patients may be fully conscious but not be introduced to residents or interns participating in the procedure.[90]

Group practice also illustrates the $n:1$ model. Some unite varying specialties, but many are expedient associations of professionals with similar training. The n on the practitioner side is a function of replaceability. Patients are never certain which physician they will see or talk with,

---

* In some orthodontists' offices, all patients are treated in a single room with multiple chairs.

† Relatives may be included in the decision-making process regarding alternative regimens.

‡ After this paper was completed, Dr. Mary Lee Ingbar, a medical economist at UCSF, suggested to me the importance of differentiating between time frames in studies of $1:n$, $n:1$, and $n:n$ relationships. The implications of simultaneous treatment of a group of patients might be quite different from sequential treatment of members of that group. In the latter case patients would actually be examined in $1:1$ situations. Analogously, it would be useful to distinguish between those situations in which a team of providers simultaneously examined and questioned a patient and those in which participants in a group practice alternated with one another.

especially on nights and weekends—thus the plural-provider image in the mind of the patient.

Other n:1 patterns might occur in encounter and lay counseling sessions where structures are fluid.[91] Several patients may join the leader in giving diagnostic and therapeutic help to one or more participants, illustrating an n:1 or n:n model. Or "patients" may collectively assume the role of therapist to the leader, paradoxically simulating the n:1 pattern.

4. The n:n model typifies emerging trends in health care. From the most depersonalizing perspective, both n's would represent masses of persons—providers and consumers. But this is hardly the only way of visualizing n:n relationships in delivery systems.

Since I have described models with n's on one or the other side of practitioner-patient interactions, one can readily extrapolate to a number of n:n situations. Families may be assigned to interdisciplinary teams or group practices.[92] Patients may be organized into therapeutic communities and treated by constellations of professionals or lay therapists.[93] Consumers may be massed for screening, immunization, or education and handled by units of health workers. Representatives of both providers and patients may collectively bargain and submit grievances in formal and informal settings; for example, unions may negotiate with employers for health benefits to be offered directly or through intermediaries.

More anomic situations are also possible where consumers resemble alienated masses associated with providers who blend anonymously into systems.[94] Clinic waiting rooms are stuffed with patients, numbered for convenience, and serviced by the next available practitioner. Professionals as well as patients rotate through drop-in clinics with a turnover that smacks of wholesale replaceability. When economic and administrative pressures bear down on providers, a "greatest-good-for-the-greatest-number" philosophy of treatment may essentially mean minimum care for maximum people provided by "professionals" who are unavoidably minimized in the process.

I believe that none of the four models is inherently depersonalizing, although contexts that involve n providers or consumers may present more obstacles than the 1:1 model.

In each ideal type, practitioners and patients are constrained in interaction. In 1:1 situations both parties are governed by role behaviors that reflect societal norms.[95] What appears to be a 1:1 interaction may occur within larger systems, constraining providers as well as consumers.[96] Furthermore, mere equivalence of numbers is no assurance that one is not master and the other slave. Nor in anomic communities is there any guarantee that 1:1 relationships go beyond superficial levels, where each treats the other in terms of stereotypic rather than unique images.

Plural providers could effect a power imbalance dehumanizing to the patient. But this would depend on their behavior. If for whatever reason they devoted themselves selflessly to the patient, more power might lie in the hands of the cared for than in the hands of the carers.[97] With respect to group practice one could argue that rotation among members does not necessarily depersonalize patients. Each provider might grasp enough of the whole patient to prevent fragmentation. If the group norms are humanistic and genuinely implemented, the result could be humanizing in spite of provider replaceability. One can also conceive of crusading endeavors where everyone on the team is so imbued with a missionary spirit that camaraderie pervades the whole and is communicated in no uncertain terms to patients.[98]

When patients themselves become practitioners in peer self-help groups,[99] some of the dehumanizing barriers between providers and consumers may be removed. Because these therapists are really laypersons who are recipients of advice one minute and advisors the next, they are likely to be more humble, less distant, less coldly powerful "experts" than usual practitioners. Analogous are interactions between mothers and their ill children. Behaviors appropriate to role of mother blend with her therapist role, warming her authoritarianism as a provider of care.

In the discussion to follow I suggest a number of necessary and sufficient conditions for humanized care. Their presence or absence is obviously influenced by the context of provider-consumer relations. However, I do not perceive a dehumanization-humanization continuum of probabilities with $n:n$ interactions at one extreme and 1:1 relations at the other. The impetus for cognitions and emotions, and the structure of interactions will differ as more or fewer people are involved. But in my opinion the ingredients of humanization transcend the variety of possible contexts.

THE INGREDIENTS OF HUMANIZED HEALTH CARE. After reviewing much of the literature relevant to personalization of care, analyzing interviews with numerous patients in various settings, and considering the biological, psychological, and sociological frames of reference mentioned earlier, I propose eight necessary and sufficient conditions for humanized health care. For heuristic purposes three can be labeled "ideological," three "structural," and two "affective" or "emotional." Whenever possible I apply the concepts to providers as well as to consumers. However, practitioners and patients are not always governed by the same set of dos and don'ts.

IDEOLOGICAL DIMENSIONS.   When I speak of ideology, I refer to cognitions based on definitions of appropriate behavior in health-care environments.

Inherent Worth.   Human beings are objects of value, to themselves if not to others. Health systems implicitly recognize the inherent worth of individuals by trying to prolong lives, reduce pain, and restore social functioning. The ideal of inherent worth is not universally accepted, however, even by "humanitarian" institutions. Providers of care often define some people as more deserving than others.[100] If the rationale for preferential treatment is based on differential medical need, the concept of inherent worth is not violated. But implicit or explicit in much discrimination is the idea that health care is a privilege rather than a right, and that eligibility is achieved rather than ascribed.[101]

If persons are forced to prove their worth, they are not accepted prima facie as fully human, or such acceptance is not sufficient to guarantee the perquisites inherently deserved. In both cases the burden of proof is dehumanizing. Institutions and practitioners may so select their constituencies that a fair degree of universal acceptance is practiced for those patients, but this is because they constitute a select in-group from which the undesirable have been excluded, voluntarily or involuntarily.[102]

Some patients we interviewed strongly emphasized that medical institutions should treat them with dignity and respect. These were usually people discriminated against in the larger society. A black woman on welfare wanted to be handled "like a paying customer." Another desired to be talked to "like you're people, not like they're high and mighty."

A hippie used free clinics because other doctors treated her like "dirt."[103] Thus, the concept of inherent worth blends with notions of equality.

The idea of ascribed worth also applies to providers. For those on the bottom of the professional totem pole, being viewed as inherently worthy is a vital key to humanized treatment from patients as well as from colleagues.[104]

A fruitful research area concerns the varying perspectives of authorities in health institutions regarding consumer eligibility[105] and the quality of care deemed appropriate for persons of differing statuses. Which providers, if any, feel obligated to accept everyone? What limiting criteria do others impose? Are some people universally discriminated against? Are others always judged worthy of first-class care? What provisions, if any, assure potential patients of being helped somewhere?[106] And what levels of care are considered minimal? Answers to these questions will suggest whether the concept of inherent worth is an empty or a viable ideal.

The frame of reference that presses us to include this variable among the ingredients of humanized care is sociological, reflecting the emergent ideology of health care as a right rather than privilege. This, of course, has implications for the fulfillment of biological and psychological needs as well as socially-induced desires, but the roots of the ideology are specifically cultural.

Irreplaceability. Humans differ from inanimate objects, other animals, and one another. We are unique and irreplaceable. When people are stereotyped and treated in terms of commonalities rather than differences, dehumanization can logically follow. The very concept of *patient* may be depersonalizing; it divests individuals of uniqueness and categorizes them by their position in a particular set of relations.

According to some scholars, the ideal practitioner takes a universalistic stance toward patients, regarding them as equally worthy of available time, skill, and interest.[107] If the practitioner differentiates, the basis is medical need, not personality or social attributes. A patient is a patient is a patient. This essentially says that persons filling the roles of physician and patient are not crucial as such. Their responsibilities and actions are predetermined by relevant norms. Individuals are replaceable.[108]

From a humanistic standpoint universalism is important, but it is not clear whether its impact is positive or negative. One can argue that the ethic is humanizing because it assumes everyone is entitled to the same level of care, the essence of the inherent worth argument above. Yet this perspective has limitations. If practitioners are not alert to individual uniqueness within an overall human framework, they will treat patients in routinized, uniform (anomic) ways, making care impersonal or falsely personal (the plastic smile.)[109]

Obviously all humans have commonalities, and health professionals recognize the importance of statistical norms in diagnosis and therapy. To maximize their value to patients they must also appreciate the significance of deviations from the norm, not all of which have adverse consequences. It is, therefore, reasonable to argue that humanized care demands an individualistic orientation toward patients,[110] superimposed on the universalistic notion that everyone has a right to receive high-quality care.

Many practitioners in large-scale institutions also feel like anomic cogs in giant machines and sense they could easily be replaced by anyone with similar credentials.[111] Thus, for professionals as well as patients, being treated as unique persons is an essential ingredient of humanization.

The concept of individuality or irreplaceability counterposes the idea of people as quantifiable or numbered things—as one respondent phrased it, "person things." It may also counterpose the concept of *patient* in any role-limiting sense. Thus, the universalism-particularism dilemma is a central research issue. We need to study conditions under which common treatment is humanizing and differentiation dehumanizing, and also situations having the opposite effect.

The ideology of individualism is accentuated by the times in which we live,[112] but throughout history humanity's failure to appreciate the special needs and wants of particular groups of people has catalyzed social criticism. It has never sufficed to say all humans are equal in the eyes of God or of society. The relative importance of individualism as a dimension of humanized behavior should be measured in rigorous ways.

Holistic Selves. Human lives are complex, embracing many behavioral milieus. At any given moment, the sum total of a person's experience influences that person's feelings, attitudes, and actions.[113] But certain aspects of the past and present are more salient than others.

Some students of professionalization suggest that the role orientation is *specific*, that practitioners are concerned only with those dimensions of their patients that are relevant to being a patient.[114] In contrast, a role such as husband or father is *diffuse*, every aspect of a wife or child being potentially relevant to the interaction.[115] This approach raises questions. What dimensions of a patient's life are irrelevant to health and disease? Is it merely a matter of those dimensions being more or less relevant? Does specificity depend on the problem involved? If variables generally deemed "nonmedical" (unemployment or divorce) are obviously affecting the patient's health, what is the practitioner's legitimate role in dealing with them?[116]

The narrower the focus, the narrower the interest and intrusion into the patient's "private" domain. Respect for privacy recognizes autonomy and freedom, and to that extent it is humanizing.[117] But specificity can also be dehumanizing if the patient is viewed as a problem rather than as a person. The patient's "whole" may be so fragmented that his or her problems become exclusive concerns of multiple practitioners who do not even communicate with one another.[118] As one respondent said: "I don't like being divided into parts like a machine, one piece sent here to be fixed and another piece there."*[119]

The more time a patient spends in a health facility, the more needs it must satisfy. Inpatients commit a greater proportion of their selves to health institutions than outpatients. If their care is to be personal, a diffuse approach is necessary, for they cannot turn elsewhere for help. In many custodial settings staff shortages force patients to humanize each other.[120]

An important question concerns the lack of symmetry in professional-patient interactions. Intrusions into the patient's life are largely at the provider's discretion, but the provider's own life remains a closed book if he or she chooses because it is presumably irrelevant to professional role behavior. Counterarguments are plausible. Since human-to-human

---

* Sometimes the complaint seems so localized that the practitioner ignores its significance for the total person. One respondent consulted a hand specialist about surgery for her finger. The office was so crowded that two patients were always seated in the examining room simultaneously. The physician was treating "detached" fingers, instead of people who are embarrassed when forced to discuss their ailments in front of others.

relations involve reciprocity or equalitarianism (see below), one-way excursions into private domains may be dehumanizing because of imbalance and implicit connotations of practitioner control. Furthermore, empathy, another ingredient of humanizing relationships, requires sharing as well as sympathy. We also know that many facets of providers' lives affect work behavior.[121] If they share with patients aspects of their total selves, mutual understanding and humanness might be enhanced.

Some physicians do reveal "private" facets of their lives when they feel that personal vignettes and reciprocity are therapeutic. This could be an insightful area for research. Treating patients as wholes may be correlated with the provider's own inclination to interact totally. Other relevant factors are probably the professional's specialty, sex, age, and ethnic background.

The next three ingredients of humanization seem associated more with the structure of provider-consumer interactions than with ideologies about them. However, the distinction is blurred because patterned relations are generally based on ideologies.

Freedom of Action. Humanized relationships are predicated on freedom of choice. Where the interaction is forced on participants and one or the other is bound against his will, the experience cannot be humanizing. Many factors restrict the freedom of practitioners and patients. Professionals are constrained by cost considerations, institutional commitments, colleague pressures,[122] and scarce resources for therapy. Patients are hamstrung by illness, ignorance, status deprivation, professional protocol,[123] and emotional investment in existing relationships.

Obviously, human beings have finite freedom.[124] Humanized relations are themselves constricting through obligations that recognize the worth and dignity of others. But the nature and extent of limited freedom are relevant considerations. Humanized persons have considerable control over their destinies. They are not merely objects of action. The quality and quantity of options available to professionals and patients in various settings are important issues for research.

Those involuntarily committed to mental hospitals (especially public facilities) are prototypes of patients with the least freedom of choice. The locked door exacerbates their degradation.[125] They may struggle for awhile to fulfill their multiple needs and test opportunities to manipulate the system.[126] But many, or most, eventually become institutionalized, offering little or no resistance to constraints upon them.[127] Outpatients are freer than inpatients, but they also have limited choices. It would be useful to know how these options vary with ethnicity, socioeconomic status, age, sex, locality, and type of illness.

Providers of care have complained bitterly about the restrictive hands of third parties such as government agencies, insurance companies, and hospital boards.[128] They feel depersonalized by constrictions on relations with patients, colleagues, and the public; constraints on procedures and regimens deemed necessary for the patient; and the red tape and paper work that accompany third-party dealings. Some complaints reflect colleague expectations and pressures, but others mirror genuine personal feelings. This area also merits systematic research.

Status Equality.   Humanized relations involve equals on some level. If either sees his or her total self as superior or inferior to the other, the interaction cannot be fully humanizing because participation of "lesser persons" destroys its human-to-human quality.

Some scholars believe that professional expertise necessarily stratifies relations with patients.[129] I challenge this interpretation on a number of grounds. Practitioners generally trade expertise for money, which can constitute a fair (or equal) bargain. When one respondent said she "wanted to be treated like a paying customer," she wished to be treated as an equal.

The universalistic ethic is also an equalizer. Professionals are supposed to accept the premise that a patient is a patient is a patient and disregard attributes extraneous to health. The service ethic is related. From a humanitarian perspective, a practitioner's knowledge is valuable only if it can be used to help patients. The instrumental focus makes the provider a kind of servant,[130] thus balancing status and lessening the symbolic significance of knowledge. Among missionary doctors, service is supposedly self-rewarding.[131]

One should also recognize that many patients hold positions in the larger world at least the equal of health professionals, and they carry their "outside" statuses into examining rooms. In fact, some physicians bemoan having to treat rich patients because these patients are so demanding they make professionals feel like "kept men."[132] The feeling of being owned may also characterize practitioners who treat organized groups of consumers. The combined power of the bargaining unit can grace individual members, enhancing their status vis-à-vis professionals supported by the collective.

Reciprocity may be still another equalizer. Some suggest that human or inhuman actions are inherently reciprocal—that the initiator is automatically affected by their quality regardless of response; thus, those who participate in depersonalizing institutions become depersonalized in the process.[133] The validity of this observation is yet to be tested. Perhaps professionals compartmentalize behavior toward certain patients to insulate themselves from dehumanization; or there may be a critical ratio for relationships such that the actor survives as a "human" as long as most interactions with patients and colleagues are personalized. This would be especially important where patients, because of illness or therapy, cannot respond to actions directed toward them.

The idea of reciprocity suggests that acts toward others feed back to their initiators and tend to equalize statuses of the parties. If practitioners treat patients or colleagues as less than fully human they function at less than full human potential and begin to conceive of *themselves* as nonpersons. When one treats another as the initiator would like to be treated, this equalizes relations by acknowledging that both participants deserve the perquisites of full human beings.

If reciprocity does in fact lead to status equality between therapist and patient, two causes would seem to be involved: the process of cognitive and emotional feedback noted above, and the tendency for situations defined as real to become real in their consequences.[134] Thus, when patients are perceived and treated as equals, some begin to so assert themselves. This conveys a greater sense of personal worth and opens the door for positive feedback to the patients themselves.

Instead of treating patients as equals many professionals accentuate the differences, speaking in the private vocabulary of their trade and relishing the mystique of their position.[135] More humanistic providers may symbolically reduce prestige and authority by adopting casual dress and permitting informal salutations.[136] Low-ranking professionals and semiprofessionals may try to counter a sense of inferiority by strategically and subtly advertising their worth—wearing white coats, name tags, and so forth. The implications of various techniques for equalizing status should be systematically explored. Investigators should study how reactions of providers and consumers to equality or inequality vary with age, sex, ethnicity, socioeconomic background, personality, and other variables.

Factors leading to patient inferiority might include nudity. Our interviews suggest that stigmas attached to being nude extend to physicians' offices and affect patient dignity. The particular impact may depend on the sex of the parties, degree of privacy, duration of nudity, professional rituals associated with body exposure, relevant subcultural values, and the patient's ability to compartmentalize views about nudity according to circumstance.

One observer believes that the horizontal-vertical dimension (patients in bed: staff standing) contributes to inequality and dehumanization of patients.[137] Proneness here is, of course, linked to dependency, which may be more important in reducing patient status than prostrate position is. Comparative studies of rich patients could be suggestive. In some situations the horizontal stance of the wealthy may enhance prestige, symbolizing leisure or rest and that others should do their bidding.

A key research area concerns the effect of fiduciary relations. Many professionals stress the importance of fee-for-service as an equalizer.[138] This reflects the cultural emphasis on money as a measure of personal worth and the historical fact that fee-for-service has been the primary method of exchange between providers and noncharity patients. We need to study the implications of various forms of payment on professional-consumer relations. Patient power may result from collective as well as from individual modes of compensation.

Consumer pressure in the health field is being recognized as legitimate and necessary to improve access to care, dignity, and quality.[139] Clinics, hospitals, and outreach programs are including consumers in advisory and policy structures. It remains to be seen if this will meaningfully affect humanization of service. On paper it has the potential of doing so through complaint and grievance mechanisms, which are at least implied in consumer representation. But paper power is often benign. If consumer participants are only figureheads, their presence may actually exacerbate dehumanization by giving existing practices a stamp of legitimacy. Genuine consumer power can also be dehumanizing where practitioners feel thwarted and manipulated by nonprofessional third hands.[140]

Shared Decision Making and Responsibility.   The concept of shared decision making logically follows from other facets of humanized relations:

inherent worth, uniqueness, wholeness of self, freedom of action, and equality. It reflects the emerging ideology that all patients, regardless of education, have a right and perhaps duty to participate as much as possible in decisions about their care.[141] Analogously, professionals and semi-professionals whose lives are increasingly controlled by large institutions are struggling for decision-making power.[142] Sensitivity and encounter groups within massive systems reflect the thrust toward broad-based input. Employees at all levels are encouraged to gripe, the implication being that they will thereby have some impact on policy.[143]

When patients share responsibility for their care, at least three assumptions are implicit: that they have behavioral options with respect to their illnesses, that the quality and quantity of *their* lives are at stake,[144] and that they deserve significant control over choices of possible regimens and life styles.

Ambulatory outpatients are virtually captains of their lives, within boundaries set by physical and social restraints. Even when they want providers to assume the total burden of decision making (and many patients do try to absolve themselves of responsibility), no practitioner can successfully play God to autonomous persons. And if it were somehow possible, the relationship would hardly be considered human-to-human, in the sense of our discussion.

If patients share in decision making about their care, they are essentially partners of providers and thus, in a way, their equals. To the extent of their competence they must be informed about prognoses, alternative therapies, and the rationales behind them.[145] Sharing truth includes sharing doubt. Practitioners who level with patients make them partners in uncertainty as well as in certainty.

Sharing knowledge can, however, present problems in humanistic treatment.[146] Patients may be too sick, anxious, or irrational to interpret facts and help make appropriate decisions, and sparing the whole truth may be more humanizing than telling all. The relevance of such caveats must be appraised by practitioners in developing cooperative arrangements with their patients.

I hypothesize that the more professionals and patients view one another as equals, the greater their propensity to share decision making. This proposition should be tested. I also feel that the self-confidence and security of providers will affect their willingness to yield authority, and that the level of education of patients will influence their desire and capacity to accept co-responsibility for their care. If education proves to be important, health professionals will have to place differential emphasis on training various types of patients to help themselves. Some consumers are already accepted as full partners in their care, while others are not even told the basic essentials for managing their condition.

The third grouping of factors in humanistic behavior is more emotional than cognitive or structural. It includes two elements: empathy and affect.

Empathy. Humans have the ability to sympathize and identify with others. The more they compare themselves to others, the more easily they put themselves in others' shoes. If one perceives a second person as less than fully human, one will have difficulty identifying with that person. This assumes that people see themselves as human, and that the reference point for empathy is self.

In stressing the importance of empathy in health care, one patient commented: "The doctor should know how my leg hurts and what it means to me." Another complained that physicians do not show enough "sympathy and concern" for patients' problems.[147] Professionals, on the other hand, are troubled by overidentification. They frequently try to control empathy to protect their psyches from sympathetic pain.[148] As one physician phrased it: "I've got to have some empathy left at day's end to take home to my wife."[149]

Astute practitioners also recognize that it may be impossible to put themselves in their patients' shoes. An orthopedist who treats paraplegics suggested the hypocrisy of projecting himself into the world of his patients. "I have two useful legs which they can see; so it's unrealistic for me to tell them how to live. They know I can't really feel what they feel. The best models for spinal cord injury patients are other spinal cord injury patients."[150]

Despite normative and psychological barriers to empathy, human commonalities will facilitate sympathy if feelings are given some free reign. A distinguishing feature of Homo sapiens is their capacity to anticipate their own death.[151] This is an important key to empathy. Another is the vulnerability of all humans, including practitioners and their families, to a vast spectrum of sicknesses. Where providers and consumers come from similar backgrounds, their needs and wants tend to be similar, and practitioners may easily see themselves when they look at their patients.

Whatever the functions of controlled empathy, constraint depersonalizes relationships among professionals and patients and among providers themselves. If practitioners contain their sympathy and avoid seeing the world from the vantage point of their patients, they cannot as readily understand the needs of those patients and appropriately respond to them as unique human beings. Yet, if they identify too freely, they can drain themselves emotionally and lose some of their own integrity as persons. Compromise is necessary, and the means of successfully achieving it is an important issue for research.

Positive Affect.   Human beings are reservoirs and conveyors of emotion. They become attached to other persons, animals, and inanimate objects. Person-to-person interactions are most likely to involve emotional commitments because reciprocity and empathy can occur.

Feelings toward others may be positive, negative, or neutral. Some believe that affective neutrality is a defining characteristic of professionalism.[152] They argue that a neutral stance protects objectivity and freedom from extraneous obligations and concerns. Presumably, one can become emotionally involved with a problem without having any special feeling for the person presenting it.

In spite of possible benefits, affective neutrality is depersonalizing for all parties and may subvert attainment of goals. Harnessed feelings can give the impression of practitioner indifference—with adverse effects on patient compliance, timely consultation, and candor. And what about the emotions of patients? Must they be neutral toward professionals they consult? This could inhibit free communication and productive dependency. Furthermore, one-sided emotional commitments can dehumanize the involved party, who gives without reciprocity.

Successful therapy may require practitioners to display varying degrees of intimacy in different contexts. Children may expect to be treated with affection. Neutrality could undermine their trust, frankness, and receptivity. Intimacy might also be used to compensate for past deprivation. Social outcasts such as alcoholics, hippies, and homosexuals have been treated as nonpersons for so long they are suspicious of almost everyone in health-care systems.[153] To prove sincerity and concern, providers may have to show genuine feelings of warmth. One black woman we interviewed was impressed with her physician because he put his arm around her and walked her down the hall.

Where patients are bereft of family and friends, health professionals cannot be oblivious to unfulfilled needs for affection. If they are unable to provide warmth and tenderness, a humanistic approach necessitates finding sincere substitutes such as the volunteer "grandmothers" in pediatric wards.

The importance of affect undoubtedly varies with type of illness as well as with the patient. In long-term treatment of mental disease, the therapist's emotional distance could thwart patient involvement, aggravate isolation, and lessen success. The degree to which professionals distinguish between problems and patients may depend on their specialty; and the more the illness engulfs the total being, the more difficult separation of emotional investment in person versus disease.

It appears that affect in humanizing relationships tends to be positive and that dehumanizing interactions involve surpluses of negative and neutral emotions for at least one participant (the initiator of depersonalization) and probably both. Perhaps negative affect is as characteristic of human-to-human relations as positive feelings, but our concept óf humanization presupposes conditions closer to the positive pole: empathy, respect for inherent worth, status equality, and shared decision making. Freedom of action is another facet of humanized relationships, and given that freedom rational consumers and providers will not subject themselves to negative abuse. Positive feeling appears necessary for continued human-to-human contact.*

Links between *empathy* and *affect* need systematic study. If practitioners really put themselves in the shoes of patients, can they remain emotionally distant? Practitioners cannot die psychologically with each patient,† but the ethic of neutrality has a strange bedfellow. Health professionals explicitly recognize the patient's need for tender loving care. Integration of these seemingly paradoxical doctrines merits investigation.

---

* Practitioners may suffer abuse from patients but continue to serve them because lives are at stake and ethics binding. Patients may continue to consult abusive providers if the talents of those providers are crucial. But these would not be considered humanizing interactions.

† A cardiovascular surgeon partly countered this idea. He says that when risk of death during surgery is high, it may be functional to grieve for the patient like family members grieve. This physician gets to know patients and allows himself to feel affect for adults as well as for children. If his patient succumbs on the table, he suffers more than if he had tried to remain affectively neutral, but his grief helps relieve the guilt he also experiences.[154]

In short-term observations of provider-consumer relations, it may be hard to determine whether plus feelings outweigh minuses or vice versa. Displays of anger may be used instrumentally to gain the patient's cooperation in therapy, and strong positive feelings can be masked by professional constraint. Thus, to measure the true emotional picture, we need in-depth studies of ongoing contact and communication.

The reader may wonder why I have not included "dedication to others" (the service ethic) among the dimensions of humanizing behavior, especially since selflessness is often cited as a distinguishing characteristic of professionals.[155] The importance of this variable is acknowledged in the discussion of status equality and balance resulting from monetary or moral bargains between providers and consumers. The concept of inherent worth and universal right to care is also related to dedicated service.

Taken at face value, professional standards probably require more self-sacrifice than is suggested by the concept of humanized interaction per se. But in any humanizing relationship, participants must be dedicated to one another to some degree. This logically follows from the conditions specified: empathy, positive feeling, equality, shared responsibility, and respect for inherent worth. One's orientation to others becomes a form of identification in accord with the Golden Rule. In essence I am saying that "selflessness" is implicit in the ingredients of humanization already set forth, not selflessness for its own sake but as an integral part of reciprocity.

Possible dehumanizing effects of self-sacrifice should not be ignored. Providers of care may so engross themselves in helping others that they fail to satisfy their own needs as whole persons and those of intimates dependent on them. Recipients of care who become obligated without opportunities to reciprocate may experience humiliating feelings of inferiority and worthlessness.

A significant research issue concerns the extent to which health professionals have internalized the ideal of selfless dedication to patients. What priorities do they place on patient needs vis-à-vis their own? Is self-sacrifice a satisfactory means of fulfilling personal expectations or is it begrudged? What, if anything, is sought in return? Answers to these questions will suggest whether the humanitarianism of providers involves special behaviors or the same responsibilities that all people acquire in human-to-human relations.

I suggested that interactions between professionals and patients may be dehumanizing because of the imbalance inherent in practitioners' discretion over what they choose to learn about their patients and not to reveal about themselves. This should be evaluated within the larger context of professional commitment. If providers are truly dedicated to their patients, the relationship might be symmetrical in a contractual sense, the patient exchanging privacy for practitioner concern.

A further research issue pertains to self-sacrifice for fellow providers. The Hippocratic ideals are perhaps more applicable to interprofessional relations than to care of the sick.[156] Under what conditions do providers behave as selfless "brothers" and "sisters" rather than as neutral colleagues, competitors, or superiors and subordinates?[157]

OPERATIONALIZING THE CONCEPT OF HUMANIZATION.   Given the proposed constellation of necessary and sufficient conditions for human-to-human behavior, the next step is to operationalize these factors so those undertaking relevant research will have objective blueprints for assessing their presence or absence.[158] I suggest some general approaches I have found useful, but not a set of procedures for measuring each concept.

First, let us distinguish between direct and indirect modes of analysis. In the direct approach the focal concept (e.g., empathy) is translated into specific actions, attitudes, and feelings. Then an instrument for observation or interviewing is designed to directly measure the reality of interest. The indirect approach is a kind of clueing and cuing. The researcher draws inferences from behavior, cognitions, or emotions and extrapolates to variables not definitively implicated. A set of observational parameters may bear upon several dimensions of humanization, not just one.

Using the indirect model as a prototype my assistants and I attempted to identify key patterns of provider-consumer interactions relevant to degrees of humanization and dehumanization. As a pilot endeavor we limited these relations to those that could be observed without questioning participants. Three indicators proved experimentally rewarding. The first concerned continuity of interaction between patients and providers. Since the contacts took place in waiting areas of health facilities, the providers were generally receptionists, nurses, and paramedical personnel. Occasionally, physicians were present.

For each interaction we counted the times providers interrupted the contact for reasons extraneous to the patient's welfare (telephone calls, irrelevant comments to and from colleagues, previously assigned tasks). We also estimated the proportion of "interruption" time over the total interaction. The assumption is that such interruptions are inconsistent with dignity, empathy, positive affect, status equality, and even freedom of action. Sometimes patients stood at the central counter for a least 20 minutes while the receptionist engaged in competing tasks.

In public clinics and one HMO this was just the beginning of a two- or three-hour wait before the patient got beyond the reception area. At some point such "thinging" of patients was defined as dehumanizing by all observers. When we interviewed the consumers involved, they acknowledged constricted options and consequent pressure to engage in trade offs. They expressed a willingness to suffer certain kinds of indignities to save money.

One problem not easily solved was determining whether interruptions were relevant to the patient's case. Some telephone calls were initiated by the professional to learn more about the patient. Our observers sat as close as possible to the locus of conversation but words were often blurred, especially where partitions intervened between patients and staff.

A second observational construct concerned body and eye contact between personnel and patients.[159] This was partly a measure of affect, but it also assessed more general attitudes of providers toward patients as human beings. Sometimes a receptionist or nurse addressed a patient by name or number and the person responded verbally or with movement without the professional ever looking in the patient's direction, let alone shaking hands or touching the person in some manner.[160] Other times the provider showed genuine affect and respect for the patient through an intimate gesture or contact.

Analogous to this approach, we took note of situations in which consumer-provider interaction was virtually absent. In some public and private waiting rooms, written signs substitute for verbal communication. Signs may refer to signs, guiding patients through the maze by telling them what floor lines to follow to their ultimate destination and stations in between, such as a cashier's office. Signs may give instructions concerning how and when to call for help if one's illness is so severe that one cannot sit upright for the duration of the usual wait.

The third technique involved a global appraisal of waiting-room environments from a humanistic perspective. Two investigators at a time independently rated the milieus on a scale of humanization-dehumanization. Then we tried to operationalize the observers' "gut" feelings to identify the criteria and valences resulting in judgments. Among the relevant factors were: adequate lighting, comfortable seats, ample and appropriate reading material or other recreational aids, warm decor to make the patient feel like a guest, convenient bathroom facilities, and "noninstitutional" furniture arrangements.[161]

Our observers were graduate students in the health and social sciences: a black woman, a male Israeli, and a white male hippie. That they closely agreed in their ratings was reassuring, but a much larger and varied sample of investigators should be used in such assessments. We would hope at least to find congruity of opinion regarding environments evaluated at the extremes of humanization and dehumanization.

One further approach was unsuccessful. We assumed that treating patients as whole persons would include interest in nontask-oriented aspects of them, that is, in dimensions not specifically health relevant. Thus, we felt that where providers of care spontaneously asked patients about their families, recreational activities, or jobs, this could be considered an index of humanism. One scholar has called such actions "voluntarism."[162]

It proved very difficult for our observers to hear entire conversations between patients and personnel; and in dealing with new patients, providers had few reference points to inquire about the total person. Where the investigators could hear most of the verbal give and take, they scored the conversation on a scale measuring "breadth of interest" in the patient or provider's life situation. When interest was holistic, other focal concepts such as empathy and affect were also identified in the conversation.

We know that only a fraction of patient-provider relations take place in reception rooms, although the verbal and nonverbal exchanges that occur there may be very important in projecting a warm or cold image of the entire facility. We were merely trying to test observational techniques in easily accessible environments. To enlarge our perspective it should be possible to gain patient and practitioner consent to tape their discussions during history taking, physicals, and postexamination conferences. Content analyses could focus on a number of relevant variables. In addition to these approaches, depth interviews with patients and providers regarding their interrelationships, and institutional analyses of health-care processes and policy making would make our battery of instruments more complete and salient.

We did successfully question a large number of patients with respect to humanizing and dehumanizing experiences in health facilities. This helped provide the theoretical framework and guidelines for choosing our eight focal concepts and evaluating subcomponents. These variables need further refinement, and their relevance to providers should also be assessed through systematic interviews. Correlations among the constellation of factors should be calculated to determine degrees of interdependence.

The magnitude of cultural relativism implicit in the dimensions we have chosen needs to be explored in greater detail, especially for such variables as freedom of action, which is obviously finite because of biological, psychological, and cultural constraints.

For convenience, I have usually illustrated my remarks by focusing on 1:1 interactions between providers and consumers. This is not meant to belittle the importance of the three other models: n:1, 1:n, and n:n. With respect to the n:1 or n:n type, an insightful study of abortion patients deserves mention. The investigator interviewed the women and medical personnel involved with them, singly or collectively in preoperative and postoperative situations. He analyzed behavior patterns, feelings, values, and interpretations of reality.[163] This seems a particularly useful approach to studying care in large institutions. It permits a number of comparisons: patient vis-à-vis patient, provider vis-à-vis provider, and patient or patients vis-à-vis provider or providers.

The proper evaluation of patient and provider comments raises another significant issue for research. How do we judge actions that are defined by recipients as real but are false by other measurements? If a practitioner feels neutral toward a given patient, but the patient feels loved by the practitioner, how do we determine whether the provider's behavior is humanizing or dehumanizing in its consequences? These knotty problems are crucial and bear on larger issues in human relations, however individuals may choose to define one another.

SUMMARY.   The major focus of this paper is to identify a set of variables that appear to be necessary and sufficient conditions for humanizing behavior in health systems. These concepts were suggested by relevant literature, interviews with patients, observations of health facilities, and theoretical speculation. It remains to be determined through further research whether humanized interaction necessitates the presence of all eight factors and if other unnamed variables must also be included.

Among critical questions are the impact of different environments on humanization of care and the extent to which human providers can be replaced by technology without totally destroying the flavor of the hand.

My assistants and I have tested several methodologies for studying personalization of care and are encouraged by preliminary results. However, this effort is still in its infancy and deserves the attention of empirically-oriented scholars from a variety of relevant disciplines. Interdependence among the eight focal variables and others that may prove cogent should be studied; and culturally-induced differences in the applicability of certain concepts to providers and consumers merit serious consideration.

This paper poses a number of theoretical and practical issues for research. The questions raised highlight important problems and dilemmas. They need systematic appraisal and screening to pave the way for fundamental parsimonious inquiry.

NOTES

1. D. E. Sobel. "Personalization in the Coronary Care Unit." *Am J Nurs*, vol. 69, July 1969, pp. 1439-1442. C. M. Brodsky. "The Systematic Incompatibility of Medical Practice and Psychotherapy." *Dis Nerv Syst*, vol. 31, September 1970, pp. 597-603.

2. J. M. Gustafson. "Mongolism, Parental Desires and the Right to Life." *Perspect Biol Med*, vol. 16, Summer 1973, pp. 532-533.

3. E. K. Caplan and M. B. Sussman. "Rank Order of Important Variables for Patient and Staff Satisfaction with Outpatient Services." *J Health Hum Behav*, vol. 7, Summer 1966, pp. 133-137. M. B. Sussman et al. *The Walking Patient: A Study in Outpatient Care*. Cleveland: The Press of Case Western Reserve University, 1967. E. Freidson. *Patient Views of Medical Practice*. New York: Russell Sage Foundation, 1961, pp. 41-70.

4. O. E. Guttentag. "Medical Humanism: A Redundant Phrase." *Pharos Alpha Omega Alpha*, vol. 32, January 1969, pp. 12-15.

5. Medical Services Division, Minnesota Department of Public Welfare. "The Attack on Dehumanization." *Hosp Community Psychiatry*, vol. 18, December 1967, pp. 34-36. T. S. Szasz. "Illness and Indignity." *JAMA*, vol. 227, February 4, 1974, pp. 543-545.

6. For a definition of "dehumanization" see D. Vail. *Dehumanization and the Institutional Career*. Springfield, Ill.: Charles C Thomas, 1966.

7. J. M. Gustafson. *Op. cit.*, pp. 529-557. C. H. Calland. "Iatrogenic Problems in End-Stage Renal Failure." *N Engl J Med*, vol. 287, August 17, 1972, pp. 334-336. D. L. Rosenhan. "On Being Sane in Insane Places." *Science*, vol. 179, January 19, 1973, pp. 250-258. D. E. Sobel. *Op. cit.*

8. R. S. Duff and A. B. Hollingshead. *Sickness and Society.* New York: Harper & Row, 1968. A. Strauss et al. *Psychiatric Ideologies and Institutions.* New York: The Free Press, 1964. I. Belnap. *Human Problems of a State Mental Hospital.* New York: McGraw-Hill, 1956. J. Roth. *Timetables.* Indianapolis: Bobbs-Merrill, 1963. B. Glaser and A. Strauss. *Awareness of Dying.* Chicago: Aldine, 1965.

9. F. J. Cook. *The Plot Against the Patient.* Englewood Cliffs, N.J.: Prentice-Hall, 1967. A. I. Solzhenitsyn. *The Cancer Ward.* New York: Harper & Row, 1969. A. Hano. "Incredible Ordeal of Chad Calland, M.D." *Redbook*, vol. 137, September 1971, p. 94. L. Bronson. "Former Patient at Agnews 'Tells It Like It Was.' " *Palo Alto Times*, June 21, 1972, p. 27. Anonymous. "Notes of a Dying Professor." *Nurs Outlook*, vol. 20, August 1972, pp. 502-506. A. M. Tao-Kim-Hai. "Orientals are Stoic." *New Yorker*, vol. 33, September 1957, pp. 105-106. D. E. Smith and J. Luce. *Love Needs Care.* Boston: Little, Brown, 1971. M. Crichton. *Five Patients.* New York: Bantam, 1970.

10. C. H. Calland. *Op. cit.*

11. K. Kesey. *One Flew Over the Cuckoo's Nest.* New York: Signet, 1962. M. J. Ward. *The Snake Pit.* New York: Random House, 1946.

12. A. Bottone. "Anatomy of a Non Strike." *N Phys*, vol. 19, October 1970, p. 836.

13. J. M. Carnoy. "Kaiser: You Pay Your Money and You Take Your Chances." *Ramparts*, vol. 9, November 1970, p. 28. H. Schwartz. "Health Care in America: A Heretical Diagnosis." *Saturday Rev*, vol. 54, August 14, 1971, p. 55. For a scholarly discussion of "crocks" and their effect on the doctor-patient relationship, see H. A. Meyersburg, S. T. Boggs, and M. B. Richmond. "The Crock—A Study of Dysfunctional Doctor-Patient Relationship in Chronic Illness." (Unpublished study.)

14. T. Thomson. "The Year They Changed Hearts." *Life*, vol. 71, September 17, 1971, pp. 56-70. J. M. Carnoy. *Op. cit.*, pp. 28-31. D. Corditz. "Change Begins in the Doctor's Office." In *The Social Organization of Health*, edited by H. P. Dreitzel. New York: Macmillan, 1971, p. 219.

15. M. Halberstam. "Liberal Thought, Radical Theory and Medical Practice." *N Engl J Med*, vol. 284, May 27, 1971, pp. 1180-1185. J. H. Knowles. "Radiology—A Case Study in Technology and Man Power." *N Engl J Med*, vol. 280, June 12, 1969, pp. 1323-1329.

16. A. I. Solzhenitsyn. *Op. cit.* E. Goffman. *Asylums.* New York: Anchor, 1961. S. M. Jourard. "To Whom Can a Nurse Give Personalized Care?" In *The Transparent Self*, by S. M. Jourard. Princeton, N.J.: Van Nostrand, 1964, p. 139. The Health Policy Advisory Committee (Health-Pac). *American Health Empire: Power, Profit and Politics.* New York: Vintage Books, 1971. R. S. Duff and A. B. Hollingshead. *Op. cit.* p. x, foreword.

17. M. Halberstam. *Op. cit.*, p. 1184. H. Schwartz. *Op. cit.*, pp. 14-17. D. Mechanic. "Human Problems and the Organization of Health Care." *Ann Acad Polit Soc Sci*, vol. 399, January 1972, pp. 1-11.

18. E. Freidson. "Review Essay: Health Factories, the New Industrial Sociology." *Soc Probl*, vol. 14, Spring 1967, p. 493.

19. For a contrasting point of view—that the whole is really more than the sum of its parts—see F. Perls, R. F. Hefferline, and P. Goodman. *Gestalt Therapy.* New York: Delta Book, 1951, p. xi. Note also that some medical information systems recognize the fact that elements interact. See *First Considerations in Selecting a Computerized Medical Information System.* Palo Alto, Calif.: Spectra Medical Systems, Inc., 1974.

20. E. Goffman. *Op. cit.,* p. 6.

21. S. M. Jourard. *Op. cit.,* p. 138 E. Fromm. *The Revolution of Hope—Toward a More Humanized Technology.* New York: Harper & Row, 1968, p. 110.

22. S. M. Jourard. "Away With the 'Bedside Manner!'" *Op. cit.,* p. 113. J. R. Guyther. "The Right to Die." *Md State Med J,* vol. 22, June 1973, p. 44. M. E. Salter. "Nursing in an Intensive Therapy Unit." *Nurs Times,* vol. 66, April 16, 1970, pp. 486-487.

23. T. Thomson. *Op. cit.,* p. 61. A. R. Jonsen. "The Totally Implantable Artificial Heart." *Hastings Cent Rep,* vol. 3, November 1973, pp. 1-4. D. Hendin. *Death as a Fact of Life.* New York: Norton, 1973. See especially Chapter 2, "Transplants—You Can Take It With You," pp. 50-65.

24. R. Hilberg. *The Destruction of the European Jews.* Chicago: Quadrangle, 1961, pp. 600-609. A. Mitscherlich. *Doctors of Infamy: The Story of the Nazi Medical Crimes,* translated by H. Norden. New York: H. Schuman, 1949.

25. J. Mitford. "Experiments Behind Bars—Doctors, Drug Companies, and Prisoners." *Atl Mon,* vol. 231, January 1973, pp. 64-73. H. K. Beecher. *Research and the Individual—Human Studies.* Boston: Little, Brown, 1970. See especially "Prisoners," p. 69. Anonymous. "Commentary: Experimental Medicine." *Br Med J,* October 27, 1962, pp. 1108-1109. G. Bach-y-Rita. "The Prisoner as an Experimental Subject." *JAMA,* vol. 229, July 1, 1974, pp. 45-46. A. C. Ivy. "The History and Ethics of the Use of Human Subjects in Medical Experiments." *Science,* vol. 108, July 2, 1948, pp. 1-5.

26. U.S. Department of Health, Education, and Welfare, Public Health Service. "Final Report of the Tuskegee Syphilis Study Ad Hoc Advisory Panel." Washington, D. C., 1973. W. J. Curran. "The Tuskegee Syphilis Study." *N Engl J Med,* vol. 289, October 4, 1973, pp. 730-731.

27. T. Thomson. *Op. cit.,* p. 69. A. R. Jonsen. *Op. cit.* D. Hendin. *Op. cit.,* pp. 35-39, 60-65.

28. T. Thomson. *Op. cit.,* pp. 56-70. C. H. Calland. *Op. cit.*

29. J. Fletcher. "Human Experimentation: Ethics in the Consent Situation." *Law Contemp Probl,* vol. 32, Autumn 1967, pp. 620-649. M. A. Meyers. "The Way of Some Flesh." *Pennsylvania Gazette,* March 1974, pp. 21-28.

30. G. G. Reader and M. H. W. Goss, eds. *Comprehensive Medical Care and Teaching: A Report on the New York Hospital—Cornell Medical Center Program.* Ithaca, N.Y.: Cornell University Press, 1967. L. Schatzman. "Voluntarism and Professional Practice in the Health Professions." In *A Sociological Framework for Patient Care,* edited by J. R. Folta and E. S. Deck. New York: John Wiley & Sons, 1966, pp. 145-155. J. A. Jackson, ed. *Professions and Professionalization.* London: Syndics of the Cambridge University Press, 1970. D. C. Brodie. "Emerging Patterns of Education and Practice in the Health Professions—Pharmacy." From the proceedings of the Pharmacy-Medicine-Nursing Conference on Health Education,

University of Michigan, February 18, 1971, pp. 23-36. R. K. Merton, G. Reader, and P. L. Kendall, eds. *The Student-Physician.* Cambridge, Mass.: Harvard University Press, 1957.

31. T. Parsons. *The Social System.* New York: The Free Press, 1964, pp. 435, 456. T. Parsons. *Essays in Sociological Theory.* New York: The Free Press, 1964, pp. 38, 39.

32. H. S. Becker and B. Geer. "The Fate of Idealism in Medical School." *Am Sociol Rev,* vol. 23, February 1958, pp. 50-56. L. D. Eron. "Effect of Medical Education on Medical Students." *J Med Educ,* vol. 10, October 1955, pp. 559-566. L. D. Eron and R. S. Redmount. "The Effect of Legal Education on Attitudes." *J Leg Educ,* vol. 9, no. 4, 1957, pp. 431-443 (includes a comparison of medical, nursing, and law students). R. M. Gray, P. M. Moody, and W. R. E. Newman. "An Analysis of Physicians' Attitudes of Cynicism and Humanitarianism Before and After Entering Medical Practice." *J Med Educ,* vol. 40, August 1965, pp. 760-766. T. F. Zimmerman. "Is Professionalization the Answer to Improving Health Care?" *Am J Occup Ther,* vol. 28, September 1974, pp. 465-468. C. P. Kimball. "Medical Education as a Humanizing Process." *J Med Educ,* vol. 48, January 1973, pp. 71-77.

33. G. G. Reader and M. H. W. Goss, eds. *Op. cit.* P. Kendall. "Consequences of the Trend Toward Specialization." In *Psychosocial Aspects of Medical Training,* edited by R. Coombs and C. Vincent. Springfield, Ill.: Charles C Thomas, 1971. pp. 498-524. R. M. Magraw and D. Magraw. *Ferment in Medicine: A Study of the Essence of Medical Practice and Its New Dilemmas.* Philadelphia: Saunders, 1966.

34. O. E. Guttentag. *Op. cit.,* p. 14. D. Ransom and H. E. Vandervoort. "The Development of Family Medicine." *JAMA,* vol. 225, August 27, 1973, pp. 1098-1102.

35. B. M. Korsch and V. F. Negrette. "Doctor-Patient Communication." *Sci Am,* vol. 227, August 1972, pp. 66-74. J. K. Skipper, Jr. and R. C. Leonard, eds. *Social Interaction and Patient Care.* Philadelphia: Lippincott, 1965. See especially Chapters 1-6. Anonymous. "Notes of a Dying Professor." *Op. cit.*

36. D. E. Smith, D. J. Bentel, and J. L. Schwartz, eds. *The Free Clinic: A Community Approach to Health Care and Drug Abuse.* Beloit, Wis.: Stash Press, 1971. D. E. Smith and J. Luce. *Op. cit.,* p. 28. I. F. Litt and M. I. Cohen. "Prisons, Adolescents and the Right to Quality Medical Care." *Am J Public Health,* vol. 64, September 1974, pp. 894-897.

37. F. Davis. *Passage Through Crisis: Polio Victims and Their Families.* Indianapolis: Bobbs-Merrill, 1963, pp. 39-43. M. B. Sussman, ed. *Sociology and Rehabilitation.* Washington, D.C.: The American Sociological Association, 1965, p. viii. R. Strauss. "Social Change and the Rehabilitation Concept." In *Sociology and Rehabilitation, Ibid.* pp. 1-34. H. H. Kessler. *Rehabilitation of the Physically Handicapped.* New York: Columbia University Press, 1947, pp. 3-15. J. Kosa, A. Antonovsky, and I. K. Zola, eds. *Poverty and Health.* Cambridge, Mass.: Harvard University Press, 1969. See especially M. B. Sussman. "The Medical Care System and the Rehabilitation of the Poor," pp. 256-260. *Poverty and Health in the United States: A Bibliography with Abstracts.* New York: Medical and Health Research Association of New York City, 1968.

38. C. Townsend. "Unloving Care." *Trial,* vol. 10, March/April 1974, pp. 16-19.

39. The Health Policy Advisory Committee (Health-Pac). *Op. cit.,* p. 15. The Boston Women's Health Collective. *Our Bodies, Ourselves: A Book By and For Women.* New York: Simon & Schuster, 1973. See especially pp. 157-159.

40. P. Chesler. "Patient and Patriarch: Women in the Psychotherapeutic Relationship." In *Woman in Sexist Society*, edited by V. Gornick and B. Moran. New York: Signet, 1972, p. 385. P. Chesler. *Women and Madness*. New York: Avon, 1973, p. 260.

41. V. Olesen and E. W. Whittaker. *The Silent Dialogue: A Study in the Social Psychology of Professional Socialization*. San Francisco: Jossey-Bass, 1968, p. 73. C. Grosser, W. E. Henry, and J. G. Kelly, eds. *Nonprofessionals in the Human Services*. San Francisco: Jossey-Bass, 1969, p. 54. For an argument that paraprofessionals are not in fact lesser beings in the health field, see A. Gartner. *Paraprofessionals and Their Performance: A Survey of Education, Health, and Social Service Programs*. New York: Praeger, 1971. An excellent bibliography is included.

42. E. Freidson. "Review Essay: Health Factories, the New Industrial Sociology." *Op. cit.* (From E. Goffman. *Op. cit.*)

43. K. Kesey. *Op. cit.* D. L. Rosenhan. *Op. cit.*, p. 256.

44. E. Goffman. *Op. cit.*, pp. 44-45.

45. M. Greenblatt, R. H. York, and E. L. Brown. *From Custodial to Therapeutic Patient Care in Mental Hospitals: Explorations in Social Treatment*. New York: Russell Sage Foundation, 1955, p. 354. D. L. Rosenhan. *Op. cit.*, pp. 254-255.

46. L. Bronson. *Op. cit.* P. Townsend. *The Last Refuge: A Survey of Residential Institutions and Homes for the Aged in England and Wales*. London: Routledge and Kegan Paul, 1962. M. Lieberman. "Institutionalization of the Aged: Effects on Behavior." *J Gerontol*, vol. 24, July 1969, pp. 330-340.

47. J. M. Carnoy. *Op. cit.*, pp. 30-31. M. Sussman et al. *The Walking Patient. Op. cit.*

48. M. Greenblatt, D. J. Levinson, and R. H. Williams. *The Patient and the Mental Hospital* Glencoe, Ill: The Free Press, 1957, pp. 234-236. A. Strauss et al. *Op. cit.*, pp. 216-217. J. C. Quint. *The Nurse and the Dying Patient*. New York: Macmillan, 1967, p. 109.

49. M. Seeman. "On the Meaning of Alienation." *Am Sociol Rev*, vol. 24, December 1959, pp. 783-791.

50. T. B. Bottomore, ed. *Karl Marx: Early Writings*. London: C. A. Watts & Co., 1963. A. W. Finifter, ed. *Alienation and the Social System*. New York: John Wiley & Sons, 1972. See especially Part IV, "Alienation from Work: The Marxian Heritage," pp. 103-179. R. Blauner. *Alienation and Freedom: The Factory Worker and His Identity*. Chicago: University of Chicago Press, 1964. C. W. Mills. *White Collar*. New York: Oxford University Press, 1956.

51. H. Gintis. "Alienation and Power in Capitalist Society." *Rev Radical Polit Econ*, vol. 4, Fall 1972, pp. 1-34.

52. H. P. Dreitzel, ed. *The Social Organization of Health*. New York: Macmillan, 1971. See especially Chapter 9, "The Organization of Hospital Care," by R. Duff and A. B. Hollingshead. A. Strauss. "Medical Ghettos." In *Patients, Physicians and Illness*, edited by E. G. Jaco. New York: The Free Press, 1958, pp. 381-388.

53. R. S. Duff and A. B. Hollingshead. *Sickness and Society. Op. cit.* R. Hurley. "The Health Crisis of the Poor." In *The Social Organization of Health. Op. cit.*, pp. 83-122. E. L. Richardson. "We Cannot Strive for Anything Less." *Soc Serv Outlook*, vol. 6, May 1971, pp. 1-3. E. Frankfort. *Vaginal Politics*. New York: Bantam, 1973.

54. E. Frankfort. *Ibid.*, pp. xviii-xxix, 217. D. L. Rosenhan. *Op. cit.*, pp. 250-258.

P. Goodman. *Growing Up Absurd: Problems of Youth in the Organized System.* New York: Random House, 1960. J. Anderson. "Those Militant New Nurses." *San Francisco Chronicle,* July 17, 1974, p. 15. State University MCHR by Stonybrook MCHR. "Parents Fight Nightmare at Willowbrook." *Health Rights News* (Chicago: Medical Committee for Human Rights), vol. 5, March 1972.

55. N. Sanford and C. Comstock. *Sanctions for Evil.* San Francisco: Jossey-Bass, 1971. The Health Policy Advisory Committee (Health-Pac). *Op. cit.* E. Freidson. "Review Essay: Health Factories, the New Industrial Sociology." *Op. cit.,* pp. 493-500.

56. T. Parsons. "Illness and the Role of the Physician: A Sociological Perspective." In *Personality in Nature, Society, and Culture,* edited by C. Kluckhohn and H. A. Murray. New York: Knopf, 1956, pp. 609-617. T. Parsons and R. Fox. "Illness, Therapy and the Modern Urban American Family." *J Soc Issues,* vol. 8, no. 4, 1952, pp. 31-44. M. M. Johnson and H. Martin. "A Sociological Analysis of the Nurse Role." In *Social Interaction and Patient Care. Op. cit.,* pp. 36-38.

57. R. Lindheim, H. Glaser, and C. Coffin. "Environments for Sick Children." Children's Hospital at Stanford, Palo Alto, Calif., November 13, 1970. (A working paper.) E. L. Brown. "Meeting Patients' Psychosocial Needs in the General Hospital." In *Social Interaction and Patient Care. Op. cit.,* p. 8. E. L. Brown. *Newer Dimensions of Patient Care: Part I—The Use of the Physical and Social Environment of the General Hospital for Therapeutic Purposes.* New York: Russell Sage Foundation, 1961.

58. D. Haire and J. Haire. *Implementing Family-Centered Maternity Care With A Central Nursery.* 3d ed. Hillside, N. J.: International Childbirth Education Association, 1971. A. D. Coleman and L. L. Coleman. *Pregnancy: The Psychological Experience.* New York: Seabury Press, 1973. See especially pp. 76-83.

59. E. L. Brown. *Newer Dimensions of Patient Care: Part I. Op. cit.,* 1965, p. 121, appendix 1.

60. E. Kubler-Ross. *On Death and Dying.* New York: Macmillan, 1970, p. 5. L. D. Hazell. *Commonsense Childbirth.* New York: Putnam, 1969, p. 139.

61. M. Halberstam. *Op. cit.,* pp. 1180-1185.

62. *Ibid.,* p. 1184.

63. E. L. Brown. *Newer Dimensions of Patient Care: Part I. Op. cit.,* 1961, pp. 30-54. C. Barnett et al. "Neonatal Separation: The Maternal Side of Interaction Deprivation." *Pediatrics,* vol. 45, February 1970, pp. 197-205.

64. R. Lindheim, H. Glaser, and C. Coffin. *Op. cit.*

65. From a 1968 lecture in Social Medicine by Dr. Paul F. O'Rourke, founding director, Charles Drew Health Center, East Palo Alto, Calif.

66. J. M. Gustafson. *Op. cit.,* pp. 556-557.

67. A. R. Jonsen. "A New Ethic for Medicine?" *West J Med,* vol. 120, February 1974, pp. 169-173. A. R. Jonsen, W. H. Tooley, and R. H. Phibbs. "Ethical Issues in New Born Intensive Care: A Conference Report." Unpublished paper, Health Policy Program, September 1, 1974.

68. D. Hendin. *Op. cit.* R. F. Drinan. "The Inviolability of the Right to be Born." *West Reserve Law Rev,* vol. 17, December 1965, pp. 465-479. J. T. Noonan. "The Constitutionality of the Regulation of Abortion." *Hastings Law Rev,* vol. 21, November 1969, pp. 51-65. D. Callahan. *Abortion: Law, Choice and Morality.* London: Macmillan, 1970. See especially Chapter 9, "The Sanctity of Life," pp.

307-348. D. F. Walbert and J. D. Butler, eds. *Abortion, Society and the Law*. Cleveland: The Press of Case Western Reserve University, 1973, pp. 63, 103.

69. O. E. Guttentag. "The Meaning of Death in Medical Theory." *Stanford Med Bull*, vol. 17, November 1959, pp. 165-170. O. E. Guttentag. "On Defining Medicine." *Christ Scholar*, vol. 46, Fall 1963, pp. 202-203. D. Hendin. *Op. cit.*, pp. 17-49. Anonymous. "Inside Judaica—At What Point Does Jewish Law Accept That Death Has Occurred?" *San Francisco Jewish Bulletin*, vol. 124, September 20, 1974, p. 4. A. R. Jonsen. "The Totally Implantable Artificial Heart." *Op. cit.*

70. J. R. Guyther. *Op. cit.*, pp. 44-45. D. Hendin. *Op. cit.* See especially Chapter 3, "Euthanasia—Let There Be Death," pp. 66-96. D. Maguire. *Death By Choice*. New York: Doubleday, 1974.

71. A. H. Maslow. *Toward A Psychology of Being*. Princeton: Van Nostrand Reinhold, 1968. E. Fromm. *Op. cit.*, pp. 58-96.

72. B. Bettelheim. "Individual and Mass Behavior in Extreme Situations." In *Readings in Social Psychology*, edited by T. M. Newcomb and E. L. Hartley. New York: Holt, 1947, pp. 628-638. O. Lengyel. *I Survived Hitler's Ovens*. New York: Avon, 1947. R. Hilberg. *Op. cit.* E. Kogon. *Theory and Practice of Hell*. New York: Octagon, 1972.

73. E. Goffman. *Op. cit.*, pp. 60-61. D. Vail. *Op. cit.* R. M. Coe. "Self-Conception and Institutionalization." In *Older People and Their Social Worlds*, edited by A. Rose. Philadelphia: F. A. Davis Co., 1965, pp. 225-243. M. Greenblatt, R. York, and E. L. Brown. *Op. cit.* See especially Chapter 2, "Eliminating Major Evils," p. 55. R. Rubenstein and H. Lasswell. *The Sharing of Power in a Psychiatric Hospital*. New Haven: Yale University Press, 1966, p. 5. A. B. Hollingshead and F. C. Redlich. *Social Class and Mental Illness*. New York: John Wiley & Sons, 1958.

74. W. I. Thomas and F. Znaniecki. *The Polish Peasant in Europe and America*. New York: Knopf, 1927. W. I. Thomas. "The Definition of the Situation." In *Sociological Theory: A Book of Readings*, edited by L. A. Coser and R. Rosenberg. New York: Macmillan, 1964, pp. 245-247.

75. R. K. Merton. "Bureaucratic Structure and Personality." In *Reader in Bureaucracy*, edited by R. K. Merton et al. New York: The Free Press, 1952, pp. 367-368. E. Goffman. *Op. cit.* See especially "The Moral Career of the Mental Patient," pp. 127-169. V. Olesen and E. W. Whittaker. *Op. cit.* See especially p. 12 and "Professional Values," pp. 123-131.

76. E. Goffman. *Op. cit.*, pp. 13–14, 62, 150, 169. R. M. Coe. *Op. cit.*

77. O. E. Guttentag. "A Course Entitled 'The Medical Attitude'—An Orientation in the Foundations of Medical Thought." *J Med Educ*, vol. 35, October 1960, pp. 903-907. O. E. Guttentag. "The Problems of Experimentation on Human Beings." *Science*, vol. 117, February 27, 1953, pp. 205-215. A. Montagu. *The Humanization of Man*. Cleveland: World, 1962.

78. K. Mannheim. *Ideology and Utopia*. New York: Harcourt Brace Jovanovich, 1936. C. W. Mills. *The Sociological Imagination*. New York: Oxford University Press, 1959.

79. A. Toffler. *Future Shock*. New York: Random House, 1971. P. Goodman. *Op. cit.*, pp. 6-11. T. Roszak. *The Making of A Counter Culture*. New York: Doubleday, 1969. F. Perls, R. E. Hefferline, and P. Goodman. *Op. cit.*

80. O. E. Guttentag. "Medical Humanism: A Redundant Phrase." *Op. cit.*

81. R. Veatch. "Updating the Hippocratic Oath." *Med Opin*, vol. 8, April 1972, pp. 56-61.

82. T. Parsons. *The Social System. Op. cit.*, pp. 455-459.

83. American Public Health Association. "Health Maintenance Organizations: A Policy Paper." *Am J Public Health*, vol. 61, December 1971, pp. 2528-2536. M. Roemer and W. Shonick. "HMO Performance: The Recent Evidence." *Health and Society (Milbank Mem Fund Q)*, vol. 51, Summer 1973, pp. 271-317.

84. H. I. Kaplan and B. J. Sadock. *Comprehensive Group Psychotherapy*. Baltimore: Williams & Wilkins, 1971, pp. 1, 515-754. R. Corsini. *Methods of Group Psychotherapy*. New York: McGraw-Hill, 1957, pp. 83-107. Z. Blyth. "Group Treatment for Handicapped Children." *J Psychiatr Nurs*, vol. 7, July-August 1969, pp. 172-173.

85. H. J. Freudenberger. "The Professional in the Free Clinic—New Problems, New Views, New Goals." In *The Free Clinic. Op. cit.*, pp. 74-75. I. Yalom. *The Theory and Practice of Group Psychotherapy*. New York: Basic Books, 1970, Preface and p. 6.

86. R. K. Merton, G. Reader, and P. Kendall, eds. *The Student-Physician. Op. cit.*, p. 89. D. C. Ransom and H. E. Vandervoort. *Op. cit.*

87. C. M. Brodsky. *Op. cit.* R. G. Faich. "Social and Structural Factors Affecting Work Satisfaction: A Case Study of General Practitioners in the English National Health Service." Paper read at the annual meeting of the Pacific Sociological Association, Honolulu, Hawaii, April 9, 1971.

88. K. S. Felix. "Total Patient Care: The Team Approach to Transplantation." *Nurs Clin North Am*, vol. 4, September 1969, pp. 451-460. G. Reader. "The Cornell Comprehensive Care and Teaching Program." In *The Student-Physician. Op. cit.*, pp. 81-90.

89. C. H. Calland. *Op. cit.*

90. This observation was made on the basis of personal experience. Also see D. R. Minor. "Psychological Interactions Between Therapeutic Abortion Patients and Their Medical Personnel: Four Case Studies." Unpublished paper, University of California at San Francisco School of Medicine, September 24, 1971, p. 8.

91. A. Burton, ed. *Encounter*. San Francisco: Jossey-Bass, 1970. See especially Chapter 11 by J. Warkentin, pp. 162-170. M. M. Berger. "Experimental and Didactic Aspects of Training in Therapeutic Group Approaches." *Am J Psychiatry*, vol. 126, June 1969, p. 845.

92. R. MacGregor. *Multiple Impact Therapy With Families*. New York: McGraw-Hill, 1961. R. Speck and C. Attneave. "Network Therapy." In *The Book of Family Therapy*, edited by A. Ferber, M. Mendelsohn, and A. Napier. New York: Science House, 1972, pp. 637-665.

93. M. Jones. *The Therapeutic Community: A New Treatment Method in Psychiatry*. New York: Basic Books, 1953. M. Greenblatt, R. H. York, and E. L. Brown. *Op. cit.*

94. L. D. Hazell. *Op. cit.*, p. xxx.

95. W. E. Moore. *The Professions: Roles and Rules*. New York: Russell Sage Foundation, 1970. S. Kasl and S. Cobb. "Health Behavior, Illness Behavior and Sick Role Behavior: Part I, Health and Illness Behavior." *Arch Environ Health*, vol. 12, February 1966, pp. 246-266. *Ibid.* "Part II, Sick-Role Behavior." April 1966, pp. 531-541. T. Parsons and R. Fox. *Op. cit.* G. Gordon. *Role Theory and Illness: A Sociological Perspective*. New Haven: College and University Press, 1966.

96. N. Sanford. "A Draft Proposal for a Comprehensive Study of Conflicts of Interest Among Psychiatrists." Unpublished proposal, The Wright Institute, Berkeley, California, August 22, 1972.

97. E. Freidson. "Review Essay: Health Factories, the New Industrial Sociology." *Op. cit.*, p. 498. T. Thomson. *Op. cit.* See especially the interactions between Alice Nye, R.N., and transplant patients.

98. D. E. Smith, D. J. Bentel, and J. L. Schwartz, eds. *Op. cit.* D. E. Smith and J. Luce. *Op. cit.*

99. T. J. Scheff. "Reevaluation Counseling: Social Implications." *J Hum Psychol*, vol. 12, Spring 1972, pp. 58-71. For a discussion of this principle in co-counseling situations, see H. Jackins. *The Human Situation.* Seattle: Rational Island Publishers, 1973.

100. J. M. Gustafson. *Op. cit.*, pp. 529-557. R. Veatch. *Op. cit.*

101. R. S. Duff and A. B. Hollingshead. *Op. cit.* A. R. Jonsen. "The Right to Health Care." *Bull San Francisco Med Soc*, vol. 46, June 1973, pp. 20-21. *Ibid.* vol. 46, November 1973, pp. 19-20. *Ibid.* vol. 47, April 1974, pp. 18-19. *Ibid.* vol. 48, January 1975, pp. 20-21.

102. T. Bodenheimer. "Dismantling California's County Hospitals." *Health/Pac Bull*, no. 51, April 1973, pp. 3-12. H. P. Dreitzel, ed. *The Social Organization of Health Care.* New York: Macmillan, 1971, pp. 223, 233. D. K. Weisberg. "And the Poor Pay More." *Synapse* (UCSF), vol. 16, December 3, 1971, p. 1. O. Hall. "The Stages of a Medical Career." *Am J Sociol*, vol. 53, March 1948, pp. 327-336. See especially Section 3, "Acquiring a Clientele," p. 332.

103. Unpublished interview data collected in the summer of 1971.

104. F. Davis, ed. *The Nursing Profession: Five Sociological Essays.* New York: John Wiley & Sons, 1966. See especially "Nursing Leadership and Policy" by W. A. Glaser, pp. 42-59, and "Problems and Issues in Collegiate Nursing Education" by F. Davis, V. Olesen, and E. W. Whittaker, pp. 138-175. A. Etzioni, ed. *The Semi-Professions and Their Organization.* New York: The Free Press, 1969. See especially Chapter 5, "Women and Bureaucracy in the Semi-Professions" by I. H. Simpson, pp. 196-265. M. Greenblatt, D. J. Levinson, and R. J. Williams, eds. *Op. cit.* See especially Chapter 12, "Vicissitudes of Psychiatric Ward Personnel" by B. H. Hall, pp. 231-236. M. Jones. *Social Psychiatry in Practice.* Middlesex, England: Penguin Books, 1968. See especially Chapter 3, "Therapeutic Communities," pp. 85-117.

105. R. S. Duff and A. B. Hollingshead. *Op. cit.* B. Stuart and R. Stockton. "Control Over the Utilization of Medical Services." *Health and Society (Milbank Mem Fund Q)*, vol. 51, Summer 1973, pp. 341-394.

106. T. Bodenheimer. *Op. cit.*

107. T. Parsons. *The Social System. Op. cit.*, pp. 454-457. T. Parsons. *Essays In Sociological Theory. Op. cit.*, pp. 40-41.

108. L. E. Moore. *Op. cit.*

109. C. W. Mills. *White Collar. Op. cit.*

110. For a similar view, see E. Freidson. *Profession of Medicine: A Study of the Sociology of Applied Knowledge.* New York: Dodd, Mead, 1973, p. 170.

111. N. H. Cassem and T. Hackett. "Sources of Tension for the CCU Nurse." *Am J Nurs*, vol. 72, August 1972, pp. 1426-1430. J. M. Carnoy. *Op. cit.*, p. 31.

112. W. H. Whyte, Jr. *The Organization Man.* New York: Doubleday Anchor Books, 1956. C. A. Reich. *The Greening of America.* New York: Random House, 1970.

113. A. Combs and D. Snygg. *Individual Behavior: A Perceptual Approach to Behavior.* New York: Harper, 1959. H. R. Wagner, ed. *Alfred Schutz—On Phenomenological and Social Relations.* Chicago: University of Chicago Press, 1970. N. Gross, W. S. Mason, and A. W. McEachern. *Explorations in Role Analysis: Studies of the School Superintendency Role.* New York: John Wiley & Sons, 1958.

114. T. Parsons. *The Social System. Op. cit.,* pp. 454-462. T. Parsons. *Essays in Sociological Theory. Op. cit.,* pp. 38, 40.

115. T. Parsons. *The Social System. Op. cit.,* pp. 65-66, 459-460.

116. D. E. Smith, D. J. Bentel, and J. L. Schwartz, eds. *Op. cit.* R. Veatch. *Op. cit.* E. L. Brown. *Newer Dimensions of Patient Care: Part I. Op. cit.,* 1961, pp. 11-17.

117. J. I. Williams. "Privacy and Health Care." *Can J Public Health,* vol. 62, December 1971, pp. 490-495.

118. T. Bodenheimer. *Op. cit.,* p. 8. C. H. Calland. *Op. cit.* R. K. Merton, G. Reader, and P. L. Kendall, eds. *Op. cit.,* pp. 81–84.

119. Unpublished interview data collected in the summer of 1971.

120. M. Greenblatt, R. H. York, and E. L. Brown. *Op. cit.,* p. 354.

121. H. J. Freudenberger. *Op. cit.,* pp. 69-78. C. R. Rogers. *On Becoming A Person.* Boston: Houghton Mifflin, 1961. See especially Chapter 1, "This is Me," pp. 3-38.

122. L. Schatzman and R. Bucher. "Negotiating a Division of Labor Among Professions in the State Mental Hospital." *Psychiatry,* vol. 27, August 1964, pp. 266-277. E. Freidson. *Profession of Medicine. Op. cit.* See especially Chapter 7, "The Test of Autonomy: Professional Self-Regulation," pp. 137-157. O. Hall. "The Informal Organization of the Medical Profession." *Can J Econ Polit Sci,* vol. 12, February 1946, pp. 30-44.

123. O. Hall, "Types of Medical Careers." *Am J Sociol,* vol. 55, November 1949, pp. 243-253. E. Freidson. "Client-Control and Medical Practice." In *Patients, Physicians and Illness. Op. cit.,* pp. 214-221.

124. O. E. Guttentag. "Man's Nature and Finite Freedom." Presented at the National Conference on the Teaching of Medical Ethics, sponsored by the Institute of Society, Ethics and the Life Sciences and by Columbia University, College of Physicians and Surgeons, New York, June 1972. O. E. Guttentag. "Medical Humanism: A Redundant Phrase." *Op. cit.*

125. M. Greenblatt and D. J. Levinson. "The Open Door: A Study of Institutional Change." In *Research Conference on Therapeutic Community,* edited by H. Denber. Springfield, Ill.: Charles C Thomas, 1969, pp. 108–125.

126. K. Kesey. *Op. cit.*

127. E. Goffman. *Op. cit.* D. Vail. *Op. cit.* See especially Chapter 5, "The Institutional Career," pp. 138-156. R. Bennett and I. Nahevow. "Institutional Totality and Criteria of Social Adjustments in Residences for the Aged." *J Soc Issues,* vol. 21, October 1965, pp. 44-78.

128. H. Schwartz. *Op. cit.,* pp. 14-17, 55. R. R. Alford. "The Political Economy of Health Care: Dynamics Without Change." *Polit and Soc,* vol. 21, Winter 1972, pp. 127-164. M. Field. "The Doctor-Patient Relationship in the Perspective of 'Fee-For-Service' and 'Third-Party' Medicine." In *Patients, Physicians and Illness.*

Op. cit., pp. 222-232. Anonymous. "Union Aims Malpractice Threat at Medi-Cal." *Am Med News*, July 29, 1974, p. 15.

129. E. Freidson. "Review Essay: Health Factories, the New Industrial Sociology." *Op. cit.*, pp. 493-500.

130. F. Kafka. "A Country Doctor." In *The Penal Colony* by F. Kafka. New York: Schocken Books, 1948.

131. T. A. Dooley. *Deliver Us From Evil*. New York: Signet, 1961. T. Allan and S. Gordon. *The Scalpel, The Sword—The Story of Dr. Norman Bethume*. New York: A Prometheus Book, 1959. W. A. Glaser. "Nursing Leadership and Policy: Some Cross-National Comparisons." In *The Nursing Profession: Five Sociological Essays. Op. cit.*, pp. 51-55.

132. A psychiatrist on the faculty at the University of California, San Francisco, voiced this opinion in a social-medicine seminar. He based his observation on personal experience.

133. N. Sanford and C. Comstock. *Op. cit.*, pp. 7, 102-124.

134. W. I. Thomas and F. Znaniecki. *Op. cit.* M. Janowitz, ed. *W. I. Thomas on Social Organization and Social Personality*. Chicago: University of Chicago Press, 1967.

135. E. Freidson. "Medicine's Mystique." A paper delivered at the Symposium on the Medical Mystique, sponsored by the Pacific Medical Center of San Francisco, March 9-11, 1973. A. Daniels. "Does the Umbrella of Medicine Shelter the Patient as Well as the Psychiatrist?" *Psychiatr Dig*, forthcoming. T. S. Szasz. *Op. cit.*, pp. 543-544.

136. D. E. Smith and J. Luce. *Op. cit.*, p. 33. D. E. Smith, D. J. Bentel, and J. L. Schwartz, eds. *Op. cit.*, p. 70. M. Jones. *Op. cit.*, p. 86.

137. M. Zborowski. "The Patient and the Hospital." A paper presented at a conference on "Developing Social Work Problems in Hospitals and Related Health Institutions," Chicago, March 1971.

138. M. G. Field. *Op. cit.*, p. 224. H. Schwartz. *Op. cit.*, p. 55.

139. G. Sparer, G. Dines, and D. Smith. "Consumer Participation in OEO Assisted Neighborhood Health Centers." *Am J Public Health*, vol. 60, June 1970, pp. 1091-1102. Health Policy Advisory Committee (Health-Pac.) *Op. cit.*, pp. 232-241. E. Freidson. *Professional Dominance: The Social Structure of Medical Care*. New York: Atherton, 1970. See especially Part III, "Problems of Organizing Medical Care."

140. Where practitioners are wary of consumer power, they try to prevent encroachment into their professional sphere. See A. W. Parker. "The Consumer as Policy-Maker: Issues of Training." *Am J Public Health*, vol. 60, November 1970, pp. 2139-2153.

141. R. Veatch. *Op. cit.* E. Frankfort. *Op. cit.*, pp. xvii-xxii.

142. A. Bottone. *Op. cit.*, pp. 833-836.

143. W. G. Bennis and E. H. Schein. "Principles and Strategies in the Use of Laboratory Training for Improving Social Systems." In *The Planning of Change*, edited by W. G. Bennis, K. D. Benne, and R. Chin. New York: Holt, Rinehart and Winston, 1969, pp. 335-357. C. Argyris. *Integrating the Individual and the Organization*. New York: John Wiley & Sons, 1964. See especially "Problem Solving and Organizational Effectiveness," pp. 136-145. E. Fromm. *Op. cit.*, pp. 105-121.

144. R. Veatch. *Op. cit.* The Boston Women's Health Book Collective. *Op. cit.*

145. E. Frankfort. *Op. cit.*, p. xxii.

146. B. G. Glaser. "Disclosure of Terminal Illness." In *Patients, Physicians and Illness. Op. cit.*, pp. 204-213. P. H Brauer. "Should the Patient Be Told the Truth?" *Nurs Outlook*, vol. 8, December 1960, pp. 672-676.

147. Unpublished interview data collected in the summer of 1971.

148. S. M. Jourard. "Away With the 'Bedside Manner'!" *Op. cit.*, pp. 111-120. J. Quint. *Op. cit.*, pp. 176-180. G. W. Tudor. "A Sociopsychiatric Nursing Approach to Intervention in a Problem of Mutual Withdrawal on a Mental Hospital Ward." *Psychiatry*, vol. 15, May 1952, pp. 193-217.

149. Statement by a pediatrician who treats cerebral palsy children. Personal communication.

150. Statement by Michael W. Chapman, M.D., Assistant Professor of Orthopedic Surgery, University of California, San Francisco, at a symposium entitled: "Do We Really Care What the Patient Thinks: Spinal Injury?", sponsored by Continuing Education in Nursing, UCSF, held at St. Mary's Hospital, San Francisco, September 23, 1972.

151. R. T. La Piere and P. R. Farnsworth. *Social Psychology.* New York: McGraw-Hill, 1949, p. 292.

152. T. Parsons. *The Social System. Op. cit.*, pp. 435, 458-459. T. Parsons. "Illness and the Role of the Physician: A Sociological Perspective." In *Personality in Nature, Society, and Culture. Op. cit.*

153. D. E. Smith, D. J. Bentel, and J. L. Schwartz, eds. *Op. cit.* See "Introduction." D. E. Smith and J. Luce. *Op. cit.*, p. 28.

154. Personal conversation with a cardiovascular surgeon at the University of California, San Francisco.

155. R. W. Tyler. "Distinctive Attributes of Education for the Professions." *Soc Work J*, vol. 33, April 1952, pp. 55-62, 94. U.S. Department of Health, Education, and Welfare, Office of Education. *Education for the Professions*, edited by L. E. Blauch. Washington, D.C.: U.S. Government Printing Office, 1955, p. 3. E. Gross. *Work and Society.* New York: Crowell 1958, p. 79, quotation from T. H. Marshall. "The Recent History of Professionalism in Relation to Social Structure and Social Policy." *Can J Econ Polit Sci*, vol. 5, August 1939, pp. 325-340. M. L. Cogan. "Toward a Definition of Profession." *Harv Educ Rev*, vol. 23, Winter 1953, pp. 33-50.

156. T. Caplow. *The Sociology of Work.* Minneapolis: University of Minnesota Press, 1954, pp. 114, 122-123. A. R. Jonsen. "Conceptual Foundations for an Ethics of Medical Care." A paper delivered at the "Conference on Human Value Issues in Health Care," Institute of Medicine, Washington, D.C., November 28-30, 1973.

157. For a discussion of norms governing relations among providers, see O. Hall. "The Stages of a Medical Career." *Op. cit.* O. Hall. "The Informal Organization of the Medical Profession." *Op. cit.* T. Caplow. *Op. cit.*

158. W. J. Goode and P. K. Hatt. *Methods in Social Research.* New York: McGraw-Hill, 1952, pp. 53-54.

159. D. L. Rosenhan. *Op. cit.*, p. 255. M. Argyle and J. Dean. "Eye Contact, Distance and Affiliation." *Sociometry*, vol. 28, September 1965, pp. 289-304. N. J. Felipe and R. Sommer. "Invasion of Personal Space." *Soc Probl*, vol. 14, Fall 1966. pp. 206-214.

160. J. DeAugustinis et al. "The Meaning of Touch in Interpersonal Communication." In *Some Clinical Approaches to Psychiatric Nursing*, edited by S. Burd and M. Marshall. New York: Macmillan, 1963, pp. 271-306. A. Montagu. *Touching: The Human Significance of the Skin*. New York: Perennial Library, 1972.

161. Unpublished observational data from pilot study, Summer 1971.

162. L. Schatzman. "Voluntarism and Professional Practice in the Health Professions." *Op. cit.*

163. D. R. Minor. *Op. cit.*

CHAPTER FIVE

A MORAL PERSPECTIVE

Commentary on Jan Howard's Conceptual View

ROBERT E. COOKE, M.D.

My discussion of Dr. Howard's thought-provoking paper is presented from a moral standpoint, not from a purely medical one. I adopt this perspective even though professionally I am a pediatrician, not an ethicist, and as department chairman I have had the responsibility for a large primary care center for children that is heavily involved with research on the delivery of care.

Although frequently not appreciated, the adequacy and distribution of medical care is an *ethical* issue rather than a professional one. Medical care is claimed as a right not because it can be clearly demonstrated that such care reduces illness or lengthens life or markedly improves health, but as a matter of justice. As moral policy, medical care of equivalent quality is owed to each person. Indeed, the very title of this book, *Humanizing Health Care*, reflects ethical considerations. In this context ethics is defined as considered reflection on human behavior, beliefs, and goals from the standpoint of what is right or wrong, what ought or ought not to be done.

The various components of humanized or dehumanized care can be readily examined from this perspective:

1. Ought patients to be treated as things?
2. Ought patients to be managed differently depending on social class or status?
3. Ought patients to be regarded as full human beings?

Basically these are moral questions, not procedural ones, although procedural approaches may be the expression of the moral policy. The sociological model, which has been emphasized, more readily relates to ethical considerations, although the biological and psychological models also have ethical aspects even though they are less obvious.

Another reason for emphasizing the ethical approach to humanized care is that ethical considerations permit a strategy for acceptance by society of the issues presented. Both professionals and laity in general claim justice as an important ethical principle even though they may be insensitive to its absence at times. The ethical approach may well be the only way to effect change when results in material terms cannot clearly be demonstrated.

Finally, the ethical perspective permits the derivation of an important factor in humanized care. If one takes a formalist approach to the series of transactions involved in medical care, trust appears to be a critical ingredient. Trust is the consequence of several basic ethical principles including promise keeping, beneficence, noninjury, and justice. Without trust the relationships between physician and patient cannot rise above that between provider and consumer. In certain respects this difference may be the difference between humanized and dehumanized care. If the physician is regarded only as a provider and the patient only as a consumer when problems so important as life and death are concerned, then medical care is dehumanized.

Although much relativism exists in society in regard to the expression of ethical principles or, in procedural terms, the ways of providing humanized care, there is considerable agreement on the moral principles underlying such care. Almost all would agree that truth telling and justice are essential moral tenets regardless of their utility. Most would agree also that such principles as gratitude, self-improvement, noninjury, and reparation are important.[1] Poor black families are owed medical care not solely as a way of improving public health and welfare or race relations for the benefit of all, but because we owe them a debt of reparation for long years of neglect.

However, if one follows the economic approach of Bentham and Mill[2] and adopts utility as the *only* criterion of right or wrong, then the only justification for the provision of humanized rather than dehumanized care would be better service at less cost. In this case there would be much disagreement as to the importance of humanized care and even greater conflict as to its ingredients, since it would be impossible to weigh all the consequences remote and immediate. It would also be impossible to decide on much good for some or a little good for all without some concept of justice, as John Rawls has frequently emphasized.[3]

Two "emotional" ingredients of humanized care suggested by Dr. Howard—empathy and affect—are also of interest to the ethicist. Their presence depends very much on the love of an individual for mankind (love of God in religious terms). The quality of the relationship between people depends greatly on what some ethicists have called "perceptivity," the degree of sensitivity of one individual to the needs of another, and on "tenacity," the extent to which one is moved by a relationship to do something on behalf of another.

Although a significant part of perceptivity and tenacity—love of mankind—may have its origin early in life, there is evidence from Kohlberg[4] that the stage of moral development on which an individual operates may be modified by exposure to ethical dilemma solving. Such studies suggest that training in moral development is important for medical education and possibly for the selection of health-care personnel.

Certain ethical principles may pose problems for the humanization of care. Individualization—the recognition of individual differences—may lead to differential treatment as in the case of a fetus or special benefits for a President. However, the justness of such an approach may be questioned. Similarly, benevolence toward others may be considered a fundamental moral principle and may be so regarded by a patient who volunteers for human experimentation. But experimentation can be dehumanizing if it counters the principle of noninjury. There is, thus, a need for caution in applying ethical standards.

The concept of philia or mutual relationship seems appropriate to describe the basic physician-patient relationship from an ethical standpoint, even though dependency is implied and is actually present.[5] It characterizes the sick adult or child because of the ego-shattering effects of illness. A mutual relationship can exist even with a high degree of dependency as in the mutuality of our relationships with our children.

Indeed, in a just and free society, there is imposed on the less dependent a greater responsibility for the rights of the more dependent. In a sense there is reciprocal association between rights and responsibilities that is necessary to maintain social balance. Consequently, professionals must assume great responsibility for the rights of their clients, even to their own discomfort.

Thus the conceptions that physicians or other professionals have of their relationships to their patients or clients are of importance from a research standpoint. My personal observations suggest a great range of conceptions. The patient may be regarded as part of self—the illness hurts the physician as well as the patient. The patient may be thought of as property under the control or ownership of the physician. At the other extreme, a relationship with a patient may be viewed simply as a technical process. This occurs, for example, in abortion procedures. Busy surgeons may think that their responsibility to the patient is best served by concentrating on the technical aspects of surgery rather than on the whole person. Good, ethical physicians differ greatly in their sense of vocation.

The sense of vocation, the ethical relationships between physician and patient, the concept of humanized care in gestalt form seem best expressed by Seneca centuries ago. This citation also summarizes my own concept of humanized care.

> Why is it that I owe something more to my physician and my teacher, and yet do not complete the payment of what is due to them? Because from being physician or teacher they become friends and we are under an obligation to them, not because of their skill, which they sell, but because of their kind and friendly good will. If, therefore, a physician does nothing more than feel my pulse and put me on the list of those whom he visits on his rounds, instructing me what to do and what to avoid without any personal feeling, I owe him nothing more than his fee because he does not see me as a friend, but as a client.
>
> Why then are we so much indebted to these men? Not because what they have sold us is worth more than we paid for it, but because they have contributed something to us personally.
>
> A physician who gave me more attention than was necessary because he was afraid for me, not for his professional reputation, who was not content to indicate remedies, but also applied them; who sat at my bedside among my anxious friends and hurried to me at times of crisis; for whom no service was too burdensome, none too distasteful to perform, who was not indifferent to my moans; to whom, although a host of others sent for him, I was always his chief concern; who took time for the others only when my illness per-

mitted him. Such a man has placed me under an obligation, not so much as a physician but as a friend.[6]

NOTES

1. W. D. *The Right and the Good*. Oxford: Clarendon Press, 1930.
2. J. S. Mill. *Utilitarianism*. New York: Liberal Arts Press, 1949.
3. J. Rawls. *A Theory of Justice*. Cambridge: Harvard University Press, 1971.
4. L. Kohlberg. "Stages of Moral Development as a Basis for Moral Education." In *Moral Education: Interdisciplinary Approaches*, edited by C. M. Back, B. S. Crittenden, and E. V. Sullivan. Toronto: University of Toronto Press, 1971.
5. P. Lain-Entralgo. *Doctor and Patient*. New York: McGraw-Hill, 1969.
6. Seneca. *De Beneficis*. VI, 16.

CHAPTER SIX

STRATEGIES FOR RESARCH

Commentary on Jan Howard's Conceptual View

EUGENE FEINGOLD, PH.D.

Dr. Howard has presented a thoughtful and sophisticated analysis of the concepts of humanization and dehumanization of health care. My comments deal with matters of emphasis and clarification.

Dr. Howard sets forth 11 different meanings of dehumanization used in the literature and then suggests 8 dimensions of humanization. This complex and sophisticated approach raises serious problems of research strategy.

The first problem is whether her analysis is too sophisticated and complex for meaningful research. Some of the dimensions she suggests are closely related to one another or, indeed, may simply be different ways of approaching the same kinds of issues and problems. If we could operationalize these dimensions adequately, we could determine whether they are independent, interdependent or perhaps, as I have suggested, just different ways of looking at the same phenomena. But the operationalization is likely to be difficult and, where done, likely to be crude and not capable of supporting the distinctions in her conceptual model.

Here we have the obvious danger, which I mention because the application of so much research ignores it: that of confusing the proxy measures used in research with the reality—or the concept—with which the research deals. I think it is significant that Dr. Howard's focus on operationalization is relatively brief and is really a discussion of research methods and strategies rather than operationalization of the concepts she presented earlier. This is partly because operationalizing those concepts is difficult and is not the major task set forth for Dr. Howard.

This difficulty of operationalization is related to the second issue of research strategy raised by Dr. Howard—the question of where we should place our emphasis. Dr. Howard has presented a series of research problems that are much more than the contributors to this book—or the larger set of interested scholars for whom we are proxies—could hope to deal with in our lifetime. How do we select from her menu of problems? Too much research seems to be done to provide employment for the researcher rather than to meet more broadly conceived social needs. I suggest that we select those problems where our research seems most likely to lead to the greater humanization of medical care. This means that we should be most concerned with variables that are subject to policy manipulation. It also means that the research problem must be carefully translated to and from the real world, lest the research findings be limited or distorted in their application to the social problems with which we are concerned.

When I say this, I do not wish to seem a philistine. I recognize the need for basic research; I recognize the need of researchers for intellectual satisfaction in what they are doing; I recognize the difficulty in determining the likely payoff from research. Yet, within those constraints, it is possible to select research problems in terms of their social significance. For example, one of the hypotheses Dr. Howard suggests might be tested is that "the more professionals and patients view one another as equals, the greater their propensity to share decision making." There is certainly intellectual interest in testing the hypothesis. It can reasonably be said to have some connection with humanizing care. However, we should be explicit in thinking through that connection. We also should assess the priority of that hypothesis—from the perspective of humanizing care—among the various hypotheses that we might want to test. That particular hypothesis would probably have a fairly low ranking in such a priority listing.

A third, and related, question of research strategy is who should define the characteristics of humanization. One who is not intimately involved in the medical-care process can provide insight and analysis that those who are directly involved—both patients and providers—cannot. Yet, presumably we are interested in actually humanizing care, not just in studying the concept. This means that we have to be responsive to those who are delivering care, and to those who are receiving it, both providers and consumers. All of us expressing our views here are, or have been, patients; some of us are also providers. However, we are certainly atypical patients, and may be atypical providers as well. Dr. Howard is correct in saying that " 'gut' interpretations" of the concept are inadequate for research, but we must be careful that we do not get too far away from an interpretation that has meaning for those who are receiving and giving care. As I pointed out earlier, I find Dr. Howard's sophisticated statement of the dimensions of humanization most attractive, but I am not sure how meaningful that complex a statement is for those who are trying to understand humanized care at the point where care is provided.

I now want to discuss some specific dimensions suggested by Dr. Howard. I am pleased that she defines humanization not only in terms of providers' attitudes toward consumers, but also consumers' attitudes toward providers and, at least implicitly, the attitudes of some providers toward others (while still pointing out that it is doubtful that providers undergo the extremes of humiliation experienced by some consumers). The attitudes of consumers toward providers, and providers toward other providers, are likely to be highly important as we move to greater use of physician extenders of various kinds, and as questions of their acceptability to patients and other health professionals are raised. Will patients want a "real" doctor? How will "real" doctors react to physicians' assistants?

Dr. Howard raises another aspect of the dehumanization of the provider when she says that "if practitioners treat patients or colleagues as less than fully human they function at less than full human potential and begin to conceive of *themselves* as nonpersons." Others may have the same thing in mind when they refer to the low morale of physicians who work in a dehumanized situation. It may be true in some philosophical sense that a provider in this setting does *become* less of a person, but this is very different from saying that such providers *conceive of themselves* as less than persons; to say that their morale is low is very different from saying that they are dehumanized.

Another dimension suggested by Dr. Howard is the treatment of the patient as a whole person. In her section on operationalization, she argues that the extent to which providers question the patient about the patient's personal life, outside of the immediate medical problem that presents itself, could be regarded as an index of humanism. Such questioning indicates an interest in aspects of the person that are not task related. Yet intrusion into the patient's private world can be patronizing and thereby dehumanizing. Thus we have a conflict between respect for privacy and the need to view the patient as a whole person. There may be similar but less obvious conflicts in the other dimensions of humanization, and we should be alert to them.

One of the variables in Dr. Howard's scheme is that of inherent worth. There is a difference between saying that all humans are beings of value, and saying that all are of equal value. It is possible to accept the inherent worth of all human beings and still say that some people are more deserving of attention than others. It seems to me reasonable, for example, that the medical needs of a person whose life or death represents a matter of great social concern, such as the President of the United States, should get more attention and greater devotion of resources than the needs of a person of whom this is less true. That may not be a popular thing to say, either in the abstract or in the case of a particular President, but our society certainly behaves that way, and we need to clarify our thinking about this question.

Perhaps all human beings are entitled to a certain level and type of care, with extra attention given to special persons. If so, can we define the level and type of care to which all are entitled? Most hospital insurance covers the cost of ward or semiprivate care, but not private rooms; rental of a television set in a hospital is typically not covered by insurance, but purchase of lotion for a back rub is covered. I suspect that we would not be satisfied with these as distinctions between that kind of care to which all are entitled and that for which the special few qualify, nor would we be satisfied with the implied basis for selection of the special few: ability to pay the extra costs. It would however, be useful to define the humanized care to which all are entitled and the characteristics that would qualify one for care beyond that level.

Another dimension of dehumanization discussed by Dr. Howard is freedom of action, freedom of choice: "Where the interaction is forced on participants and one or the other is bound against his will, the experience cannot be humanizing." I am not so sure that freedom of action is a dimension of humanization. I think it is possible to have constraints on freedom and still have a humanizing or humanistic experience. Perhaps this is a matter of the range or extent of constraints. Or perhaps there is a threshold beyond which constraints precipitate dehumanization, although some constraints may not be inconsistent with humanization.

My earlier comments about the difficulty of operationalization are supported by Dr. Howard's report of her own research. The three indicators used in that research (the extent of interruption of relationships between patients and providers, the use of signs, and the comfort of the environment) are not related to any of the eight dimensions or, at least, the association is not self-evident. This is important because it suggests she is returning to the " 'gut' interpretation" that we started with, and it may not be possible or desirable to get away from that.

Moreover, I am not certain whether any of those three indicators actually measures dehumanization. I will focus particularly on written signs. I find signs humanizing. In a strange setting, I am always concerned about information. The more information I get, the happier I am; if there is a sign that tells me where to go and how to get help and so on, I am happy with that. I do not know if I would be happier if a human being told me this orally; but, for me at least, information presented on written signs is not necessarily an indication of dehumanization. If the signs are necessitated by crowding that makes it difficult for the individual to get attention, it is not the signs that are dehumanizing, but rather the crowding. The same may be true about the frequency of interruption in contact. It is not necessarily inconsistent with the patient's inherent dignity to have interruptions, if they are courteous. Again, it may be a matter of the extent of interruptions.

Finally, let me comment on the general social setting within which we are working. Dr. Howard started by saying that there seems to be an idea that health-care systems should not replicate the impersonality of the larger social system and culture within which they exist. I do not know whether that is possible; I suspect it is not a realistic expectation. We may try to work in that direction, but one of the reasons why health care is so dehumanized is that our whole culture is to a large extent dehumanized. It may be unrealistic to try to change the medical-care system without changing the social system as a whole. This may be one of the more important topics we should deal with in our research.

PART THREE

CONSEQUENCES

J an Howard summarizes the many ways humanization and dehumanization have been conceptualized and portrayed in relevant literature. She presents a framework for achieving greater clarity and doing more pertinent research on these issues. Next, Howard Leventhal, a professor of psychology at the University of Wisconsin, sets forth a social-psychological model whereby the consequences of dehumanization in health-care systems can be traced and the process and content of interaction possibly altered. Because effects are inextricably bound to causes, he also discusses certain conditions that lead to depersonalization and dehumanization of patients. His perspective differs considerably from that of Jack Geiger who places greater emphasis on social structure than on social psychology.

Leventhal first considers what might be the various components of dehumanization from the patient's viewpoint. He distinguishes between the psychological process of self-depersonalization and dehumanization— the feeling that one is isolated from others. Then he offers a schematic model of how information is processed when one is perceiving, interpreting, and reacting to the environment. Next Leventhal describes linkages between the informational inputs from illness and treatment settings, and the development of self-depersonalization and the feeling of being dehumanized. Finally, he suggests how this model can be applied to research and medical practice. In doing so, he uses some of his own experimental studies, noting that they have already influenced medical practice in settings where his research was carried out.

Professor Leventhal's model grows directly out of his own investigations. His most recent work includes: "Changing Attitudes and Habits to Reduce Risk Factors in Chronic Disease," *Am J Cardiol*, vol. 31, May 1973, pp. 571-580; (with R. Mazen) "The Influence of Communicator-Recipient Similarity Upon the Beliefs and Behavior of Pregnant Women," *J Exp Soc Psychol*, vol. 8, July 1972, pp. 289-302; "The Emotions," in *Social Psychology*, edited by C. Nemeth, Chicago: Markham, 1974; "Attitudes, Their Nature, Growth, and Change," *ibid.*; and (with J. Johnson) "Effects of Accurate Expectations and Behavioral Instructions on Reactions During a Noxious Medical Examination," *J Pers Soc Psychol*, vol. 29, no. 5, 1974, pp. 710-718.

The two commentators on Howard Leventhal's paper, Irving L. Janis and Jeanne Benoliel, are respectively teachers and researchers in psychology and nursing. Each discusses Leventhal's paper from a perspective influenced by personal research. Irving Janis has taught for many years at Yale University, where he holds a professorship in the Department of Psychology. He has had a long-time interest in psychological stress, one of the most important research areas in personality and social psychology and, of course, one that is highly relevant to illness and health care. His book, *Psychological Stress* (New York: John Wiley & Sons, 1958), was a pioneering work, and 13 years later he followed this with *Stress and Frustration* (New York: Harcourt Brace Jovanovich, 1971). His most recent volumes are: *Victims of Groupthink: A Psychological Study of Foreign Policy Decisions and Fiascos,* Boston: Houghton Mifflin, 1972 and *Changing Behavior Through Counseling*, in press.

Janis's research is based on what he calls, in the closing paragraph of his discussion, "a free-wheeling methodological approach that combines the best of the clinical and experimental traditions." His books contain materials of direct and indirect relevance to the psychological reactions of the ill. His discussion of Leventhal's paper reflects his interests both in social-psychological research and in community problems. Janis points to what he believes is a somewhat broader approach than Leventhal's and emphasizes the role of the psychological "helper." He stresses theory and research bearing on the potential functions of paramedical personnel who will be trained in giving the kind of psychological care that will reduce patients' tendencies toward isolation and self-depersonalization.

Jeanne Quint Benoliel is professor and chairman of the Department of Comparative Nursing Care Systems at the University of Washington. She previously taught at the University of California at Los Angeles and the University of California at San Francisco, where she also received her doctoral degree. She has a wealth of personal experience in clinical nursing, as well as many years of research experience employing field methods in hospitals and patients' homes. Dr. Benoliel is best known, perhaps, for her publications on various aspects of dying and terminal care: for instance, (Jeanne Quint) *The Nurse and the Dying Patient,* New York: Macmillan, 1967; "Nursing Care for the Terminal Patient: A Psychological Approach," in *Psycho-Social Aspects of Terminal Care,* edited by B. Schoenberg et al., New York: Columbia University Press, 1972, pp. 145-161; "The Concept of Care for the Child with Leukemia," *Nurs Forum,* vol. 2, no. 2, 1972, pp. 194-204; and "Impact of Life-Threatening Disease on Family Interaction," in *The Patient, Death, and the Family,* edited by S. Troup, New York: Charles Scribner's Sons, in press. But her writings also include more general issues involving patient care—for instance, her dissertation on the social aspects of diabetes in children, and her article, "Institutionalized Practices of Information Control," *Psychiatry,* vol. 28, May 1965, pp. 118-132. Her discussion of Howard Leventhal's paper flows naturally from her research and clinical experience in hospitals.

CHAPTER SEVEN

THE CONSEQUENCES OF DEPERSONALIZATION DURING ILLNESS AND TREATMENT

An Information-Processing Model

HOWARD LEVENTHAL, PH.D.

A STRATEGY FOR DEALING WITH THE CONCEPT OF DEHUMANIZATION. The term "dehumanization" has two major shortcomings as a guide to the scientific analysis of patients' feelings and behavior during illness and treatment: (1) it fails to specify the covert feeling and overt actions that accompany dehumanization, and (2) it does not show how these feelings and actions are produced. Thus, the process of dehumanization is poorly understood because there is no analytical model that defines its essential components and helps to explain its origin and development. Only with

The ideas developed here reflect my work on grants from the National Science Foundation (GS-31450X) and the Robert Wood Johnson Foundation, and my participation on a Committee for Reviewing Research in Health Behavior sponsored by the American Sociological Association.

the development of such a model will it be possible to understand and possibly ameliorate the experience of dehumanization.

As Jan Howard's review of the literature reveals, the lack of such a model impedes scholarly analysis. To remedy this, a "bootstrap" strategy[1] must be adopted to provisionally define the phenomenon, propose a conceptual model of the underlying process, and modify the conceptualization as more is learned.

This paper is divided into four parts. The first uses a speculative, phenomenological approach to define the components of dehumanization as the patient might experience them. Many of the components might be better understood as aspects of the process of self-depersonalization, the division of self into psychological and physical parts.[2] By contrast, "dehumanization" might be defined as the feeling that one is isolated from others and is regarded as a thing rather than as a person. Second, a schematic model of how people process information in perceiving, interpreting, and reacting to the world is presented. In the third part, it is suggested that self-depersonalization and dehumanizing experiences are caused by the interaction of this processing system with the informational inputs from both the illness and the treatment setting, and that the experiences and behaviors characteristic of dehumanization are "natural outcomes" of this interaction. This does not mean that these experiences are necessary or unavoidable, nor that they occur because of deliberate planning by malicious others. These dehumanizing experiences can be avoided or reduced if *specific actions* are taken to redirect the ongoing interplay between individuals' processing systems and their environments. This section also examines some of the effects of self-depersonalization and dehumanization on the patient's decision to seek and follow through with medical advice.

The last section introduces a model that suggests a distinctive approach to research and medical practice, and that can be used to generate clinical research to test hypotheses with direct relevance to clinical practice. As an example, I describe some experimental work that has already influenced practice in endoscopy. An important goal of this section is to show that experimental studies, which vary situational conditions to produce changes in specified behaviors, offer the richest reward for both theory and practice, as they increase the confidence in the validity of conceptual models and provide a direct route for introducing change in the clinical setting.

COMPONENTS OF SELF-DEPERSONALIZATION AND DEHUMANIZATION. A set of six factors is proposed to describe the process of self-depersonalization and dehumanization during illness. Whether these six factors exhaust the domain, or whether they are distinct or overlapping, is not of immediate importance. This list was developed from clinical material and from the literature of medical sociology and psychology. A source that deserves special mention is Janis's *Psychological Stress*.[3] We should view the six factors as a starting point for conceptual and empirical analysis, and they will be used to pose questions about the information processing model presented in the following section.

1. SEPARATION OF THE PHYSICAL AND PSYCHOLOGICAL SELF. A component common to most reports of self-depersonalization is the experience of one's self as a physical object or thing. In extreme cases a patient seems to report a complete separation of the conscious, psychological self from the physical self.[4] This experience may well be the basis for the entire complex of experiences that can be grouped under self-depersonalization *and* dehumanization.

2. ISOLATION OF THE PSYCHOLOGICAL SELF. The sense that one's conscious psychological self is isolated from other conscious, psychological selves seems to be a second important factor in both self-depersonalization and dehumanization. This feeling may reinforce the belief that one is treated as a thing, that people are indifferent to one another's private experiences, and exaggerate the feeling of a split between the psychological self and the physical world.

3. UNCERTAINTY AND CYCLIC THOUGHT. Doubt, confusion, and uncertainty will appear when the individual encounters internal events (e.g., pains, symptoms) and external events (e.g., diagnostic tests) that are novel and inadequately labeled and understood. Because patients are unable to explain the causes of these events and cannot, therefore, anticipate their consequences, they may become uncertain about what they are actually experiencing, whether it is real, or whether it is purely subjective.

4. PLANLESSNESS AND LOSS OF COMPETENCY. The separation of psychological and physical self, the difficulty in labeling events, perceiving causes and anticipating consequences, the sense of isolation, and the appearance of uncertainty and repetitive thinking create for patients a deep sense of incompetence and loss of ability to plan and cope with their immediate situation. They may feel totally incapable of influencing their situation, and this feeling can be intensified by the institutional imposition of roles such as the sick role,[5] whereby individuals are treated as persons to be acted upon and are denied the authority and knowledge to act on their own behalf and participate in their treatment.[6]

5. EMOTIONAL DISTRESS, HOPELESSNESS, AND DESPAIR. Negative emotions —fear, terror, and depression—often accompany acute experiences of depersonalization and dehumanization and may eventually result in chronic states of anxiety, despair, and hopelessness. These emotional responses are both a consequence and another cause of the cognitive aspects of self-depersonalization and dehumanization.

6. BARRIERS TO COMMUNICATION. The experience of self-depersonalization may lead patients to believe that they cannot communicate with others, and thus their feelings of dehumanization increase. These barriers to communication may be either cognitive or motivational. They are cognitive when individuals are unable to categorize and describe their experiences. The split between the psychological and physical self, the complex internal physical stimuli, and the endless cycle of self-stimulating fantasies and ever-fluctuating shades of negative emotion may defy description. Motivational barriers may exist if patients believe that others are indifferent to their psychological experiences, and if they anticipate criticism and negative self-appraisal for attempting to describe or for referring to their novel and confusing private experiences.

The Conceptual Status of the Components. The above factors are tentative descriptions of attributes of conscious experience. It is not clear that the six variables are completely independent, and they may well be redundant under some environmental circumstances. Their interdependence is both a theoretical and an empirical issue. An empirically-oriented factor analyst might urge us to develop measures for each factor and then assess their interdependence,[7] but I believe that such advice would be premature. Stable, independent factors are more likely to be observed if we have a clear idea about *how* and *when* to measure them. To answer the questions about how and particularly when to measure them, a provisional model that explains the underlying process of these experiences must be developed.

By assuming that each of these tentatively identified factors reflects a particular outcome of the interaction between situational conditions and the person's information-processing mechanism, it is possible for us to see that a descriptive or correlational study may show a high degree of association between two of these factors. This is because the factors are either produced by the same underlying component of the information-processing mechanism, or because they are produced by two closely linked components of the information-processing sequence. A true test of the independence of these two factors requires an experimental rather than a correlational examination; that is, manipulations must be designed that would separate the parts of the information-processing mechanisms to which the two experiences are linked.

A second suggestion of the hypothesis of an underlying mechanism is that not all aspects of the process will be conscious. But this does not mean that the conscious experience of dehumanization is a surface factor and has no causal significance; such an extrapolation is unnecessary and false.[8] Conscious experience (thingness, isolation, uncertainty, and so on) is a product, but one that can serve as a cause in a system that is partially closed so that consciousness feeds back into the system and influences the subsequent actions of the information-processing mechanism.[9] Our goal is to understand the processes creating these feelings and to introduce situational changes that will alter the information-processing sequence.

AN INFORMATION-PROCESSING MODEL. Most people follow an epistemology of naive realism. Taking the world for granted, they believe that what they see and hear they see and hear because of what *is there*. The perceived environment provides a structured framework for behavior, and experience and action are treated as facts or simple givens. When in a philosophic and reflective mood, however, individuals may realize that both experience and action depend on their own activity. An information-processing model attempts not only to describe the activities that produce experience and to explain how experience comes into being, but also how planning and action take place. The goal is to describe the active process that exists both between input and experience and between experience and action.

The Construction of Perceptual Experience. Momentary experience seems to be a product of two clearly interrelated, yet distinguishable, steps: (1) decoding the distinctive features of the stimulus input, and (2) synthesizing or enriching the input with a hypothesis or schema.

DECODING. Decoding involves a sequence of steps in the selective abstraction of environmental features. The decoding or abstracting system is highly organized, and the development of its physical structure is guided by innate processes. First, it is divided into receptor systems (e.g., visual, auditory, and kinesthetic) that are sensitive to a particular type and range of physical energy. Abstracting continues within a system as signals are transmitted from the periphery to the brain. For example, successive layers of the visual system respond to abstracted *distinctive features* of the input, for example, retinal units may respond to light onset or light offset. These signals are used to build contrast and define edges. Cells in specific layers of the cortex respond to features of this retinal output, for example, some cells respond only to dark lines and others only to bright lines. Further on in the system some cells respond only to horizontal lines and others only to vertical lines.[10] Different parts of the nervous system, therefore, are responding to specific features of the stimulus input.

SYNTHESIS OF FEATURES AND HYPOTHESIS. We see a world of things, events, and meanings, not a collection of lines, edges, and corners. Synthesizing the abstracted elements by means of hypotheses or neural schemas is a key step in the completion of a perceptual experience. Synthesis takes time, that is, it is an active process with a beginning and an end,[11] but it is so rapid that it is usually entirely unconscious. That synthesis occurs outside of awareness may explain why we experience our perceptual worlds as external to ourselves.

What is the evidence for synthesis? Common sense provides some, as when we "sense" that an object, while hidden, still exists, or recognize that different reflected images belong to the same object.[12] Strong evidence for the role of synthesis in perception has emerged from cross-cultural studies of people from non-Western cultures lacking experience with perspective in drawing. These people make incorrect judgments about the distances of objects in photographs because they interpret all of the size differences between objects in a photograph as cues to the relative size of the objects and not as cues to their relative distance.[13] Another striking example of synthesis is seen in the perception of the rotating trapezoid. Because Western observers of the trapezoid see it as a window, they incorrectly see it as oscillating when it is in fact rotating. But non-Western viewers who lack experience with windows do not synthesize the trapezoid with the concept of windows and do not see the illusion.[14]

Finally, each of us can become acutely aware of the active synthetic process when it is slowed or disrupted, for example, by very brief presentations of stimulus inputs,[15] by reversible, illusory, or other novel and impossible forms,[16] or by drugs.[17] Under these conditions the ambiguity of the input and the discrepancy between schema and input stretches out the synthesis process, and we must make an effort to organize the perceptual field. In summary, our moment-by-moment experience is the product of an active integration of the inputs ordered by external reality with hypotheses or schemas that are products of our past experience.[18]

The process of integrating hypothesis and distinctive features, although not well understood, is clearly more complex than a simple process of matching an input pattern to one of a set of templates.[19] Some psychologists think of the features of the abstracted sensory input as actively seeking their appropriate schema, but this view omits the fact that the schema also seems to reach out and seek its appropriate input.[20] How else can we account for our sometimes seeing what we expect to see?[21]

An important aspect of the synthetic process is the effect of hypotheses on the rate and quantity of information that we can handle in a unit of time. Complex hypotheses are capable of integrating large units of experience. Learning to read provides a good example of how schemas can change and grow in order to speed the rate of information processing.[22] In the early stages we learn each of the 26 characters and painfully spell out words so that we can recognize them. When we develop word hypotheses, recognition shifts to word units, and we no longer need attnd to individual letters; indeed, when the schemas for words are well formed, it is dfficult to notce errors in spelling or omission of letter elements (as in attend, difficult, and notice in this sentence). Highly skilled readers anticipate what is coming and reach out for large chunks of meaning;[23] as they scan the material, they may ignore word and phrase components.

Plan and Action Units. Information processing serves as the basis for planning overt, goal-oriented action. Indeed, synthesized perceptions and conceptions seem to produce direct pressure toward action. William James in his ideomotor theory of action hypothesized that thought automatically gives rise to an impulse to act. This hypothesis has been verified in a number of experimental studies.[24] One can recognize two clear functions of overt instrumental responses: (1) they are useful in moving toward and obtaining goals, and (2) they serve to validate and to sustain our perceptual and conceptual experience. This testing function of action is extremely important as a means of building the complex schemas that organize our perceptual world.[25]

PLANS AND PERCEPTION.   Plans are often treated as products of perception and interpretation. Thus, the perception of a situation, the particular threats and rewards offered, and the means of obtaining the rewards and avoiding the threats determine the selection of particular instrumental actions. Decision theories deal with act selection by developing models where the choice of an action is based on a combination of the *values* (positive and negative) of the goals and *probabilities* of achieving (or avoiding) them.[26] It is important to recognize that plans do not emerge solely from externally induced perceptions: we may plan to act on the basis of internal states, feelings, images, verbal associations and ideas, as well as because of external reality.[27] In *Principles of Psychology*, James[28] suggested that behavioral plans may be linked to different external and internal stimulus events. This may be one reason for the difficulty experienced in controlling behavior under certain circumstances, for example, when a verbally stored self-controlling, antismoking plan fails to be retrieved by the sights and sounds of a party, whereas the desire to smoke and smoking behavior is readily activated by these same social stimuli.[29] Evidence has supported the idea that behaviors may be linked to quite different sources of antecedent stimulation.

Plans, however, are not simply a product of externally and internally generated perceptions and feelings; they may also influence perception and feeling. Because action seems to follow perception it appears illogical to argue that a person's actions or plans for action can influence what that person sees. Action and action plan (sets or behavioral readiness) can maintain or change experience by focusing attention on one or another stimulus input, making some things more clear and salient than others, strengthening some perceptual structurings while discouraging others, and by altering or maintaining features of the external world.[30] This dual aspect of action plans—their dependence on and ability to influence perceptual experience—produces many of the complications in information processing observed during illness.

The Validation of Experience. I have given a brief version of the complex sequence of steps that gives rise to what is typically called "objective" experience and the acts chosen to cope with the "real" external world. An important feature of objective experience is our expectation that it be shared by others. On most occasions, the inputs that initiate information-processing activity are available to all the participants in a given environment, and their sensory decoding systems are nearly always reactive to the same distinctive features of the stimulus input, thus providing a common basis for perceptual organization. Also, within the bounds of a single culture, there is a high degree of similarity between hypotheses or schemas that are used in perceptual synthesis. Thus, our perceptual experiences usually agree with those of others.

SUBJECTIVE EXPERIENCE. The feeling that experience is shared enhances the belief that there is another domain in which perception is experienced as "subjective." Dreams and fantasy best define the subjective end of this dimension. Subjective and objective experiences are not always sharply distinguished; children under four or five years of age think their dreams so real that they can be seen by others. In certain cultures no sharp distinctions exist between dream and reality.[31] The distinction between objective and subjective modes of experience should not be confused with the distinction that defines objective events as independent of an observer and subjective events as dependent upon an observer.[32] This distinction drawn with regard to modes of experience is phenomenological. Thus, both objective and subjective experience are dependent upon individual observers, who refer their objective experiences to the external world and their subjective experiences to an internal world.

Often experience is a blend of the objective and the subjective. For example, while examining a new car in a showroom, one may simultaneously perceive the realities of its shape, color, and mechanical design but also experience the private fantasy of speeding along narrow, winding roads in thrilling pursuit of an exotic rendezvous. The degree to which we are aware of one or the other modes depends on the salience or attention given to each.

Without defining cues, we would never learn to distinguish between objective and subjective events and would confuse the two more frequently than we do. What cues enable us to make this differentiation? One possible cue is that external events usually produce *changes in several modalities*;[33] for example, when we hear a voice we expect to see a speaker and if we do not see the speaker we are likely to regard the experience as subjective or "strange." *Vividness and clarity* provide a second source of cues. "Real" events also have their own, well-defined pace. Further, *mental effort* may provide a cue to subjectivity; for example, if experience changes are concomitant with willful changes in the direction of thought or with the awareness of a shift in one's hypotheses, the contingency will suggest that the variation in experience is dependent upon internal rather than external inputs. Finally, the close link between perception and action may provide a motor signal that helps differentiate external from internal information.

SOCIAL VALIDATION.   There are occasions, however, when the synthesis of objective features and hypotheses slows or falters, and the person becomes aware of himself or herself as a "junction at which sensory ideas terminate and from which motor ideas proceed, [the self] forming a kind of link between the two."[34] Awareness of our role in synthesis makes us conscious that we must weigh and decide whether experience reflects variation in input or variation in hypothesis and whether experience is real and of something "out there" or subjective and of something "internal."

When doubts arise about experience a person may turn to others for clarification and validation. The need to validate experience is the basic proposition of social psychological theories of consensual validation[35] or social comparison.[36] The events leading to social validation are occasionally depicted in bold relief by situations that spread the validation process over time. A recent and vivid personal example occurred late one night when I heard a rattling sound from the gravel on the roof of our house. The noise sounded like the wild running about of dozens of squirrels, but this hypothesis was quickly rejected when a distant rumble suggested that a convoy of heavy trucks had passed. Although this suggestion was inconsistent with usual street traffic and with the time of day, it was not impossible, so I conducted a simple test; I looked out the window and saw nothing. I was now more than slightly curious about the cause of the sounds and even wondered if I had imagined them. There seemed to be two alternatives: to forget the issue or to seek confirmation of my initial experience. I asked my wife if she had heard any noise. She confirmed my initial observation and added to my data by reporting a tremor in the concrete foundation. Two new causal hypotheses came to mind: (1) a violent explosion, and (2) an earthquake.

To test these new hypotheses I sought additional social validation. Now I had to reach out to "experts" who had special information because of their training, geographic location, or access to others. My source was the radio. I tuned to a local talk show and heard others calling in because they had detected the tremors. Since no explosion was reported, the quake hypothesis seemed increasingly likely. For a definitive test, I turned to a station 140 miles to the southeast and heard that tremors had been reported there and further south. The announcer attributed the disturbance to a jet breaking the sound barrier but I rejected this hypothesis because it seemed inconsistent with the fact that the tremor was felt along a line of more than 200 miles. I felt no surprise the next morning to read that a Richter-level 4 quake had hit the Midwest.

Social validation played a key role in structuring this experience. I began with an evaluation of the initial input by confirming that it was experienced by someone in the same environment. Initial attempts at validation are directed toward individuals who share important characteristics with the person needing the information; that is, the other must be in a similar environment[37] or have similar characteristics[38] to insure that the comparison will produce relevant information. When comparisons validate but fail to explain the input, information is sought from experts. The sequence is similar to that reported in studies of response to disaster.[39]

VALIDATION BY ACTORS AND OBSERVERS. The earthquake experience is an example of an unusually orderly series of hypothesis tests moving from efforts at direct validation of reality to efforts at social validation. The testing process, however, can be far less orderly and can result in a far less clear and satisfactory conclusion, as often occurs when the event initiating the sequence of hypothesis tests is internal or nonpublic. Establishing consensus under these circumstances requires that persons acting upon and testing reality communicate with someone who is external to their own situation. Such efforts at social validation may fail because: (1) the observers lack information about the features to which the actors are responding; (2) the actors have difficulty in communicating or raising questions about their observations because they are unable to describe what they saw or because they are unwilling to communicate because of embarrassment or fear of criticism; or (3) the actors cannot understand the observers' responses to their questions. Breakdowns in communication, problems in interpersonal and mutual labeling can arise in these circumstances. These processes are crucial to the illness setting and are discussed in detail in the next section.

PROCESSING INFORMATION DURING ILLNESS AND TREATMENT.   In applying the model to illness and treatment, material previously discussed is repeated and expanded. Thus, additional features are added to our model and new complexities arise.

Illness.   Sickness generates a variety of inputs, from those caused by internal symptoms to those arising from social interactions with members of the helping profession. Often, these inputs are processed and responded to quickly and smoothly. On occasion, however, processing and decision making are ambiguous and conflicting and may lead to strong feelings of self-depersonalization, dehumanization, and stress.

SYMPTOMS.   Symptoms are often the initial clue to illness and can serve as an important focus for hypothesis testing. Symptoms have two characteristics that differentiate them from other inputs: (1) they tend to be ambiguous, and (2) they carry clear implications of threat. Ambiguity is high because symptoms are often novel, of sudden onset, located well within the physical self, experienced through only a few senses (e.g., felt kinesthetically but not seen), fleeting in occurrence (appearing and disappearing with suddenness), hard to localize, and of varying severity. These characteristics make it difficult to evaluate a symptom; it is not clear what it is or if it is getting better or worse. Moreover, the threat implied by the symptom is indeterminate until one can account for and classify it as to an underlying causal process.

The ambiguity, novelty, and potentially threatening implications of symptoms make them a good focus for active hypothesis testing. In an unpublished study, Leventhal and Quinlan[40] asked a number of students what they would think, feel, and do if they noticed each of six different symptoms. Even in this hypothetical setting in which no symptoms were actually present, the protocols revealed a rich set of imagined actions that could be classified into three categories: (1) efforts to identify the antecedent causes of the symptom, (2) efforts to locate additional correlated symptoms to help identify the underlying problem, and (3) attempts to define potential consequences and to evaluate future implications of the disturbance.

Because symptoms serve as a focus for hypothesis testing, they are likely to lead to feelings of self-depersonalization. The body becomes a focus of attention, and ambiguities of the symptom slow a person's processing and lead to conscious, active hypothesis testing, producing a heightened awareness both of one's thoughts and of one's body as an object of thought. This is the basic condition involved in the creation of a division of the mental and physical self. The stage is set, therefore, for self-depersonalization and dehumanization.

HYPOTHESES.   Although the average symptom may be more ambiguous than the average external cue, the ambiguity of any cue—the difficulty in defining its nature, obtaining positive confirmation of its causes, and being aware of its potential consequences—depends on the individual's hypothesis system. A person with many hypotheses about a symptom's meaning can engage in more testing than a person with a limited set of hypotheses who is likely to arrive at a speedy integration of the information, whether this integration is true or false. The range of hypotheses depends on the individual's past history—what he or she has read; the illnesses suffered by self, family, and friends; and the illnesses that are part of family and community folklore. We must not forget, however, that experience can narrow as well as broaden the range of hypotheses applied to threat events. Thus, an illness that is encountered under unusual circumstances (for example, when one is too young to comprehend the situation, or when one lacks the ability or is untrained to cope)[41] can have a strong impact, and later life situations may tend to stimulate worry about the recurrence of this same illness.[42]

But the main generalization seems clear: when an ambiguous input is interpreted by a complex hypothesis system under conditions of threat, active self-evaluation will take place. Unless the individual is especially skilled in completing definitive tests, each interpretation is as likely to generate negative as positive outcomes, and negative outcomes will stimulate alternative hypotheses, with new tests leading to additional negative feedback. The testing process is likely to be *self-stimulating* and may resemble that seen in chronic hypochondriases.[43]

AFFECTIVE RESPONSES.   The ambiguity of a symptom, the multiplicity and threat value of some of its interpretations (e.g., is it cancer?), and the overload of attending simultaneously to an internal event and an objective environment will provoke stress as well as acute and chronic emotional responses. Emotional responses, or felt or perceived subjective reactions, add two important factors to symptom evaluation: (1) they are an additional source of information, and (2) they stimulate behavioral tests or plans.

There are two ways in which the emotional responses may generate information. First, felt emotion provides its own goal. Persons who are frightened or sad will want to reduce their fear or sadness; persons who are angry will want to satisfy their anger. Affects inform and suggest particular actions.[44] For example, if fear and pain lead to the avoidance of a diagnostic test—as seen in studies by Kornzweig[45] and Leventhal and Watts[46]—fear and doubt may be strengthened because the avoidance maintains the uncertainty about one's condition and keeps alive the thoughts of unknown threats. Second, affects may create bodily reactions that can confuse or intensify symptoms. Specific attitudes and emotional states have been shown to influence cooling or warming of the hands, flushing of the face,[47] or heart-rate acceleration, and these can be confused with skin irritation, fever, and heart trouble. Thus, emotions generated by the threat and ambiguity of a symptom may intensify the existing symptom or create new symptoms that add to the perceived threat.

ACT PLANS OR TESTING ROUTINES.   How persons respond to their symptoms and to their subjective affects depends on their specific acquired response plans. If individuals have learned to seek medical help for most symptoms,[48] their particular subcategorization of the symptoms (for example, heart disease, cancer, or stomach upset) and their emotional reactions will have little effect on their behavior. But, in the absence of help-seeking responses, the chosen act will be affected by the cultural, familial, and idiosyncratic interpretations and plans used to cope with the threat.

If persons who know about infections and cancers notice a hard swelling in their neck, they have two possible interpretations of the event, one far less threatening than the other. Since they are likely to have had many infections and few cancers, infection is the more likely interpretation and it may generate various expectations and test plans; for example, if it is an infection, the lump should be sore (feel it); it might feel more sensitive at night than in the morning, there should be other signs of infection (search); there may be an antecedent source of infection (search for memory of injury, fatigue, and so forth); and it should respond to medication.

While these interpretations and tests may be appropriate (lead to desired outcomes) for some conditions, they are unlikely to be relevant to all infectious conditions and rejection of any one possibility may increase the likelihood of interpreting the event as a cancer. Unless the individual knows a good deal about cancer and the means to validate a diagnosis, the tests suggested by the cancer interpretation are even more likely to fail validation than the tests of the infection hypothesis. The ambiguity of the situation may be sufficiently great and the threat sufficiently strong to make the entire system self-stimulating, with mental activity subsiding only when the symptom disappears of its own accord. Failure to stop this mental activity can generate feelings of incompetence and despair. If these feelings become sufficiently intense, they may lead to feelings of isolation and entrapment within a private world.

SYMPTOM AS SUBJECTIVELY EXPERIENCED. A symptom's combination of privacy, ambiguity, and concrete features places it in an ambiguous middle ground between experiences that are objective and subjective. The inability to focus all senses on the symptom, variations in its characteristics, and the presence of other competing external events, for example, insure that much of its existence is outside focused awareness. It has been shown that messages and signals outside of focused awareness often have strong impacts on attitudes[49] and feelings, and may be integrated with complex fantasies and images in ways not observed when material is directly attended to.[50] When patients do not directly attend to the symptom, they place it in the same position as an overheard or partially ignored message. If in these circumstances the symptom connects more easily with fantasies and dangerous thoughts it is neither fully objective nor fully subjective. The patients may then begin to question their ability to distinguish the real from the unreal and be uncertain whether they are acting out of an objective perception, a subjective concern, a confusion of the two, or some other pressure that is produced by the conflict and ambiguity of the setting. We should not be surprised if simple reassurances, such as "everything will be fine," fail to eliminate such hypochondriacal worries and fears.

The "mystery" of the hospital, the white coats, instruments, strange vocabulary, and the instruction to call when help is needed, can sustain fear by creating ambiguity and by *suggesting* that patients are expected to be frightened and unable to cope with their situation. A parallel case arose in psychological investigations of sensory deprivation.[51] Data from early studies suggested that the disintegration of structured, objective experience caused by sensory deprivation was sufficient for the creation of stress,[52] but later studies failed to confirm these findings.[53] It now appears that sensory deprivation caused stress because it combined with situational factors that implied threat (e.g., giving the subject a button to push to call for help).[54]

Delay in Treatment. Persons predisposed to seek medical help for any symptom will be highly predictable in their health behavior, but in the absence of such programming their decision to seek help will depend on the interaction of symptom interpretations, emotional reactions, and the action plans elicited by each. This interactive process could lead to immediate responses or could involve lengthy delays. Blackwell[55] reviewed an unpublished thesis by Roberts[56] that illustrates these effects. In 71 women with breast cancer symptoms, awareness of symptoms combined with anxiety led either to very prompt or to delayed seeking of care. Thus, objective interpretations of a symptom and subjective, affective reactions to it can stimulate action plans that are congruent, in which case there will be little conflict, few false moves and immediate seeking of help, or stimulate action plans that are incongruent, in which case we can expect false starts, conflict, delays of varying durations, and other irrelevant behaviors. A simple example would be seen in two contra-dictory emotional reactions to severe stomach pain. If individuals assume they have appendicitis (objective interpretation) and are afraid they might die before being treated (subjectvie affect), the two motives would combine to elicit immediate help seeking. But if they are afraid they might die during surgery, the goals of the subjective affect and the objective interpretation are incongruent and their behavior will be erratic, delaying, and irrational.

COGNITIVE FACTORS IN DELAY.   A wide range of cognitive variables may affect symptom interpretation and cause delay in treatment. Initially, the availability of plausible, competing interpretations is an important factor. Individuals who entertain a set of interpretations of a symptom are likely to delay action until they attain some clarity as to which inter-pretation is most plausible. Delay is especially likely where there is a difference in the action implications of the different interpretations. For example, persons experiencing cardiac arrhythmia may believe they are suffering serious cardiac disease or temporary disturbance from over-exertion or anxiety-induced hyperventilation. The first interpretation clearly implies immediate, costly medical visits, tests, and so on; the sec-ond requires the inexpensive, self-treatment of sleep, rest, and relaxation.

In most instances, delay and benign neglect verify the less serious of our interpretations. The expectation of benign outcomes, a second and powerful source of delay in help seeking, emerges from such experiences. But competing interpretations and expectation of benign outcome can combine to cause delays fatal to well-being. For example, heart-attack symptoms often imitate symptoms of gastrointestinal disturbance. Symp-tom overlap, or shared features, creates interpretive (diagnostic) diffi-culty, and the fact that a person usually has more stomach upsets than heart attacks makes the benign interpretation more reasonable. Data strongly suggest that the above factors are critical causes of delay in seeking care in the initial, critical minutes and hours following a heart attack.[57]

The very act of *interpreting and testing* a symptom can also create additional delays in seeking medical help. People who assume that a pain is a sign of stomach distress and take an antacid to cure it must wait a reasonable period of time to evaluate the adequacy of their act. Unless they experience increased pain after the self-medication, they are highly likely to wait an hour or more to "see what happens." If new symptoms seem mild in comparison to those initiating the self-treatment, the wait may be extended.[58]

Interpreting and testing can create barriers to help seeking and be hazardous to health for less serious threats than that of death due to heart attack. When self-diagnosis and treatment prove wrong, the individual can attempt a second and a third diagnosis and treatment. With each diagnosis and effort the individual may become increasingly committed to self-medication. The longer one lives with a symptom, and the more one denies its immediate severity and continues self-treatment, the less likely one is to seek help until the repertory of self-medication procedures has been exhausted. The longer the self-treatment period the greater the potential for embarrassment upon seeking help, because one may feel compelled to explain the delay and the self-treatment steps to a doctor.

Curiously enough, symptoms may eventually be disregarded if they are stable and easily categorized. Delay in seeking diagnosis of a lump or a discolored patch of skin may initially arouse competing interpretive hypotheses (is it an infection or is it cancer?), but stability in the symptom features, or failure to notice additional changes, can lead the symptom to be accepted as part of the natural order of things. Mechanic[59] has discussed this normalization process in detail and has suggested that it is likely to occur when the symptom is painless, stable, and highly visible. Studies of delay in seeking diagnosis for cancer have found that highly visible tumors, especially tumors that are seen by other people, are overrepresented in delay.[60]

EMOTIONAL FACTORS.   Emotionally-based denial is so frequently mentioned as the cause of delay in the diagnosis of cancer and heart disease that its mention here seems almost unnecessary.[61] Blackwell[62] makes clear that good health education practice requires that we distinguish denial from mere ignorance. The information-processing model also suggests that it is critical to distinguish delay due to emotionally-based denial from delay that is based on cognitive interpretations unrelated to fear. Denial is present when increasing a person's fear of a disease leads that person to reject a diagnosis in the presence of the disease symptoms, and when the reduction of threat-induced fear leads the person to accept the diagnosis. The distinction is important, because in those instances where treatment is delayed due to misinterpretation or ignorance, behavior can be changed by giving the individual accurate and detailed information on how to identify and to react to the potential threat.

It is also important to recognize that emotionally-based reactions may find support in "realistic" or objective expectations. Thus, while fear may be responsible for the strengthening of an expectation of benign outcome, the expectation may well be plausible. Health workers may undermine their own creditability if, when they strive to change health behavior by using dramatic messages to attack the "emotional basis" of health-belief systems, the information they use exaggerates the likelihood that an individual has a given disease.

It is worth repeating that strong emotions can intensify barriers to communication by adding to the difficulties of defining bodily states and by strengthening feelings of isolation. Communication is difficult enough within a shared external framework; communication may seem impossible, however, if it originates in patients' unshared, internal subjective states. Besides the difficulties of verbalizing the complexities of their symptoms and the fears the symptoms generate, patients may feel it self-demeaning to discuss their condition or the time spent and the techniques used to evaluate and test it. The longer the isolation exists, the larger the set of private experiences, and the greater the individual's absorption in his or her private world, the more difficult it is for communication to take place. The barriers become more formidable because health professionals and health consumers define the physician's role as excluding concern with subjective ideas and emotions. This may explain why patients often prefer to focus on physical symptoms and problems, although their difficulties involve life stress and emotional disturbance.[63] By talking about their subjective lives, patients risk being labeled as mentally disturbed.

SOCIAL FACTORS. Both medical experts and friends and relatives play critical roles in speeding or delaying the use of health-care facilities. Telling the latter about one's symptoms often elicits new interpretations and suggestions for tests and self-treatment, and this causes further delay in seeking expert care. Of course, social contacts can be a source of pressure for immediate help seeking; this has been found for those who seek care following myocardial infarctions.[64]

A common outcome of the social validation process is learning that one's symptoms are shared by another. This may reduce distress by shifting experience from a subjective to an objective frame of reference. There is also a "fallacy of sharing"; if others have it, it could not be all that bad. Of course, in most instances the "fallacy" is true; if everyone in one's environment has a symptom, it is most likely to reflect a benign infectious process. But that is a matter of time and place; shared symptoms undoubtedly failed to relieve distress during times of plague. In most instances, however, discovering shared symptoms would seem to *reduce* threat and alleviate the pressure for seeking medical advice.

ACT PLANS.   Patients with a history of effective medical behavior are less likely than other patients to delay in seeking care. But there are times when awareness of symptoms and appreciation of their danger does not lead to action even in patients who might usually be expected to show effective utilization patterns.[65] This occurs when patients experience symptoms they suspect point to a serious disease, such as cancer, and believe that the medical-care system lacks effective means of dealing with the disorder. Goldsen, Gerhardt, and Handy[66] report delay in seeking diagnosis for suspected cancer in patients who have low scores on a test of knowledge of cancer symptoms and also in patients who had high knowledge scores but who were "generalized cancer worriers." For these patients "knowledge seemed to increase the tendency to delay."[67] Resistance to acceptance of recommendations to take tetanus innoculations[68] and to stop smoking[69] have also been found when subjects low in self-esteem or high in reported susceptibility to disease were exposed to highly threatening messages. These individuals resist the recommendations because they doubt their ability to carry out effective, preventive health practices.[70]

Giving and Following Medical Advice—Actor and Observer in Interaction.   The patient-physician interaction brings two people together in a common setting to focus on a common problem: the patient's illness. Because of this, they are likely to assume a common world, even though there are substantial differences between these two perspectives, and this may affect what is communicated and the degree to which the patient follows the doctor's recommendations. First, the perspective of doctor and patient are different because each is attending to a *different set of cues*, and the cues available to one may be unavailable to the other. Second, the interpretative frameworks of the participants are vastly different. Laypersons use a folk-medical system based on the general knowledge of their culture and ethnic group and the assumptions acquired in their personal and family experiences. Physicians use a medical-scientific frame of reference. Because of the differences in cue input and interpretative system, each party *acts* from a relatively unique frame of reference, and each party is an *observer* of only some of the factors that are influencing the other's behavior. There are three cases that we should now consider: (1) the patient as actor and the doctor as observer, (2) the doctor as actor and the patient as observer, and (3) the case of a third party as actor and observer.

PATIENT AS ACTOR AND DOCTOR AS OBSERVER. Although patients are asked to describe their symptoms and to tell the doctor what is bothering them, they may fail to communicate because of difficulty in describing their ambiguous body state, and because of embarrassment in exposing their feelings and interpretations of their illness. By keeping these concerns to themselves, patients sustain their sense of involvement in a private, subjective reality and prevent the physician from removing groundless fears and correcting many of their misconceptions about their condition. If untreated, these private events may interfere with acceptance of necessary medical procedures. For example, if a patient is suffering from two different conditions and reports the symptoms and is treated only for the more serious of the two, only part of the symptoms will respond to treatment. And if the patient fails to recognize that two disorders are present, he or she may become anxious and think the worst when some of the symptoms remain. Such patients may also lose confidence in their doctors and discontinue what they see as an unsuccessful treatment of their conditions.

Another frequently reported problem is the tendency for patients to discontinue treatment as soon as their most serious or painful symptoms are alleviated. In these cases the doctor is treating a disease agent, but the patient is treating subjective discomfort.[71] The failure to continue treatment poses threats to the patient's health, creates strains on the health-care system because of the requirement for repeated treatment, and increases the patient's sense of dehumanization. Real or apparent failure of treatment can intensify feelings of dehumanization for many reasons. Failure can be taken as a sign of indifference or incompetence of the health-care authorities. To modify these feelings is difficult because patients must report their dissatisfaction either to the offending authority or to another authority when explaining their reasons for change. To have to criticize individuals who are responsible for the management of one's illness can be very stressful, and the patient may fear angering the authorities and risking retribution.[72]

Finally, failure of treatment raises doubts about one's eventual recovery and imposes days of doubt and discomfort. And continued participation in a treatment situation as a less-than-equal partner can erode the patient's self-esteem, and enhance feelings of worthlessness and dehumanization.

The perspective of the physician-observer with respect to the symptomatology and behavior of the patient should be considered in greater detail. Doctors can directly observe overt physical signs of patients' disorders and can obtain additional evidence by means of special instruments and tests. Second, physicians can directly observe the behavior of patients; they hear the patients' words and see their expressions and actions. But although doctors can hear patients' reports of their pains, and can see their anxious expressions, jumpy movements, and external signs of doubt, hesitation, depression, and despair, *the doctors are largely ignorant of the situational and internal cues and ideas that elicit them.* And when patients express fear, pain, and anxiety, the patients themselves are seen as the cause of this behavior, and these causal perceptions are exaggerated when the behavior of these patients differs from that of other typical patients.[73]

Doctors are likely to explain such behavior by applying labels to the source, the patients. The patients' reports of distress, their failure to carry out prescribed treatments, and so forth reflect the fact that they are neurotic, uneducated, or lacking the motivation to be concerned for themselves and their families. Physicians will explain the actions of these patients on the basis of observed variance between patients and will attribute permanent personality characteristics to them.[74]

The fact that the doctor's attention is on the patient's behavior and away from its eliciting conditions does not appear to be a sufficient explanation for labeling. Observers could observe without inferring cause, but explanations are necessary if observers must communicate or act upon their observations.[75] Threats to life and the role demands for precise testing and firm action can force physicians to seek convenient explanations or labels.

Labeling patients can have reasonably clear and predictable consequences. If a patient is defined as neurotic, nervous, and/or unmotivated, the doctor is dealing with a relatively permanent, difficult-to-change set of inner determinants of behavior. By ignoring the environmental events that elicit and become integrated with the patient's hypotheses, the physician defines the task of behavior change as a problem of changing personality traits. This attribution has serious implications for treatment. Because traits seem a sufficient explanation of the action, doctors believe they can do little to influence patients' behavior. Indeed, the physician's role defines their competence as disease directed; they are *not* personality psychologists or psychiatrists, and they are not supposed to meddle with personality or education. They may conclude, therefore, that they can do little more than treat the disease, repeat their recommendations, and throw in an occasional reassuring remark. A consequence is the disruption of communication with those patients who most need information about their conditions. The disruption of communication can intensify patient dissatisfaction and failure to follow medical advice; both responses can probably be taken as signs of dehumanization.[76]

DOCTOR AS ACTOR AND PATIENT AS OBSERVER. Let us reverse the perspective and consider the doctor as actor and the patient as observer. Physicians see and feel some of the things that directly affect patients' experiences, and they also detect events that the patients cannot see and feel. Thus, although there is some sharing of external events, doctors will pay close attention to things outside patients' awareness, and they will ignore many aspects of patients' reports, since they are uninterested in patients' interpretations of their symptoms and those symptoms that do not fit the disease interpretation suggested by objective data.

Physicians also communicate conclusions and recommendations; they may present a diagnosis or request additional technical tests and give some rationale for doing them. Physicians often use technical language or simple phrases that incompletely describe complex, technical procedures. Even if patients are fully aware of the medical implications of their diagnoses, they may not connect the diagnoses to their personal experiences. There are several things physicians can do to connect their statements to the patient's world. The first is to make clear *how medical tests and therapeutic procedures will feel.* "Feel" subsumes the full range of sensory experiences elicited by a test or treatment procedure: coldness, numbness, tingling, sharpness, and so forth. The second concerns *how the procedure will change one's body and its ability to do things.* The third concerns *the full range of implications of these changes for one's future life.* These three types of statement (sensory feeling, bodily changes, future self) form a dimension of information about the self which ranges from concrete sensory experience to abstract issues of self-definition. The usual process of informing patients, for example, naming a medical procedure, or describing how it is performed, does not tell patients how the procedure will affect their experiences and their lives.

The physician's behavior can assume an air of mystery and threat when the patient fails to understand the cues and hypotheses guiding it. This can lead to the following difficulties: (1) provoking fear and suspicion that things are being held back (there must be something else wrong with me—that test means I really must have cancer); (2) creating expectations of miraculous cures that, when frustrated, will lead to doubt, disappointment, and anger; and (3) causing excessive passivity (the doctor will do it all) when active patient participation is desirable or necessary.

Patients may also begin to pay close attention to irrelevant actions that they believe they can understand. Variations in expressive behavior and in tone of voice and facial expression are cues that patients can observe and comprehend. Thus, each smile, frown, or worried look becomes a clue to patients that their conditions are hopeless or curable. Studies of terminally ill patients report that subtle expressive cues from the staff often induce shifts and changes in expectations about the curability of an illness and the expected duration of one's life span.[77] The same process is likely to occur during diagnostic examinations. Patients who are concerned about the outcome of a test and are unable to assimilate statements about the probability of their having a certain disorder may be convinced by a worried or harried look on the face of the doctor, caused perhaps by overwork or some other problem, that they have a fatal illness. Indeed, even the professional manner, with its controlled expressiveness, can be read as an effort to conceal the truth.

Finally, if the doctor's behavior is governed by a system that is neither visible nor understandable, and the doctor makes an effort to eliminate or control emotional and expressive cues, the patient will see the doctor's behavior to be entirely controlled by some impersonal professional role or a defective personality (e.g., the physician seems stiff, inhuman, and machinelike). Under these circumstances, patients feel that they are nothing more than objects diagnosed and treated, and keep their subjective worlds to themselves.

THIRD-PARTY ACTORS/OBSERVERS. A multitude of third parties can function as actors and observers in relation to both the doctor and the patient. Three-party relationships are interesting at both a theoretical and practical level. They are important in demonstrating that some roles encourage the observer to seek situational rather than dispositional explanations of the actor's behavior, an effect that, if real, is inconsistent with the assumption that the observer's explanations of behavior are always biased toward attributing personal dispositions to actors.[78] At a practical level, the three-party relationships illustrate the growing complexity of communication and the barriers to communication in an expanded social-psychological network. I comment briefly on two triads: (1) the child, mother, and doctor, and (2) the patient dealing with two (or more) doctors.

The mother in the first triad brings a third perspective to an already complex interaction; she observes the behavior of both child and doctor and shares some of the physician's informational biases toward the child. But physicians are exposed to many children in a common setting, and comparisons between children will lead them to account for behavioral differences by attribution of variation in personality or behavior traits. The role of mother, however, demands that one pay attention to environmental variation in order to control the exposure of the child to risk (both disease and interpersonal). The mother, therefore, attends to variation in the child's environment. She asks: "Where was he immediately prior to contracting his illness? What was he wearing? Who did he see? What did he do?" Since the mother believes she can and should control exposure to health risks, her explanations and intervention behaviors are likely to be directed toward external events.

We have the interesting case, therefore, of the child's behavior being viewed from both the medical and the maternal frame of reference. Some outcomes of this situation illustrate the difficulties people have in shifting between the actor and observer perspective. For example, when the mother is ill, she will frustrate the physician because the premature clearing of her symptoms often leads her to terminate treatment. But as an observer, she will insist that the child adhere to self-denying acts that she believes necessary to cure the child's illness. These action strategies are consistent with her attributions of the illness to antecedent environmental factors. Of course, this does not mean that the mother will do better in following the doctor's recommendations for the child than she does for herself. If she fails to understand the cause, risk, and treatment of disease she will treat according to her own presuppositions.[79] For example, she may decide to keep her child away from the beach but not take him or her for polio vaccination. Elling, Whittemore, and Green[80] found that 30 percent of their sample of mothers failed to follow prescribed penicillin dosages for children with rheumatic fever. Mostly the failure to follow treatment was related to a lack of understanding of therapy; the mothers did not see how the therapy was related to the agent causing the disease and did not understand what tests were needed to evaluate when treatments could be successfully terminated. For example, one mother gave her child only some of the penicillin prescribed by the doctor because she believed strong drugs should be used sparingly.

Pediatricians often claim their most difficult patients are mothers. From the mother's vantage point the child's environment provides the critical source of variance to account for the onset of the child's illness, and because these events are presumed to be susceptible to control, the child's illness implies that the mother has been derelict in her duty. If the physician fails to respond to her perceptions of cause and her possible feelings of guilt, the physician leaves her highly motivated to cure the child's illness with her own separate, private system of beliefs. This private belief system will affect her execution of the doctor's prescribed treatment. Her evaluation of the child's medical progress is especially likely to control her behavior if that evaluation is reinforced by friends or family members with similar beliefs. Once a social reality is established for an irrelevant and medically unsound belief system, it may be extremely difficult to obtain compliance with needed treatment alternatives.

The second multiple-party arrangement—patient and two or more doctors—appears with increasing frequency in large medical establish-

ments such as university hospitals and private or public clinics that are
staffed by a full complement of specialists. Patients are referred from
doctor to doctor, each of whom examines them through the microscope
of a particular specialty. As Zola[81] has pointed out, patients may have little opportunity to communicate about their private concerns under these
conditions because specialists are not concerned with the total person.
In addition, the difficulty of forming a relationship with each new examining physician arouses fears that one is a number or an object rather
than a person. This perception is readily reinforced by the doctor or
nurse who fails to remember the patient's name, repeats a question
asked by another doctor, and/or appears ignorant of what was said by
some other staff member. If no single person is responsible for care,
patients may wonder to whom they should report new symptoms, and
may begin to feel responsible for coordinating their own care. Such a
thought is not reassuring if they are afraid they are seriously ill and feel
unable to make appropriate decisions. Bold patients may attempt to
manage their own care, but more timid souls may flee from the treatment
setting if this responsibility becomes too frightening.

IMPLICATIONS FOR RESEARCH AND PRACTICE.   The information-processing
model attempts to account for the major aspects of self-depersonalization
and dehumanization experiences during illness and treatment. The
model deals with both the evaluation of internal, illness-based cues and
with the effects of social validation on the evaluation process. Although
a number of the hypotheses derived from the model have been tested in
the laboratories of perception and social psychologists, the extensions to
medical problems are largely unverified. To make these extensions, some
investigators might feel it important to conduct detailed, descriptive
studies of the factors comprising dehumanized experience in different
medical settings and then proceed to locate groups of environmental and
personality variables related to these experiences. It is my belief, however, that the primary approach to testing the model in the medical
area should be experimental; that is, studies should be conducted where
patients are randomly assigned to groups and where the material to
which each group is exposed is carefully prepared to achieve specific
behavioral effects predicted from theory. An experimental approach has
two distinct advantages. First, it allows us to discover causal relationships,

and to learn that one variable temporally precedes another. For example, in a descriptive correlational study relating dehumanization and stress to an impersonal style of interaction, we never can be sure whether the style of interaction is the cause of dehumanization and emotion or whether the dehumanization and emotion cause the style of interaction. In an experimental study we can see if interaction style actually causes or precedes these feelings. Second, the outcomes of the experimental study can be used most easily to change practice. For example, if we know that a particular format of interaction or a particular mode of patient preparation produces less dehumanization and fear than do two alternative procedures, we can put the best procedure to immediate use.

Of course, my preference for the experimental method should not be taken as a blanket endorsement of experimentation. Descriptive work may be needed prior to experimentation, to identify conditions in which dehumanization is most severe, to discover the classes of variables that may cause dehumanized feelings, and to develop measures of dehumanization and distress.

The experiment also has shortcomings, among them the difficulty of isolating those features of a treatment or preparation procedure that are necessary and sufficient for the experimental outcomes. Often the mere introduction of change is sufficient to produce therapeutic effects,[82] and the behavior of staff members may produce demands that bias experimental findings.[83] In either instance, we will be unable to tell which component of a procedure is important, and we may mistake irrelevant factors as necessary conditions for successful delivery of care. Unfortunately, the most complex, costly, and dramatic part of a treatment is likely to be seen as the necessary component; the critical element may be a more subtle factor that is less costly to introduce. To decide which factor is likely to be relevant, we need theories that suggest what to change and what to measure, and we need careful controls to determine precisely which factor is responsible for outcomes. If our theories are precise we can take full advantage of modern procedures of regression analysis and add to the explanatory power of our experiments. Although many problems can be investigated within our information-processing framework, only two will be discussed here.

Creating Shared Expectations. The model stresses the importance of keeping patients oriented to shared objective experiences and providing meaningful action plans or tests for coping with their health problems. Subjective reactions, fears, doubts, and false interpretations are a threat to both treatment and the doctor-patient relationship. Three factors appear to impede the shared communication. First, it may seem necessary to engage in the time-consuming process of in-depth exploration of the patient's subjective world. Any benefits derived from such a costly procedure could readily be offset by reductions in the number of ill people who could be treated. This argument should not be accepted, however, without comparing time spent in treatment with time gained by avoiding repeated visits for improperly treated illness. A second problem concerns which private expectations and feelings should be made public; some may be more therapeutic to share than others. Free expression or ventilation of emotions such as anger, fear, sadness, and disgust may intensify rather than minimize dehumanization.[84] This may occur because (1) expressing emotion serves as a stimulus to more emotion, (2) expression eliminates inhibitions that check unacceptable behavior, and (3) aggression can increase fear and guilt by increasing expectations of justified counterresponses from important figures in the environment.

The third barrier is the fact that the physician tends to ignore the situational component in the patient response and to overemphasize individual differences in hypothesis system, coping strategies, and emotional response that are part of the patient's constitution and past history. These aspects of the processing system are less changeable and discourage intervention.

COMMON DISTINCTIVE FEATURES. My model suggests that in any given treatment situation, the variance in the distinctive features synthesized with each individual's hypotheses may be substantially less than the variance in the individual hypotheses themselves. The model also suggests that identifying these features and preparing patients to interpret them in an appropriate way will eliminate much of the individual variation in patient perception and action.

On the basis of several years of experience in surgical nursing, Jean Johnson[85] suggested that the tactile, kinesthetic, auditory, and visual cues produced by a doctor or nurse when manipulating the patient during diagnosis and treatment were the critical sources of sensory features that generated subjective fear and inappropriate interpretation. The sticking of needles, stretching of skin, abrasions, sounds of cutting, discoloration of skin, and so on[86] were starting points for subjective interpretation.

If virtually all patients experience the same sensations, they can be prepared for the sensations in order to short-circuit this private hypothesis testing. Features that are identified beforehand become part of the normal experience of treatment and do not attract attention or stimulate complex private testing that leads to intense emotional distress.

LOCATING DISTINCTIVE FEATURES.   There are several ways in which specific sensory features can be identified. First, if medical practitioners have themselves undergone an examination or procedure they can use their experience to identify the noticeable pains, the tactile and kinesthetic sensations generated by the procedure, and the sounds or sights that attracted their attention. Whether these features frightened them is unimportant; what is critical is the identification of salient features. A second method of isolating a potential feature is to interview patients. Questions should focus on the particular sensory features noticed while experiencing particular procedures; the interpretation of the features and the affective responses they elicit are of less importance. In short, it is the common sensory material we wish to identify.

Finally, we can carefully observe the setting and patients' responses to it. What do patients stare at? What makes patients flinch? When do they back off? What is done to the patient and how is it likely to feel? From these types of data we can compile a comprehensive list of the sensory features attended to during a treatment or diagnostic procedure. This information can then serve for preparation. We can tell patients what they will feel, see, and hear during a procedure, for example, and we can provide them with interpretations of these events and with plans for responding to them.

THE ENDOSCOPIC STUDY.   Johnson and Leventhal[87] have used the above model to evaluate a procedure to prepare patients for an endoscopic examination. The examination involves a series of potentially threatening and noxious steps: throat swabbing with a novocainelike preparation to achieve local anesthesia, intravenous puncture, swallowing of a fiber optic tube 12 millimeters in diameter and 90 centimeters long, retention of the tube for 15 to 30 minutes, and tube removal. An image of a section of the gastrointestinal tract is projected on one end of the tube and transmitted along the tube to an eyepiece for direct observation. A camera can also be attached to the tube and the image recorded on film.

Because the examination can be safely and successfully conducted only if patients follow a number of instructions, such as breathing through the mouth when the throat is swabbed and numbed, making swallowing motions when the tube is passed, and changing position during the examination, the patients are sedated but not anesthetized. Mouth breathing and swallowing motions are particularly important to throat swabbing and tube swallowing, and if patients faithfully perform these acts, they are likely to gag less and to control the rate at which they swallow the camera tube. Thus, gagging and swallowing time are indicators of successful adaptation to the setting. The amount of tranquilizer given prior to the exam, the increases in heart rate from before to after the tube is swallowed, and the efforts to resist tube swallowing (such as pushing the doctor away) serve as measures of emotional upset and fear.

Johnson and Leventhal hypothesized that the distinctive sensations produced by the procedure were the critical source of negative affective response, and that persons would be less fearful if they accurately anticipated each of these experiences. To do this, a preparatory message was developed that described the private, sensory experiences generated by the endoscopic examination. This message was expected to reduce emotional behavior. A second message was developed to maximize patients' ability to execute the behaviors (mouth breathing and swallowing) requested by the physician.

Four treatment groups were formed so that we could examine the separate and the interactive effects of the two types of preparatory messages: (1) a *sensory-descriptive* group, (2) a *behavioral-instruction* group, (3) a *combined* group-sensory description and behavioral instruction, and (4) a *control* group that received no preparatory information. The sensory description was expected to eliminate idiosyncratic interpretations of the experience and to reduce emotional responses (reduce heart rate, gagging, and the need for tranquilizers). Behavior instruction was expected to change ability to cope with the stress setting and to affect gagging and time for tube swallowing. Together the two messages were expected to reduce fear and facilitate coping.

Patients were accepted into the study if they had not previously received an endoscopic examination, were not disoriented, and were not blind or deaf. Males and females were separately assigned to conditions. Within sex groups, assignment to conditions was in a fixed order; this assured that all four conditions were run within a reasonably short period of time. Even so, eight months were required to obtain complete data on 48 patients.

Care was taken to guard against bias or context-induced effects that would reduce the validity of the experiment by using double-blind procedures for informing patients and measuring patient behavior. The preparatory messages themselves were tape-recorded to eliminate biases introduced by reading. The information on the tape described the specific sensations the patient would experience during the examination. A booklet of 11 photographs accompanied the message; it showed patients in different phases of the examination. When possible, specific sensory experiences were related to similar past events. For example, the message described the painting of the throat as similar to having an examination with a tongue depressor, and photographs showed a patient's face and position while the throat was being painted. The message also described the positions the patient would be asked to assume during the examination, what the patient would feel (a needle stick and drowsiness) during the administration of the intravenous medicine, and the size of the camera tube in relation to a thimble and a pencil. The message also indicated that the physician would insert a finger into the patient's mouth to guide the passage of the tube, that air would be pumped into the stomach and cause a sensation of fullness as though one had eaten a large meal, and that the level of room lighting would be varied to facilitate observation. The message was designed to be an objective description of sensory features (what was seen, felt, tasted, and heard).

There were two parts to the behavioral message. The first gave specific instructions for rapid mouth breathing and panting to reduce gagging during throat painting. The second gave specific instructions on how to swallow while the tube was being inserted, that is, patients were told to make swallowing motions with their mouths open and their chins down. Patients tried each of the actions while listening to the tape and were given additional instructions by the experimenter when the tape concluded.

The analysis of the group differences in patient behavior showed that patients in the *sensory-description* group received significantly less tranquilizer (diazepam) and had more stable heart rates than control patients. Sensory information also significantly reduced the number of patients gagging but by itself had no effect on time for tube passage. The *com-*

bined condition, sensory description plus behavioral instruction, showed more stable heart rates (for patients under 50), very marked reductions in gagging, and a sharp *increase* in time for tube passage. The *combined* message had equivocal effects on miligrams of tranquilizer.

The results show that preparatory communication based on sensory expectations and coping skills can reduce distress and increase compliance with recommended actions. The sensory information reduced distress but did not by itself facilitate action. But the combination of sensory information and behavior instructions had effects on behavior; they reduced gagging and increased the time for tube swallowing by allowing the patients to control the rate of swallowing. To achieve this level of control both fear reduction and instruction were necessary. We did not initially expect the combined message to slow the time required for tube swallowing (the time actually doubled). In retrospect we can see that we should have anticipated the effect because achieving voluntary control of what is usually an automatic act will slow and exaggerate the act's performance.[88] Finally, it is worth emphasizing that these beneficial effects were observed even though the physicians had already given some kind of preparatory information to each patient.

THE PROCEDURE-ILLNESS MATRIX. The model used for the endoscopic study can be extended to a large number of health-care settings. Indeed, it may be useful to think of health care as a matrix of illnesses and procedures (diagnostic and treatment) in which each cell defines a particular illness and procedure and has a set of sensory features. These might be easier to locate in some cells than in others, and there may be procedure-illness combinations where common features are nonexistent. But the hypothesis of common features, that is, that most patients being treated for the same illness have the same sensory experiences, seems the most plausible and potentially most productive. Initially, descriptive work is necessary to identify the sensory features and effective coping reactions. The second step would be experimental studies using carefully constructed preparatory messages to vary patient expectations.

It is worthwhile to reemphasize the role of theory in understanding the preparation process. Both the investigator and the practitioner who know the informational model will attempt to observe and locate common distinctive features and will make use of them in practice. But, in the absence of a theoretical orientation to help raise questions about their experiences, even intelligent professionals may ignore and fail to observe the obvious, common features that initiate interpretations. This point was brought home to me by a resident anèsthesiologist's letter recounting his experiences with the psychoactive anesthetic, ketamine. Having experienced the drug firsthand, he was totally impressed and engrossed by his interpretations and emotional reactions and strongly believed the drug should be avoided at all costs. But he did not provide a detailed report of the sensory changes introduced in his sensorium nor did he think of using such features as a means of patient preparation. Having had the drug myself during a brief hospitalization, I could not help being impressed by the contrast in our reactions. Engrossed in information models, I could not avoid separating and largely ignoring my interpretations and feelings because of my absorption in the intriguing sensory changes induced by the drug. On questioning other patients we discovered that, although their feelings and interpretations differed sharply from my own, they too had experienced these features. How we formulate an experience and what we retain from it is greatly influenced by prior theoretical conceptualization. To prepare individuals we must utilize, where possible, conceptualizations based in empirically tested psychological theory and be prepared to discard our personal interpretations of reality.

Other directions can be taken in research on the process of sharing private experience. For example, we have paid little attention to aspects of the behavior of the health professional. Doctors and nurses differ in personal "warmth" and ease in interpersonal settings,[89] but it is not clear whether a warm and attentive attitude can do as much to eliminate distress and dehumanization as preparation with information on distinctive features, which seems to eliminate idiosyncratic interpretations of stressful events. But these questions can be phrased in experimental form and the data generated could have important effects upon practice.

Institutionizing Change. Since it is not my intention to discuss dehumanization from an institutional framework, my remarks on institutional change are brief. The first point to emphasize is that the informational model requires consideration of the physical and social environment for the sharing of information so that it is not exclusively intrapsychic or patient-oriented. I confined the discussion of social interaction to the traditional doctor-patient dyad and analyzed this interaction by treating each as an actor and an observer. The analysis can be extended, however, to other role relationships such as nurse and patient, nurse and doctor, dietitian and patient, doctor and administrator, and relative and patient. For each relationship one must analyze the kinds of inputs and conceptualizations available to actor and observer with regard to both their own behavioral plans and their expectations regarding the behavior of the other. A role consists of a set of hypotheses that bias one to attend to particular inputs and that specify interpretations and actions suitable for each input.

There are two points I would like to make about the relationship of our information-processing model to roles. First, there may be greater demand for highly structured roles in settings where there is difficulty in sharing private experience, where complex decisions and acts must be performed quickly and where one or both parties are threatened. When many cues are private and when those cues that are public are susceptible to differential interpretation, there is a high probability of incompatible perception and conflict. This conflict cannot be tolerated if speedy decisions are needed to control threat. The consequence is rigid role training to minimize conflict, training to take an annual medical examination, training to be a good and uncomplaining patient, and so forth.

These roles regulate behavior and keep subjective factors out of the interaction. While formalizing relationships can be valuable in creating orderly human interchange, such procedures "dehumanize" the treatment process as the patients are regimented, ignored as persons, and denied their accustomed autonomy.

However, I do not think dehumanization is a necessary consequence of clearly defining the role of doctor and patient and their expectations respecting the roles of the other. Indeed, when situations are structured and the participants understand what they are doing and how to do it, they can predict the outcomes of their interactions and develop a sense of trust. Structuring produces dehumanization when it excludes crucial cues and behaviors; for example, when the doctor's role excludes attention to and fails to train the doctor to uncover the situational features that steer the patient's behavior, or when it leads the doctor to ignore or deny the idiosyncratic interpretations elicited by these factors.

My second point concerns the often made comment that major institutional changes are needed to improve the delivery of health care and to eliminate the evil of dehumanization. A serious problem provokes calls for major change. It is conceivable, of course, that a major social overhaul might solve our problems, although past efforts at drastic, utopian changes seem to have created as many or more new problems than the old problems they were purported to solve.[90] In this instance, however, it is extremely important to examine the claims of those who advocate institutional change and to ask if the elimination of old positions and the creation of new ones, or the alteration or elimination of status hierarchies will solve the problems created by the process of private feature interpretation and the problems encountered in communicating these private processes. To minimize self-depersonalization and dehumanization *it is necessary to alter the content and process of person-to-person interaction and not simply to change the labels applied to the participants.*

Asking for change at the person-to-person level is arguing for changes in the actor-observer framework to increase the access of each observer to the private world of the other actor. Changes of this kind will insure that actors make decisions about themselves based on the best available information regarding their illness and its implications for the economic and social aspects of their lives. While human goodness may help to motivate such change, it is not a sufficient mechanism to initiate and to preserve change once it occurs. Something must penetrate the role definitions of the participants; that is, the doctor role must include rules that guide the doctor to detect the patient's hypotheses and the cues to which the patient is responding. And this holds for many roles in the health-care system. The redefinition of roles may be included or omitted in a wide variety of publicly and privately financed health-care systems, and it must be understood that institutional change is no guarantee of role change, as the role characteristics necessary to reduce dehumanization have been lacking in both privately and publicly financed systems.[91] Basic additions are needed on the medical curriculum and basic redefinitions are needed of the daily tasks legitimate to the roles of those involved in health care.

But if roles are to be redefined to include the task of reducing dehumanizing experience, role participants need to be instructed in how to identify dehumanizing situations and how to act to change them. To learn these things requires theories and practice; just as students learn theories of chemistry and cellular growth so they can better diagnose and treat illness, they need to learn theories about the generation of dehumanizing experience. Theory is needed so they can grasp the structure and dynamics of these situations. Once students have learned the theory they can learn to cope with these situations by practicing specific action paradigms that can be applied to these and to other situations. The model in the present paper is presented as a step in this direction; it is an analytical tool that focuses the user's attention on both the environmental inputs and the personal hypotheses of the perceiver, on the environmental supports and personal skills that sustain the perceiver's decisions, and on the perceiver's problems in sharing inputs, hypotheses, and plans with an observer who has access to different information. The model is a paradigm for both research and practice. But it is neither complete nor the only model available to improve patient care. It is compatible, however, with a wide variety of models of institutional process.

SUMMARY. I have presented a simple model of the experience of self-depersonalization and dehumanization during illness and the consequence of these experiences for seeking and following medical advice. The basic assumptions are that self-depersonalization begins with a separation of the psychological and physical selves and an increased awareness of the privateness of one's own experience. This experience involves an increasing absorption with private events and focuses one's consciousness on bodily and physical processes. This self-evaluation process is self-stimulating rather than self-terminating, because the cues observed are ambiguous both in their sensory and in their interpretive aspects, and the ambiguity leads to repetitive efforts at evaluation.

The social setting can intensify the individual's absorption with his or her private world, or it can encourage the individual to make private matters public and to share key features with others. Pressures against sharing create a sense of dehumanization and alienation from others, and many factors in the doctor-patient relationship create barriers to sharing and encourage dehumanization. For example, both doctor and patient respond to cues that are unavailable to the other, and each may place different interpretations on the cues they do share. This creates barriers to communication ranging from problems in language usage to the absence of shared external referents. This interaction was analyzed in terms of actor-observer relations.

Observers see others' behavior without perceiving or understanding the cues that elicit it; this creates a strong tendency to explain the behavior by attributing characteristics or traits to the actor (i.e., trait labeling). The doctor sees the patient as neurotic, anxious, and dull, for example, and the patient sees the doctor as heartless and unconcerned. Because these attributes take the form of traits or class characteristics, the behavior they explain is not attributed to manipulable, situational cues. As a consequence, neither party feels that it is useful or possible to communicate to the other. This outcome may increase the patient's sense of isolation and dehumanization and lead to serious breakdowns in medical care. If patients' key private cues are made public, they can obtain adequate definition of their situation, terminate repetitive self-evaluative processes, and learn to cope with a relatively well-defined problem.

Finally, an effort was made to develop some of the model's implications for research, practice, and teaching. It was suggested that medical practices can be understood in terms of a matrix of illnesses and procedures, each of which has its own set of common sensory cues (such as aches, pains, movement sensations, sights, and sounds) that are likely to be experienced by all people in that specific setting. By preparing patients for these cues, that is, by telling them what they will see, feel, and hear beforehand, by providing interpretations for the cues (e.g., this is just a sign of . . .), and by providing clear behavioral instructions on how to respond to these cues, one can short-circuit the process of self-stimulating tests and eliminate fear, stress, and individual differences in response to the procedure. A controlled study was described where patients were prepared in this way for an endoscopic examination. The study serves as a model for preparation in other settings. A few comments were made on institutional and role changes needed to insure change in doctor-patient relationships to eliminate dehumanizing experiences.

NOTES

1. R. B. Cattell. "Psychological Theory and Scientific Method." In *Handbook of Multivariate Experimental Psychology*, edited by R. B. Cattell. Chicago: Rand McNally, 1966, pp. 1-18.

2. H. C. Shands, et al. "Psychological Mechanisms in Patients with Cancer." *Cancer*, vol. 4, November 1951, pp. 1159-1170. I would like to thank Irving Janis for suggesting this clarification.

3. I. Janis. *Psychological Stress*. New York: John Wiley & Sons, 1958.

4. H. C. Shands, et al. *Op. cit.*

5. T. Parsons. "Illness and the Role of the Physician." *J Orthopsychiatr*, vol. 21, July 1951, pp. 452-460.

6. S. W. Bloom. *The Doctor and His Patient: A Sociological Interpretation.* New York: Russell Sage Foundation, 1963.

7. R. B. Cattell. *Op. cit.*

8. R. W. Sperry. "A Modified Concept of Consciousness." *Psychol Rev*, vol. 76, November 1969, pp. 532-536.

9. M. A. Arbib. *The Metaphorical Brain: An Introduction to Cybernetics as Artificial Intelligence and Brain Theory.* New York: John Wiley & Sons, 1972. W. T. Powers. "Feedback: Beyond Behaviorism." *Science*, vol. 179, January 1973, pp. 351-356.

10. P. H. Lindsay and D. A. Norman. *Human Information Processing: An Introduction to Psychology.* New York: Academic Press, 1972.

11. N. Neisser. *Cognitive Psychology.* New York: Appleton-Century-Crofts, 1967.

12. T. G. R. Bower. "The Object in the World of the Infant." *Sci Am*, vol. 226, October 1971, pp. 30-38.

13. J. B. Deregowski. "Pictorial Perception and Culture." *Sci Am*, vol. 227, November 1972, pp. 82-88.

14. G. W. Allport and T. F. Pettigrew. "Cultural Influence on the Perception of Movement: The Trapezoidal Illusion Among Zulus." *J Abnorm Soc Psychol*, vol. 55, 1957, pp. 104-113.

15. J. S. Bruner and L. Postman. "On the Perception of Incongruity: A Paradigm." *J Pers*, vol. 18, December 1949, pp. 206-223.

16. R. L. Gregory. *Eye and Brain: The Psychology of Seeing.* New York: McGraw-Hill, 1966. M. C. Escher. *The Graphic Work of M. C. Escher.* New York: Ballantine, 1971. W. H. Ittelson. *The Ames Demonstrations in Perception.* Princeton: Princeton University Press, 1952.

17. A. Huxley. *The Doors of Perception and Heaven and Hell.* New York: Harper & Row, 1956.

18. J. S. Bruner. "On Perceptual Readiness." *Psychol Rev*, vol. 64, March 1957, pp. 123-152. D. O. Hebb. *The Organization of Behavior.* New York: John Wiley & Sons, 1949.

19. P. H. Lindsay and D. A. Norman. *Op. cit.*, pp. 1-8.

20. J. S. Bruner. *Op. cit.* R. L. Gregory. *Op. cit.* N. Neisser. *Op. cit.*

21. J. S. Bruner and L. Postman. *Op. cit.*

22. E. J. Gibson. "Learning to Read." *Science*, vol. 148, May 1965, pp. 1066-1072.

23. G. A. Miller. "The Magical Number Seven, Plus or Minus Two: Some Limits on Our Capacity for Processing Information" *Psychol Rev*, vol. 63, March 1956, pp. 81-97.

24. W. James. *The Principles of Psychology.* New York: Holt, 1890, vols. I and II. A. G. Greenwald. "Sensory Feedback Mechanisms in Performance Control: With Special Reference to the Ideo-Motor Mechanisms." *Psychol Rev*, vol. 77, March 1970, pp. 73-99.

25. R. L. Gregory. *Op. cit.*

26. J. W. Atkinson. "Motivational Determinants of Risk-Taking Behavior." *Psychol*

Rev, vol. 64, November 1957, pp. 359-372. W. Edwards, H. Lindman, and L. D. Phillips. "Emerging Technologies for Making Decisions." In *New Directions in Psychology II*, edited by T. M. Newcomb. New York: Holt, Rinehart and Winston, 1965, pp. 258-325.

27. H. Leventhal. "Findings and Theory in the Study of Fear Communications." In *Advances in Experimental Social Psychology*, edited by L. Berkowitz. New York: Academic Press, vol. 5, 1970, pp. 119-186. H. Leventhal and D. B. Lindsley. "Subjective States." In *Human Factors in Long-Duration Spaceflight*, edited by D. B. Lindsley et al. Washington, D.C.: National Academy of Sciences, 1972, pp. 144-159.

28. W. James. *Op. cit.* Vol. II, Chapter 22.

29. H. Leventhal. "Changing Attitudes and Habits to Reduce Risk Factors in Chronic Disease." *Am J Cardiol*, vol. 31, May 1973, pp. 571-580. H. Leventhal. "Attitudes: Their Nature, Growth, and Change." In *Social Psychology*, edited by C. Nemeth. Chicago: Markham, 1974.

30. D. Kahneman. *Attention and Effort*. Englewood Cliffs, N. J.: Prentice-Hall, 1973.

31. L. Kohlberg. "Stage and Sequence: The Cognitive-Developmental Approach to Socialization." In *Handbook of Socialization Theory and Research*, edited by D. A. Goslin. Chicago: Rand McNally, 1969, pp. 347-480.

32. B. Russell. *An Outline of Philosophy*. New York: Meridian, 1960. (Original publication in United States by Norton, 1927.)

33. H. H. Kelley. "Attribution Theory in Social Psychology." *Nebraska Symposium on Motivation*, vol. 15, 1967, pp. 192-238.

34. W. James. *Op. cit.* Vol. I, p. 298.

35. H. S. Sullivan. *The Interpersonal Theory of Psychiatry*, edited by H. S. Perry and M. L. Garvel. New York: Norton, 1953.

36. L. Festinger. "A Theory of Social Comparison Processes." *Hum Relat*, vol. 7, no. 2, 1954, pp. 117-140. G. H. Mead. *Mind, Self, and Society*. Chicago: University of Chicago Press, 1934.

37. S. Schachter. *The Psychology of Affiliation*. Stanford: Stanford University Press, 1959.

38. L. Festinger. *Op. cit.* R. Mazen and H. Leventhal. "The Influence of Communicator-Recipient Similarity Upon the Beliefs and Behavior of Pregnant Women." *J Exp Soc Psychol*, vol. 8, July 1972, pp. 289-302.

39. L. M. Killian. "The Significance of Multiple-Group Membership in Disaster." *Am J Sociol*, vol. 57, January 1952, pp. 309-314.

40. H. Leventhal and D. Quinlan. "Perceptual and Cognitive Component of Symptom Testing: A Model for the Evaluation of Danger." Mimeo, University of Wisconsin, 1969.

41. L. A. Pervin. "The Need to Predict and Control Under Conditions of Threat." *J Pers*, vol. 31, December 1963, pp. 570-587. J. H. Geer, G. C. Davison, and R. I. Gatchel. "Reduction of Stress in Humans Through Nonveridical Perceived Control of Stimulation." *J Pers Soc Psychol*, vol. 16, December 1970, pp. 731-738. M. E. P. Seligman. "Phobias and Preparedness." *Behav Ther*, vol. 2, July 1971, pp. 307-320.

42. J. S. Bruner. *Op. cit.*

43. D. Mechanic. "Social Psychological Factors Affecting the Presentation of Bodily Complaints." *N Engl J Med*, vol. 286, May 1972, pp. 1132-1139.

44. L. Berkowitz. "The Concept of Aggressive Drive: Some Additional Considerations." In *Advances in Experimental Social Psychology. Op. cit.* vol. 2, 1965, pp. 301-329.

45. N. D. Kornzweig. "Behavior Change as a Function of Fear Arousal and Personality." Unpublished doctoral dissertation, Yale University, 1967.

46. H. Leventhal and J. Watts. "Sources of Resistance to Fear-Arousing Communications on Smoking and Lung Cancer." *J Pers*, vol. 34, June 1966, pp. 155-175.

47. D. T. Graham, J. K. Kabler, and F. K. Graham. "Physiological Response to the Suggestion to Attitudes Specific for Hives and Hypertension." *Psychosom Med*, vol. 24, March-April 1962, pp. 159-169. D. T. Graham, J. A. Stern, and G. Winokur. "The Concept of a Different Specific Set of Physiological Changes in Each Emotion." *Psychiatr Res Rep*, vol. 12, January 1960, pp. 8-15.

48. D. Apple. "How Laymen Define Illness." *J Health Soc Behav*, vol. 2, 1961, pp. 219-225. R. K. Goldsen, P. R. Gerhardt, and V. H. Handy. "Some Factors Related to Patient Delay in Seeking Diagnosis for Cancer Symptoms." *Cancer*, vol. 10, January 1957, pp. 1-7. D. Mechanic and E. H. Volkart. "Stress, Illness Behavior, and the Sick Role." *Am Sociol Rev*, vol. 26, February 1961, pp. 51-58.

49. R. S. Baron, P. H. Baron, and N. Miller. "The Relation Between Distraction and Persuasion." *Psychol Bull*, vol. 80, October 1973, pp. 310-323.

50. F. Pine. "Incidental Stimulation: A Study of Preconscious Transformation." *J Abnorm Soc Psychol*, vol. 60, January 1960, pp. 68-75.

51. D. O. Hebb. "The Motivating Effects of Exteroceptive Stimulation." *Am Psychol*, vol. 13, March 1958, pp. 109-113.

52. W. H. Bexton, W. Heron, and T. H. Scott. "Effects of Decreased Variation in the Sensory Environment." *Can J Psychol*, vol. 8, June 1954, pp. 70-77. J. P. Zubek, W. Sansom, and A. Prysiazniuk. "Intellectual Changes During Prolonged Perceptual Isolation (Darkness and Silence)." *Can J Psychol*, vol. 14, December 1960, pp. 233-243.

53. J. P. Zubek. "Urinary Excretion of Adrenaline and Noradrenaline During Prolonged Immobilization." *J Abnorm Psychol*, vol. 73, June 1968, pp. 223-225. J. P. Zubek and W. Schutte. "Urinary Excretion of Adrenaline and Noradrenaline During Prolonged Perceptual Deprivation." *J Abnorm Psychol*, vol. 71, October 1966, pp. 328-334.

54. M. T. Orne and K. E. Scheibe. "The Contribution of Nondeprivation Factors in the Production of Sensory Deprivation Effects: The Psychology of the Panic Button." *J Abnorm Soc Psychol*, vol. 68, January 1964, pp. 3-12.

55. B. Blackwell. "The Literature of Delay in Seeking Medical Care for Chronic Illness." *Health Educ Monogr*, no. 16, 1963, pp. 3-31.

56. B. J. Roberts. "A Study of Selected Factors and Their Association with Action for Medical Care." Unpublished doctoral dissertation, Harvard University, 1956.

57. S. H. Croog and S. Levine. "Social Status and Subjective Perceptions of 250 Men After Myocardial Infarction." *Public Health Rep*, vol. 84, November 1969, pp. 989-997. T. P. Hackett and N. H. Cassem. "Factors Contributing to Delay in Responding to the Signs and Symptoms of Acute Myocardial Infarction." *Am J Cardiol*,

vol. 24, November 1969, pp. 651-658. H. S. Olin and T. P. Hackett. "The Denial of Chest Pain in 32 Patients with Acute Myocardial Infarction." *JAMA*, vol. 190, December 1964, pp. 977-981.

58. T. P. Hackett and N. H. Cassem. *Op. cit.*, p. 656.

59. D. Mechanic. *Op. cit.*

60. R. K. Goldsen, P. R. Gerhardt, and V. H. Handy. *Op. cit.*

61. B. Cobb et al. "Patient Responsible Delay of Treatment in Cancer." *Cancer*, vol. 7, September 1954, pp. 920-924. T. P. Hackett and N. H. Cassem. *Op. cit.*

62. B. Blackwell. *Op. cit.*, p. 19.

63. P. Kuriloff. "Towards a Viable Public Practice of Psychology: A Psychoecological Model." Doctoral dissertation, Harvard University, 1970.

64. T. P. Hackett and N. H. Cassem. *Op. cit.*

65. B. Kutner and G. Gordan. "Seeking Care for Cancer." *J Health Hum Behav*, vol. 2, no. 3, 1961, pp. 171-178.

66. R. K. Goldsen, P. R. Gerhardt, and V. H. Handy. *Op. cit.*

67. *Ibid.*, p. 5.

68. N. D. Kornzweig. *Op. cit.*

69. P. Niles. "The Relationships of Susceptibility and Anxiety to Acceptance of Fear-Arousing Communications." Unpublished doctoral dissertation, Yale University, 1964.

70. B. Cobb et al. *Op. cit.* H. Leventhal. "Findings and Theory in the Study of Fear Communications." In *Advances in Experimental Social Psychology. Op. cit.*

71. D. Mechanic. *Op. cit.* M. Zborowski. *People in Pain.* San Francisco: Jossey-Bass, 1969.

72. I. Janis. *Op. cit.*, p. 135.

73. E. E. Jones and R. E. Nisbett. *The Actor and the Observer: Divergent Perceptions of the Causes of Behavior.* Morristown, N.J.: General Learning Press, 1971.

74. E. E. Jones and K. E. Davis. "From Acts to Dispositions: The Attribution Process in Person Perception." In *Advances in Experimental Social Psychology. Op. cit.*, pp. 219-266. E. E. Jones and R. E. Nisbett. *Op. cit.* H. H. Kelley. *Op. cit.*

75. H. Leventhal and R. P. Singer. "Affect Arousal and Positioning of Recommendations in Persuasive Communications." *J Pers Soc Psychol*, vol. 4, August 1966, pp. 137-146. R. B. Zajonc. "The Process of Cognitive Tuning in Communication." *J Abnorm Soc Psychol*, vol. 61, September 1960, pp. 159-167.

76. M. H. Becker, R. H. Drachman, and J. P. Kirscht. "Predicting Mothers' Compliance with Pediatric Medical Regimens." *J Pediatr*, vol. 81, October 1972, pp. 843-854. E. Charney et al. "How Well Do Patients Take Oral Penicillin? A Collaborative Study in Private Practice." *Pediatrics*, vol. 40, August 1967, pp. 188-195. M. S. Davis. "Variations in Patients' Compliance with Doctors' Advice: An Empirical Analysis of Patterns of Communication." *Am J Public Health*, vol. 58, February 1968, pp. 274-288. M. S. Davis. "Variation in Patients' Compliance with Doctors' Orders: Medical Practice and Doctor-Patient Interaction." *Psychiatry Med*, vol. 2, January 1971, pp. 31-54. M. S. Davis and R. P. von der Lippe. "Discharge from Hospital Against Medical Advice." Paper read at the annual meeting of the American Sociological Association, Chicago, September 1965. B. M. Korsch, E. K.

Gozzi, and V. Francis. "Gaps in Doctor-Patient Communication." *Pediatrics*, vol. 42, November 1968, pp. 855-871. V. Francis, B. M. Korsch, and M. J. Morris. "Gaps in Doctor-Patient Communication: Patients' Response to Medical Advice." *N Engl J Med*, vol. 280, March 6, 1969, pp. 535-540.

77. H. C. Shands et al. *Op. cit.*

78. E. E. Jones and R. E. Nisbett. *Op. cit.*

79. M. H. Becker, R. H. Drachman, and J. P. Kirscht, *Op. cit.*

80. R. Elling, R. Whittemore, and M. Green. "Patient Participation in a Pediatric Program." *J Health Hum Behav*, vol. 1, Fall 1960, pp. 183-191.

81. I. Zola. "Problems of Communication, Diagnosis, and Patient Care." *J Med Educ*, vol. 38, October 1963, pp. 829-838.

82. D. T. Campbell. "Reforms as Experiments." *Am Psychol*, vol. 24, April 1969, pp. 409-429. H. Leitenberg. "The Use of Single Case Methodology in Psychotherapy Research." *J Abnorm Psychol*, vol. 82, August 1973, pp. 87-101.

83. M. T. Orne. "On the Social Psychology of the Psychological Experiment: With Particular Reference to Demand Characteristics and Their Implications." *Am Psychol*, vol. 17, November 1962, pp. 776-783.

84. L. Berkowitz. "Two Cultures of Violence: Some Opposing Views of Aggression in Therapy." Presidential address to Division 8, Personality and Social Psychology, American Psychological Association, Honolulu, Hawaii, September 1972.

85. J. E. Johnson. "Effects of Accurate Expectations About Sensations on the Sensory and Distress Components of Pain." *J Pers Soc Psychol*, vol. 27, August 1973, pp. 261-275.

86. I. Janis. *Op. cit.*, pp. 361-363.

87. J. E. Johnson and H. Leventhal. "Effects of Accurate Expectations and Behavioral Instructions on Reactions During a Noxious Medical Examination." *J Pers Soc Psychol*, vol. 29, no. 5, 1974, pp. 710-718.

88. G. A. Kimble and L. C. Perlmuter. "The Problem of Volition." *Psychol Rev*, vol. 77, September 1970, pp. 361-384.

89. B. Freeman et al. "Gaps in Doctor-Patient Communication: Doctor-Patient Interaction Analysis." *Pediatr Res*, vol. 5, July 1971, pp. 298-311.

90. K. R. Popper. *The Poverty of Historicism*. New York: Harper & Row, 1964.

91. J. T. Shuval. *Social Functions of Medical Practice*. San Francisco: Jossey-Bass, 1970.

As general references for this chapter, the reader should also see I. L. Janis and H. Leventhal, "Human Reactions to Stress." In *Handbook of Personality Theory and Research*, edited by E. Borgotta and W. Lambert. Boston: Rand McNally, 1968, pp. 1041-1085. I. L. Janis and H. Leventhal, "Psychological Aspects of Physical Illness and Hospital Care." In *Handbook of Clinical Psychology*, edited by B. Wolman. New York: McGraw-Hill, 1965.

CHAPTER EIGHT

PREVENTING DEHUMANIZATION

Commentary on Howard Leventhal's Information-Processing Model

IRVING L. JANIS, PH.D.

Howard Leventhal gives a rich account of a relatively neglected aspect of human stress reactions: the self-dehumanization process that occurs when people become ill. He calls attention to two major sets of antecedent factors that give rise to self-dehumanization in afflicted persons.

One set of factors involves psychological changes induced by the state of being ill. The salience of pain, of unusual sensations, and of all sorts of distressing inner cues creates a sense of separation between the conscious self and the bodily self, as Leventhal puts it. This separation provides the groundwork for perceiving oneself as an object or as a thing.

The second set of variables that foster self-dehumanization pertains to the treatment that the ill person receives from the social environment, particularly from those responsible for the patient's care. It is this set of factors that we can do something about. From a humanistic point of view it is crucial that we try to prevent dehumanizing treatment, both

---

The latter half of this paper is based on material from a forthcoming book, on *Changing Behavior through Counseling*, edited by I. L. Janis. New Haven: Yale University Press.

directly and indirectly. For example, physicians and nurses might compensate for the natural tendencies toward self-dehumanization created by the illness itself. In this respect, Leventhal's analysis in terms of an information-processing model generates practical implications for the way medical care should be organized, as well as some fresh theoretical leads for basic research on stress behavior.

I shall concentrate first on the practical implications, not only because of their inherent social importance but also because they enable us to see clearly what is at stake when we come to the theoretical implications for the psychology of stress. At the end of my paper, I try to show how Leventhal's analysis links up with some new theoretical developments that I believe will lead to innovative research.

At first I visualized the dissemination of the messages of Leventhal and other contributors to this book as bringing about a significant improvement in the direction of humanizing treatment. Right now, I do not think it will. I do not believe it will eliminate the worst evils. One reason for this relatively pessimistic judgment is precisely the factor that David Mechanic raises in his introduction: the time factor. Doctors and nurses are kept extremely busy just by carrying out their prime functions of giving medical care and managing the wards in hospitals. They simply do not have the time to develop the kind of relationship with their patients that is needed to prevent self-dehumanization and demoralization. Preventing the unfavorable emotional consequences that Leventhal talks about is going to be costly, because it will take up a lot of staff time in hospitals and clinics. But I suspect that the costs would somehow be bearable.

The problem of avoiding dehumanization is going to be greatly complicated by technological advances that we are becoming increasingly aware of. Consider what it will mean to patients when it becomes standard practice to use computers to automate diagnosis and prognosis, a development that is now in the wings. When automation takes over it will save a lot of personnel time, and it may well be a blessing from the standpoint of increasing the accuracy of diagnosis and even increasing equity in the distribution of medical resources. But it will certainly augment the problems of dehumanization and therefore become a mixed curse unless we can develop a psychologically sophisticated plan to transform it into an unmixed blessing. Let me briefly allude to the main components that together might constitute a potential solution.

First, we would need to have in every medical setting a full library of sound and videotapes, with messages similar to those on the sound tapes used by Leventhal and his collaborator, Jean Johnson, in their field experiment with patients undergoing endoscopic examination. Their results showed that certain types of preparatory communications can help patients cope more successfully with a distressing medical procedure.[1] I can visualize a whole new industry—hopefully not dominated by Madison Avenue or Hollywood—producing videotapes for use in TV consoles at the patient's bedside. In these tapes a kindly doctor might explain each distressing procedure in a way that would help eliminate disruptive ambiguities and misconceptions about the disease. The tapes might also contain other material designed to help patients carry out the "work of worrying" so as to prepare them psychologically for subsequent stressful experiences—for example, by warning them about temporary episodes of pain and giving them realistic reassurances and a basis for hope that takes account of the typical course of the illness.[2]

But how hopeful can we be, as social scientists, about curing or at least mitigating the psychological consequences of dehumanization that are likely to beset large numbers of people in medical clinics and hospitals? It seems to me that the problem cannot be fully solved even if a videotape industry provides the essential messages and even if doctors, nurses, and hospital administrators acquire all the right kinds of attitudes and values. There is a third factor that is also essential. From what we now know about psychological stress, it seems highly probable that a necessary condition for preventing the self-dehumanization process that typically occurs when a patient is seriously ill is direct human contact with a supportive authority figure. Put another way: patients have powerful social and emotional needs that cannot be filled unless they can interact with a trusted, protective person. Leventhal discusses patients' needs to share their private worlds with a physician or with somebody else involved in their care. He speaks about two factors that contribute to the tendency toward self-dehumanization: the patient's fear of being ignored by the powers that be and the patient's sense of isolation.

If we take seriously the problem of preventing depersonalization and related disruptive reactions that occur under conditions of severe stress, the only practical solution for providing sufficient staff time for direct interaction with patients is to recruit and train paramedical personnel. What we need, in effect, is a new paramedical profession. I emphasize the word "profession" because I think the auxiliary staff must be carefully selected and trained. The degrees they hold are less important than certain human qualities that hit off the values Jan Howard discusses. But good values and good intentions are not enough. We need to develop a well-validated blueprint for effective selection and training.

What specific types of persons ought to be recruited to fulfill these much needed and neglected functions in our present medical-care system? What type of instruction and guided practical experience should these persons be given? What kind of interaction should they have with patients? This is where theory and research come into the picture, because we do not have dependable answers yet.

At this point, we have to remind ourselves of the classic statement made by Kurt Lewin that nothing is so practical as a good theory. Leventhal provides some highly relevant theoretical ideas, although I regard his analysis as incomplete, as I explain shortly. The approach in terms of an information-processing model has considerable merit. The ways that afflicted people label themselves and their physicians and nurses undoubtedly influence the decisions they make about the best course of action to pursue. One of the most intriguing aspects of Leventhal's analysis has to do with the tie-in between information processing and the specific decisions that have to be made by the patient. We do not ordinarily think of the patient as a decision maker. In middle-class America and Europe, the patient role is defined as a passive one. Ill persons are supposed to put themselves into the hands of medical authorities and do whatever they say without complaining very much. (Perhaps that is part of the more general social context that fosters dehumanization in our culture.) But, in fact, patients are active decision makers, as Leventhal points out. First, they must decide whether to seek medical treatment and from whom. Then they must decide whether to accept the treatment the doctor recommends. After that, they must make a series of decisions, sometimes every day, as to how conscientiously they are going to follow all of the rules laid down for them in the recommended medical regimen.

We are just beginning to understand the conditions under which people will adhere to difficult decisions that entail a temporary increase in suffering. When we examine the decisions that must be made by physically afflicted patients, we discover that many of them require the acceptance of short-term losses, such as the physical discomforts of orthopedic exercises, nauseating medicines, or surgery, in order to attain long-term goals—counteracting a structural defect or a disease that might get worse but has not yet created much suffering.

In these cases the positive incentives for adhering to the course of action recommended by the medical authorities are relatively weak, since they involve rather remote, problematic gains in the distant future that can hardly offset, psychologically, the threat of immediate discomfort and suffering. To compensate for the relatively weak incentive value of long-term goals in the face of more immediate and vivid short-term losses, some additional here-and-now incentives to adhere to the stressful decision must be introduced. This is the context in which social support from paramedical professionals can serve a crucial practical function. And it is in this context that I try to explain why, from a theoretical standpoint, I have characterized Leventhal's analysis as valuable but incomplete.

It seems to me that there are fundamental motivational and emotional variables that should be added to Leventhal's information-processing analysis in order to account for the differences between those afflicted patients who steadfastly adhere to difficult therapeutic regimens and those who start off trying to do so but become demoralized and fail. I have in mind variables involving the quality of the patient's interpersonal contact with one or more members of the medical staff, which has a marked effect on feelings of alienation and self-depersonalization. My own studies suggest that such contacts determine the degree to which the patient is influenced by preparatory communications—authoritative recommendations, reassurances, coping instructions, and sensory-descriptive messages.

In observing patients suffering from neurological damage to the spinal cord and various other back injuries, I have noticed that some of them rapidly become hopeless, depersonalized invalids, similar to the patients Leventhal describes. Others, who are suffering from disorders just as severe, actively struggle against becoming demoralized. The latter patients vehemently reject being labeled as permanent cripples. They work day in and day out to carry out all the prescribed procedures and exercises, whether or not the medical staff is around. Sometimes they end up amazing their physicians with the extraordinarily large number of seemingly lost functions they have been able to get back.

One situational variable that seems to loom large in these successful cases is the presence of a warm, dependent relationship with at least one member of the medical staff, a relationship that entails considerable social support during the most stressful periods, as well as bolstering self-confidence. Often I have been reminded of the buddy system and of similar helping relationships in Alcoholics Anonymous and Synanon, which undoubtedly play an important part in enabling some addicted individuals to adhere to the stressful decision of giving up alcohol, nicotine, or other drugs.[3]

This type of observation led me to develop a program of research on helping relationships. My recent studies are directed toward understanding how and why the communication interchanges that occur in counselor-client relationships influence the client's adherence to a stressful decision. As a starting point, I make the following assumption, derived from a considerable body of social psychological research on affiliative needs: when people face a stressful dilemma—including decisional conflicts—they generally become motivated to affiliate with others in order to satisfy a number of important needs. These may involve seeking for social comparison, obtaining reassurance, or bolstering self-esteem.[4]

The central question the studies address is one about which we know relatively little as yet: *How can this need for affiliation be channeled in the direction of heightening the decision maker's responsiveness to a particular type of social support that will strengthen his or her decision to carry out a difficult course of action?*

Although designed primarily to illuminate basic theoretical issues in social psychology, the research bearing on this question could lead to practical improvements in the effectiveness of face-to-face counseling, particularly for clients who seek help in carrying out personal decisions oriented toward future gains in their health, competence, or welfare. Such applications might represent a significant contribution in a variety of community settings—including hospitals and clinics where members of the staff try to help patients cope with discouraging setbacks in carrying out medical recommendations.

Various reports describing the work of community clinics that attempt to help people stop smoking, stay on a diet, undergo painful medical treatments, or carry out other stressful courses of action suggest that contact with a sympathetic counselor, in individual or group sessions, can help people tolerate subsequent stresses or deprivations.[5] These studies provide only remote clues, however, when we ask the key question of interest to social psychologists: What factors make a difference in producing either temporary or sustained positive effects?

I would like to share with you the tentative answers to this question that have emerged from research to date. I focus on key theoretical ideas that are supported by findings from a variety of social psychological investigations. Of special relevance in this connection are the numerous studies in experimental social psychology bearing on the concept of *social commitment* and its effects on stability of attitudes and decisions.[6] Also relevant—as will be seen shortly—are certain findings from research on *interpersonal attraction*[7] and *self-esteem dynamics*.[8]

Much of this prior research indicates that powerful new incentives to adhere to behavioral norms can be introduced through direct interaction with a highly valued person. In terms of the decision-making model I have been developing, certain forms of social support from a counselor or some other norm-transmitting communicator can change the person's decisional balance sheet by inserting a powerful new positive incentive that was not there before.[9] This new incentive involves anticipated social approval from a "significant other." As I suggested earlier, there is a here-and-now reward value in signs of social approval that can, to some extent, compensate for the relative weakness of anticipated long-term gains, especially at crucial times when here-and-now negative feedback is so salient that it can negate the person's readiness to carry out good intentions.

Given the strong affiliation motivation of persons in a stressful dilemma, the question of whether they will develop strong affiliative ties with another person depends partly on whether they receive positive social reinforcement, as Bercheid and Walster[10] point out. One type of social reinforcement from a communicator that is expected to be extraordinarily powerful involves the communicator's making "acceptance" statements that enhance the person's self-esteem.[11] Dittes and Kelley[12] have provided some experimental evidence that a person's attraction toward other persons or groups will rapidly increase when he or she is given accepting comments that raise self-esteem.

Other variables affecting the degree to which a decision maker will be influenced by a would-be helper are suggested by my theoretical analysis of self-esteem dynamics during critical phases of dyadic relationships.[13] This analysis is based on observations of subjects who have come to our

Yale psychology clinics for people who seek help in carrying out health-oriented decisions (e.g., staying on a low-calorie diet). I single out three critical phases in a dyadic relationship that must be successfully surmounted when a counselor, a "buddy," or someone else helps a person adhere to a stressful decision:

1. In the first phase, the helper must surmount the subject's wariness or indifference and acquire motivating power as a significant "reference person," comparable to the motivating power of a reference group.[14] This occurs when the decision maker develops an attitude of reliance on the helper for enhancing and maintaining self-esteem. Such reliance is facilitated when the helper: (a) encourages the decision maker to reveal his or her personal strengths and weaknesses and (b) responds to each self-disclosure with explicit acceptance statements.

2. In the second critical phase, the helper must become a norm-transmitting communicator by endorsing the norms that are implicated by the decision and by eliciting from the decision maker a commitment to live up to those norms. These demands, however, will impair the relationship built up during the first phase, with a consequent loss of the helper's motivating power, unless the helper conveys two important points: that the demands are very limited in scope and that failure to comply with them will not change the helper's basic attitude of acceptance toward the ·decision maker. Helpers are most likely to retain their motivating power as norm setters if they use a selective pattern of social reinforcement whereby they give negative reinforcement, in a nonthreatening way, only for specifically counternorm assertions and give positive reinforcement for all other assertions, including all other admissions of personal shortcomings.

A vivid illustration of a patient's response to a helper who has become a powerfully motivating norm-setter can be cited from the pioneering work of Neal Miller and Barry Dworkin on biofeedback training. These investigators use the techniques of instrumental conditioning with verbal rewards to help patients suffering from hypertension gain control over their blood pressure. A young woman who wrote down her impressions of an arduous 10-week training period during which she temporarily succeeded in lowering her diastolic pressure from a dangerously high average of 97 to a satisfactory average of about 80 had this to say about her trainer:[15]

I always depend very heavily on Barry Dworkin's encouragement and on his personality. I think he could be an Olympic coach. He not only seems aware of my general condition but he is never satisfied with less than my best, and I cannot fool him. I feel we are friends and allies—it's really as though *we* were lowering my pressure.*

Incidentally, if biofeedback training ultimately proves to be effective for large numbers of patients suffering from hypertension and other pathologies of visceral functioning, a whole new area of psychological medicine will open up requiring the services of yet another group of paramedical professionals. Like Dworkin, they will have to be skilled trainers and, at the same time, highly motivating norm setters, similar to Olympic coaches.

3. In the third critical phase, the influence of the helper as a norm setter persists despite the termination of all direct contact with the decision maker. This requires that the decision maker internalize the norms that the helper had been advocating, which will not occur if the decision maker interprets the termination of contact as a sign of rejection or indifference. Adverse reactions to separation are likely to be minimized when the helper, in addition to giving assurances of continual positive regard, arranges for gradual rather than abrupt termination of contact. For example, the helper can offer the decision maker the opportunity to maintain symbolic contact via letters or phone calls.

This brief summary of the theoretical framework indicates the type of considerations that have guided the selection of variables for a number of research investigations that my collaborators and I have recently completed.[16] Confirmatory evidence in support of key hypotheses in the foregoing theoretical analysis has been obtained from our field experiments, which are carried out in clinical settings where people are offered genuine psychological help. The clients who participate in our investigations are mature men and women who are having typical troubles sticking to their decision to go on a diet, to stop smoking, and so forth. The field experiments use factorial designs to investigate main effects and interaction effects predicted by hypotheses that specify the mediating processes whereby a given treatment or combination of treatments by a "helper" will give rise to: (a) immediate changes in the subject's attitudes

* G. Jonas, "Profiles: Visceral Learning I." Copyright © New Yorker Magazine.

and behavior during the period of dyadic contact, and (b) persistent changes in the subject's attitudes and behavior after contact has terminated. The main treatment variables that have been found to be effective include: (1) inducing *self-disclosures* concerning personal weaknesses and misgivings, (2) responding to admissions of personal shortcomings with *explicit acceptance*, (3) using a *selective pattern of social reinforcement*, after presenting action recommendations, and (4) eliciting a *commitment* to the action recommendations.

The findings provide at least tentative support for the theoretical account of the first and second critical phases in a successful helping relationship. We are now carrying out further studies bearing on the third critical phase by investigating variations in the way the relationship is terminated, such as comparing gradual versus abrupt terminations. In this way we hope to fill some of the gaps in existing knowledge about the conditions for counteracting discouragement and inadequate coping behavior in carrying out stressful decisions.

One final point concerning methodology: the most productive research, in my opinion, comes from a freewheeling methodological approach that combines the best of clinical and experimental traditions. Leventhal's contributions, for example, are based on phenomenological descriptions from case studies as well as on statistical data from survey research and social psychological experiments. This type of combined approach should enable us, sooner or later, to obtain evidence for the empirical generalizations that are crucial both for developing a sound theory of stress behavior and for blueprinting effective practical programs to prevent self-dehumanization and demoralization among afflicted people.

NOTES

1. J. E. Johnson and H. Leventhal. "Effects of Accurate Expectations and Behavioral Instructions on Reactions During a Noxious Medical Examination." *J Pers Soc Psychol*, vol. 29, no. 5, 1974, pp. 710-718.

2. I. L. Janis. *Stress and Frustration*. New York: Harcourt Brace Jovanovich, 1971, pp. 93-105.

3. I. L. Janis and D. Hoffman. "Facilitating Effects of Daily Contact Between Partners Who Make a Decision to Cut Down on Smoking." *J Pers Soc Psychol*, vol. 17, January 1970, pp. 25-35.

4. W. G. Bennis et al., eds. *Interpersonal Dynamics: Essays and Readings on Human Interaction*. Homewood, Ill.: Dorsay Press, 1964, pp. 207-225. L. Festinger. "A

Theory of Social Comparison Processes." *Hum Relat*, vol. 7, May 1954, pp. 117-140. J. M. Darley and E. Aronson. "Self-evaluation vs. Direct Anxiety Reduction as Determinants of the Fear-Affiliation Relationship." *J Exp Soc Psychol Suppl*, vol. 1, January 1966, pp. 66-79. R. L. Helmreich and B. E. Collins. "Situational Determinants of Affiliative Preference Under Stress." *J Pers Soc Psychol*, vol. 6, May 1967, pp. 79-85. I. L. Janis. "Group Identification Under Conditions of External Danger." In *Group Dynamics: Research and Theory*, edited by D. Cartwright and A. Zander. New York: Harper & Row, 1968. S. Schachter. *The Psychology of Affiliation*. Stanford: Stanford University Press, 1959. P. G. Zimbardo and R. Formica. "Emotional Comparison and Self-Esteem as Determinants of Affiliation." *J Pers*, vol. 31, January 1963, pp. 141-162.

5. G. Caplan. *An Approach to Community Mental Health*. London: Tavistock, 1961. M. Grant. "The Group Approach for Weight Control." *Group Psychother*, vol. 4, December 1951, pp. 156-165. I. L. Janis and H. Leventhal. "Psychological Aspects of Physical Illness and Hospital Care." In *Handbook of Clinical Psychology*, edited by B. Wolman. New York: McGraw-Hill, 1965, pp. 1360-1377. H. Leventhal. "Changing Attitudes and Habits to Reduce Risk Factors in Chronic Disease." *Am J Cardiol*, vol. 31, May 1973, pp. 571-580. B. Mausner. "Report on a Smoking Clinic." *Am Psychol*, vol. 21, March 1966, pp. 251-255. J. C. Miller and N. Trieger. "Personal and Situational Determinants of Presurgical Stress." Mimeo, Yale University, 1971. M. Rosenbaum. "Group Psychotherapy and Psychodrama." In *Handbook of Clinical Psychology*. Op. cit., pp. 1254-1274. N. Sanford. "The Prevention of Mental Illness." In *Handbook of Clinical Psychology*. Ibid., pp. 1378-1402.

6. L. Festinger, ed. *Conflict, Decision and Dissonance*. Stanford: Stanford University Press, 1964. C. A. Kiesler. "Commitment." In *Theories of Cognitive Consistency: A Source Book*, edited by R. P. Abelson et al. Chicago: Rand McNally, 1968, pp. 21-32. K. Lewin. *Field Theory in Social Science: Selected Theoretical Papers*, edited by D. Cartwright. New York: Harper & Row, 1951.

7. E. Berscheid and E. H. Walster. *Interpersonal Attraction*. Reading, Mass.: Addison-Wesley, 1969. D. Byrne. *The Attraction Paradigm*. New York: Academic Press, 1971. M. Deutsch and L. Solomon. "Reactions to Evaluations by Others as Influenced by Self-Evaluation." *Sociometry*, vol. 22, June 1959, pp. 93-112. J. E. Dittes. "Attractiveness of the Group as a Function of Self-Esteem and Acceptance by Group." *J Abnorm Soc Psychol*, vol. 59, 1959, pp. 77-82. S. M. Jourard. *Disclosing Man to Himself*. Princeton: Van Nostrand, 1968. S. M. Jourard. "Healthy Personality and Self-Disclosure." In *The Self in Social Interaction*, edited by C. Gordon and K. J. Gergen. New York: John Wiley & Sons, vol. 1, 1968, pp. 423-433. G. Lindzey and D. Byrne. "Measurement of Social Choice and Interpersonal Attractiveness." In *The Handbook of Social Psychology*, edited by G. Lindzey and E. Aronson. 2d ed. Reading, Mass.: Addison-Wesley, vol. 3, 1969. A. Sigall and E. Aronson. "Opinion Change and the Gain-Loss Model of Interpersonal Attraction." *J Exp Soc Psychol*, vol. 3, April 1967, pp. 178-188.

8. W. G. Bennis et al., eds. *Op. cit.* C. Rogers. *On Becoming a Person*. Boston: Houghton Mifflin, 1961.

9. I. L. Janis. "Motivational Factors in the Resolution of Decisional Conflicts." In *Nebraska Symposium on Motivation*, edited by M. R. Jones. Lincoln: University of Nebraska Press, 1959, pp. 198-231. I. L. Janis and L. Mann. "A Conflict-Theory Approach to Attitude Change and Decision-Making." In *Psychological Foundations*

of Attitudes, edited by A. Greenwald et al. New York: Academic Press, 1968. I. L. Janis, ed. *Changing Behavior Through Counseling*. New Haven: Yale University Press, in press.

10.   E. Berscheid and E. H. Walster. *Op. cit.*

11.   W. G. Bennis et al., eds. *Op. cit.* C. Rogers. *Op. cit.*

12.   J. E. Dittes and H. H. Kelley. "Effects of Different Conditions of Acceptance Upon Conformity to Group Norms." *J Abnorm Soc Psychol*, vol. 53, 1956, pp. 100-107.

13.   I. L. Janis. *Op. cit.*, in press.

14.   B. E. Collins and B. H. Raven. "Group Structure: Attraction, Coalitions, Communication and Power." In *The Handbook of Social Psychology*. Op. cit., vol. 4, pp. 102-204.

15.   G. Jonas. "Profiles: Visceral Learning I" (on Neal E. Miller). *New Yorker*, vol. 48, August 19, 1972, pp. 34-57.

16.   I. L. Janis. *Op. cit.*, in press.

CHAPTER NINE

THE REALITIES OF WORK:

Commentary on Howard Leventhal's Information-Processing Model

JEANNE QUINT BENOLIEL, D.N.Sc.

In a thoughtful and persuasive argument, Howard Leventhal invites us to examine the influence of one type of personal experience—illness—on the development, maintenance, and alteration of certain interrelated psychological states. His model of depersonalization provides both a theoretical perspective on the meaning of dehumanization and a conceptual framework for implementing empirical research in practice settings. Specifically, it offers a method for designing experiments to study the effects of planned communication on patient behaviors under specified and restricted circumstances. In keeping with this goal, Leventhal provides a narrow rather than a global perspective on the meaning of dehumanization.

It is not my intent to offer a detailed and rigorous critique of the model itself or of the research that has been reported. Instead, I comment briefly on what I consider to be (1) the usefulness of the model for increasing knowledge about the process of depersonalization as it pertains to patients in contact with medical authority, and (2) some of its limitations for investigating depersonalization as a social phenomenon

175

within the context of organized health care. Concerning the depersonalizing influences of social context, I give one example regarding nursing
personnel—the dehumanizing effects of working under conditions that
offer few if any social rewards or that are high in conflicting expectations
about proper nurse performance.

STRENGTHS OF THE MODEL. The strength of Leventhal's conceptual
model rests in its usefulness for experimental investigation of the antecedents and consequences of caretaker-patient interactions under selected and limited sets of conditions. Study of such problems implies the
need for effective collaboration by health-care practitioners and social
scientists. This approach has been used quite successfully at the Yale
School of Nursing in studying the effects of nurses' actions on the situa-
tionally derived needs of patients.[1] In the context of these studies, situa-
tionally derived needs are those that result from patients' reactions to
the situations in which they find themselves, rather than from their
pathology per se, since the latter is considered the province of the physician.

A second strength of the model is the unusual opportunity it offers
for combining the conceptual and research orientations of psychology,
sociology, and other disciplines to study commonly recurring situations
that depend on patient cooperation with medical authority. Studies of
this nature can help clarify effective and noneffective modes of communication between caretakers and patients under different conditions
of wellness and illness. They might also be used to identify and specify
differences in expectation and response among groups of patients with
different social and cultural characteristics.

LIMITATIONS OF THE MODEL. Useful as the model is for examining
certain aspects of the patient-physician relationship, it is limited in
application to others. For one thing, it assumes the traditional doctor-
patient relationship, with the doctor occupying the position of all-
powerful authority and the patient in the dependent status of person
asking for help. In a sense, assumption of the medical model implies
that the judgment of the physician about "what is right" in a given
situation is proper. Yet acceptance of this assumption by investigators

can effectively bias them against designing research that examines the consequences of medical practice from the client's perspective. For example, the somewhat common practice of nondisclosure of diagnosis and prognosis in the case of cancer can readily be rationalized by medical authority as being in the best interests of patients. Yet people who are living with cancer report wanting more information about their condition than they are able to obtain from their doctors.[2]

If humanization of care means access to information about the true state of illness and well-being, perhaps painful to hear but highly relevant to the individual's present and future plans, a model oriented around the medical perspective about information exchange is unlikely to be adequate from the patient's point of view. It will not permit a full understanding of patient perspectives about their contacts with the medical-care system, especially when the disease is chronic or life-threatening in nature.

Let me illustrate the complexity of the problem with one example. A patient with a life-threatening illness chooses the route of noncompliance with medical instruction because of his own beliefs about how he wants to end his final days. Because the medical-care system is organized around the primacy of cure goals, however, should he be admitted to the hospital the patient may well be denied his desire for a dignified death— that is, a death unimpeded by the application of heroic lifesaving interventions. I use this example because it suggests that personalization of care for this man would include respect for his choice to engage in noncompliance with medical recommendations. Yet it also shows that respect for his choice (personalization of care *by his standards*) does not fit in well with the accepted and usual practices of medical and nursing personnel in the hospital setting.

Furthermore, the example points to a serious matter that I believe is central to any investigation concerned with the causes and consequences of humanized and dehumanized care. Today's health-care services, by and large, are provided not by individual practitioners in isolation but by collectivities of practitioners grouped together into organizations having various sizes and purposes. Notwithstanding their differences in size and goals, the dilemma faced by each collectivity, it seems to me, centers around the difficulties of offering personalized care on a mass scale, that is, to large numbers of clients.

At this point I should offer a definition of personalized care that moves beyond the construct of one-to-one practitioner-patient transactions to include the social reality that patient care (especially for inpatients) takes place in a context of multiple transactions involving patients and a range of personnel. Within the framework of this broader context, I think of *personalized care* for each patient as having three components: *continuity of contact* with at least one person who is interested in the patient as a human being, *opportunity for active involvement* in social living to the extent that the patient is able—including participation in decisions affecting how he or she will die, and *confidence and trust* in those who are providing the care.[3]

PERSONALIZED CARE AND SOCIAL VALUES. As Glaser, Strauss, and I have reported, medical and nursing practitioners face serious and difficult problems when the threat of death is a critical and frequent feature of their work.[4] The evidence at hand suggests that the care presently available to those who are dying is a direct reflection of the primary values of our society. Thus, terminal care—the provision of daily services to people who are living through their final days—is essentially a form of low-status work delegated to workers in the lower echelons of the status hierarchy in health care. An examination of staffing patterns in nursing homes generally provides support for this statement.

The problem for nursing personnel in these essentially custodial settings centers around the achievement of job satisfaction from work with patients whose main need is human concern, when the primary rewards in society are granted for lifesaving activity and technical achievement. More than one observer of the nursing-home scene has commented on the limited and superficial communication that takes place between the staff and their aged clientele and among the patients themselves.[5] In a very real sense, the patients in these settings become victims of depersonalizing practices because they no longer have social worth. The influence of perceived social worth on staff evaluations of clients who come to the hospital for emergency services has been shown by Roth to reflect the concepts of social worth common in the larger society. For example, patients labeled as drunks are more consistently treated as undeserving than any other category of patient.[6]

Although conditions of work in intensive-care settings are markedly different from those found in nursing homes, communication between staff and patients appears to be remarkably similar: impersonal, detached, and superficial in nature. One might hypothesize that people who work in these settings objectify their interactions and relationships with patients in response to work conditions that are socially dehumanizing for them, the staff. To generalize, I suggest that a situation can be defined as socially dehumanizing if its structural conditions are such that they encourage one set of individuals to depersonalize their interactions and relationships with another set of persons.

SOCIAL VALUES AND STRUCTURAL CONDITIONS OF WORK. My thinking about the effects of external and structural conditions on behavior patterns has been stimulated by Lifton's work, beginning with his reports of the psychological aftermath of being a survivor of the Hiroshima holocaust and the "psychological numbing" that followed exposure to death on a mass scale.[7] More recently, I have been impressed by his description of the war in Vietnam as an "atrocity-producing situation," a dehumanized and meaningless experience that left many young American veterans with a sense of absurd evil. Lifton reported the situation in these words:

> Beyond just being young and having been asked to fight a war, these men have a sense of violated personal and social order, of fundamental break in human connection, which they relate to conditions imposed upon them by the war in Viet Nam.*[8]

The crux of his argument rests with the assumption that these young men found themselves in a war that had no purpose, that nobody really believed in, and that created a set of conditions that caused men of very different backgrounds to enter together into a "psychology of slaughter," such as took place at My Lai.[9]

Over the past few years I have talked with a number of young nurses who have returned to school because they could no longer tolerate working in intensive or coronary care settings. To judge from their remarks, they experienced a sense of purposelessness about their work similar to that which Lifton observed in his conversations with veterans of Viet-

* Robert Jay Lifton, "Home From the War: The Psychology of Survival." Copyright © 1972, *Atlantic Monthly*.

nam. Perhaps conditions of work on intensive care wards are similar to the situation in Vietnam. In a recent study of the psychological stresses of intensive care nursing, Hay and Oken compared the nurses' situation to that of soldiers serving in an elite combat group.[10]

This study and another have described, in some detail, the situational and psychological strains experienced by nurses who are assigned to intensive care wards.[11] The work situation is marked by these conditions: repetitive exposure to death and dying, daily contact with mutilated and unsightly patients, formidable and demanding work loads, limited work space, intricate machinery, and communication problems involving physicians, staff, and families. My observations suggest that nurses who cannot tolerate continuous assignment to the intensive care setting feel caught between the task of "lifesaving at all costs" and a desire to provide the patient a humane and dignified death. Especially upsetting to many are decisions to prolong the patient's life when he or she is obviously not going to survive.[12]

Influenced by Lifton's observations about the psychological effects of being in combat in Vietnam, I have pondered about the psychological and social consequences for nurses of continued exposure to situational pressures that, it seems to me, create a *conflict-producing situation* of high intensity. Utilizing several standard psychological tests, Gentry, Foster, and Froehling compared nurses working on three intensive care settings with nurses on three nonintensive wards and showed these findings. In general, ICU nurses reported more depression, more hostility, and more anger than was reported by non-ICU nurses. No differences in terms of guilt, self-esteem, and general personality were found. CCU nurses at a medical center hospital reported more negative affect than CCU nurses at a veterans' hospital. The psychological stresses appeared to be tied to situational stresses of work overload, poor communication, and too much responsibility.[13]

It is my contention that intensive care nursing creates dehumanizing circumstances for the staff in that they must constantly deal with four critical conditions of work: conflicting expectations and demands, frequent decisions of life and death and their aftermath, information overload, and patients who are highly dependent on them for both lifesaving activity and personalized care.[14] The question that I raise for consideration is as follows: Are the structural conditions of work on intensive care units such that they breed dehumanized practices under the guise of the cure goal?

IMPLICATIONS FOR RESEARCH. To judge from the literature that is accumulating, the experience of intensive care is high in stress for patients and for staff alike. To date, research bearing on this matter has dealt with the consequences of the experience for one group or the other, but not for both simultaneously. If one assumes that work on intensive care wards contains dehumanizing elements for the personnel who provide services to patients, logic suggests that the consequences for patients will be in a similar vein. I argue that assessment of the consequences of dehumanization (and humanization) requires a research design that examines the outcomes of particular experiences—such as intensive care —for the providers of services as well as for recipients.

In addition to the need for a complex design that takes account of both the receivers and the givers of health and medical care, any assessment of the consequences of humanization/dehumanization requires definitions of results that go beyond the *cure* outcome that is so dominant in this society. Let me illustrate with the findings produced by an analysis of the results of using cardiopulmonary resuscitation techniques in seven community hospitals over a period of one year. Of the total of 214 patients included in the study, 171 (79.9 percent) died during or within 24 hours after the resuscitation and were classed as permanent failures. Seventeen (7.9 percent) survived 24 hours postresuscitation but were discharged as dead (classed as temporary successes). Twenty-six (12.1 percent), classed as permanent successes, survived the arrest and were discharged.[15]

These data also showed that patients under 50 years of age had a better chance of surviving than did those over 50. Ten of 37 patients under 50 survived (27 percent) compared to 9 percent of the over-50 group; yet 83 percent of the patients on whom resuscitation was attempted were 50 years of age or over.[16] Such findings tell us something about the application of life-prolonging medical technologies to a group of hospitalized patients. They say very little about the personal meanings of these experiences for the patients (both those who lived and those who died), their families, and the staff who took care of them.

Research that attempts to shed light on humanizing and dehumanizing experience within the health-care system must begin by identifying ways of "measuring" the results of human interactions and relationships in terms that reflect a different set of values than those espoused by the cure goal in isolation. Kass believes that the greatest danger associated with expanding biomedical technology will come from a general tendency

for people to submit to voluntary self-degradation (willing dehumanization). They tend to accord specialists unlimited freedom and power to
utilize their knowledge and skill, without necessarily taking account of
the wishes of the patient or subject.[17] In my opinion, research that is
concerned with the outcomes of service relationships characterized by
unequal distribution of power among the interactants needs to focus
explicitly on the influence of different structural conditions and value
orientations on decision-making opportunities and processes available to
the recipients as well as to the providers.

SUMMARY. Where compliance with medical authority is not a useful
criterion for judging the effectiveness of provider-client interactions,
Howard Leventhal's model has limited applicability. Thus, I have identified two circumstances that critically affect the experiences of people
who enter the medical-care system as patients and that facilitate the
development of depersonalizing behaviors by members of the hospital
staff. The primary value attached to the cure goal in this society estab-
lishes a high priority for recovery-oriented medical activity and encourages the indiscriminate use of life-prolonging technology. Health-care
services are delivered by collectivities of practitioners to large numbers
of people, a phenomenon that makes the provision of personalized care
almost impossible to achieve.

The intensive care ward is described as an example of health-care
activity that creates dehumanizing conditions and high levels of situational and psychological stress for the personnel who work there. It is
my thesis that social values and structural conditions of work in some
settings can be such that providers as well as recipients of care undergo
dehumanization. Research concerned with identifying the causes and
consequences of humanized and dehumanized practices in these settings
must take account of what happens to both givers and receivers of services and emphasize the impact of social values on decision-making opportunities and processes available to each group.

NOTES

1. P. J. Wooldridge, J. K. Skipper, and R. C. Leonard. *Behavioral Science, Social
   Practice and the Nursing Profession*. Cleveland: The Press of Case Western Reserve
   University, 1968.

2. J. C. Quint. "Institutionalized Practices of Information Control." *Psychiatr*, vol. 28, May 1965, p. 119.

3. J. Q. Benoliel. "Nursing Care for the Terminal Patient: A Psychosocial Approach." In *Psychosocial Aspects of Terminal Care*, edited by B. Schoenberg. New York: Columbia University Press, 1972.

4. B. G. Glaser and A. L. Strauss. *Awareness of Dying*. Chicago: Aldine, 1965. J. C. Quint. *The Nurse and the Dying Patient*. New York: Macmillan, 1967.

5. E. Gustafson. "Dying: The Career of the Nursing Home Patient." *J Health Soc Behav*, vol. 13, September 1972, p. 226. J. Birren. *The Psychology of Aging*. New Jersey: Prentice-Hall, 1964. A. D. Weisman and R. Kastenbaum. *The Psychological Autoposy: A Study of the Terminal Phase of Life*. New York: Community Mental Health Journal, 1968. (Community Mental Health Journal Monograph No. 4.)

6. J. A. Roth. "Some Contingencies of the Moral Evaluation and Control of Clientele: The Case of the Hospital Emergency Service." *Am J Sociol*, vol. 77, March 1972, p. 839.

7. R. J. Lifton. "Psychological Effects of the Atomic Bomb in Hiroshima: The Theme of Death." *Daedalus*, vol. 92, Summer 1963, p. 462.

8. R. J. Lifton. "Home from the War: The Psychology of Survival." *Atl Mon*, vol. 230, November 1972, p. 56.

9. *Ibid*.

10. D. Hay and D. Oken. "The Psychological Stresses of Intensive Care Unit Nursing." *Psychosom Med*, vol. 34, March-April 1972, p. 109.

11. *Ibid*. R. Vreeland and G. Ellis. "Stresses on the Nurse in an Intensive-Care Unit." *JAMA*, vol. 208, April 14, 1969, p. 332.

12. J. C. Quint. "When Patients Die: Some Nursing Problems." *Can Nurse*, vol. 63, December 1967, pp. 12-33.

13. W. D. Gentry, S. B. Foster, and S. Froehling. "Psychologic Response to Situational Stress in Intensive and Nonintensive Nursing." *Heart and Lung*, vol. 1, November-December 1972, p. 793.

14. D. Hay and D. Oken. *Op. cit.* J. C. Quint. "When Patients Die: Some Nursing Problems." *Op. cit.*

15. R. Scheuer. "Cardiopulmonary Resuscitation in Seven Community Hospitals." *Heart and Lung*, vol. 1, November-December 1972, p. 810.

16. *Ibid*.

17. L. R. Kass. "The New Biology: What Price Relieving Man's Estate?" *Science*, vol. 174, November 1971, p. 779.

PART FOUR
CHANGE

Donald Kennedy, who was trained as an anthropologist, has worked for many years in educational and clinical health settings. Formerly in the Department of Health Services Administration of the School of Public Health at Harvard University, he is now a professor and Director of the Division of Research in the Department of Family and Community Medicine at Pennsylvania State University College of Medicine. His writing during the past five or six years has considered problems in planning medical-care settings, teaching medical students, and dealing with issues in community health. His paper displays this broad range of interests as well as his familiarity with many current trends and innovations in health care. He makes a great many detailed recommendations for reducing the dehumanization that he sees in health settings. He also is very specific in setting forth tasks that need to be carried out, while criticizing current practices of various functionaries. Among his suggestions are those that pertain to the creation of new health roles and the training of new health personnel.

Professor Kennedy's most recent publications include: "Planning a New Children's Hospital," in *Red is the Color of Hurting*, edited by

M. Shore, Washington, D.C.: U.S. Government Printing Office, 1967; (with A. Yerby) "The Organization of Health Services," in *Report of the National Advisory Commission on Health Manpower*, Washington, D.C.: U.S. Government Printing Office, vol. 2, 1967; (with R. Olmsted) *Behavioral Sciences and Medical Education: A Report of Four Conferences*, Washington, D.C.: NICHD, Pub. no. (NIH) 72-41, 1972; and "Community Health and the Urban Environment," in *The Effect of the Man-Made Environment on Health and Behavior*, edited by L. Hinkel and W. Loring, Washington, D.C.: U.S. Government Printing Office, 1974.

The commentators on Dr. Kennedy's paper are academicians. Elliot Studt, a social worker by training, is a professor in the School of Social Welfare at UCLA. She was previously at the University of California in Berkeley, where she was engaged for several years in studies of prisons and parole. Her discussion of Dr. Kennedy's views demonstrates her interest in service organizations, in how they function and how they might be improved. Her research publications include: *People in the Parole Action System*, 1971, and *Surveillance and Service in Parole*, 1972, both published by the Institute of Government and Public Affairs, UCLA; also (with S. Messinger and T. Wilson) *C Unit: Search for Community in Prison*, New York: Russell Sage Foundation, 1968. Dr. Studt's recent teaching and guidance of research students is especially in the area of organizational planning.

The second commentator is Eliot Freidson. He began his teaching career at the City University of New York but has for many years taught at New York University, where he is a professor of sociology. Freidson gained early recognition for his research, *Patients' Views of Medical Practice*, New York: Russell Sage Foundation, 1961, which introduced the well-known concept of "patient referral system." His long-term interest in the medical profession and in medical institutions is evidenced in numerous publications, including his editing of the widely read *The Hospital in Modern Society: Eleven Studies of the Hospital Today*, New York: Free Press, 1963, and four more recent publications: *Professional Dominance: The Social Structure of Medical Care*, New York: Atherton, 1970; *Profession of Medicine: A Study of the Sociology of Applied Knowledge*, New York: Dodd, Mead, 1970; *Medical Men and Their Work*, Chicago: Aldine, 1972; and *The Professions and Their Prospects*, Beverly Hills: Sage Publications, 1973.

Professor Friedson's work has made him a leader both in medical sociology and in the general area of the sociology of occupations-professions. Using his broad and sometimes highly critical perspective, he not only points to certain positive aspects of dehumanized health care but notes the negative aspects of professionalism (whether it concerns licensed professionals or paramedical personnel). He suggests that professionalism may increase the dehumanization of health care.

CHAPTER TEN

ADAPTATION TO MORE HUMANIZING FORMS OF HEALTH CARE

DONALD A. KENNEDY, PH.D.

In the sense in which a man can ever be said to be at home in the world, he is at home not through dominating, or explaining, or appreciating, but through caring and being cared for.[1]*

In *The Active Society*, Amitai Etzioni[2] argues that our society must find ways to make large social organizations more responsive to the personal needs of consumers and employees. At the same time, these large organizations must become more strongly controlled by fundamental human values as translated into continuing revisions of laws and social norms by legitimate political processes. He proposes that larger and larger numbers of people become involved in these political activities. The learning associated with extensive political participation will generate improved levels of solidarity and adaptability within the population at large. The "active society" is our society in control of itself and

---

* Milton Mayerhoff, "Introduction" from *On Caring* by Milton Mayerhoff, Vol. XLIII of World Perspectives Series, edited by Ruth Nanda Anshen. Copyright © 1971 by Milton Mayerhoff. Reprinted with permission of Harper & Row, Publishers, Inc.

operating in conformity with recently discovered ecological and humanitarian requirements.[3]

Etzioni is optimistic about the possibility of generating significant
humanizing improvements in basic social institutions if one can increase
the level of political participation throughout the system. Goodenough,
after studying many community modernization programs, comes to a
similar conclusion.[4] To achieve effective reforms, it is essential for both
ethical and practical reasons to obtain broad participation and cooperation in the process of change itself. I assume that these principles hold
in making improvements in patterns of health care. Physicians, nurses,
patients, and families will have to engage in more active and more politically effective change-oriented discussions if we are to achieve desirable
improvements.

Another major principle guiding this analysis is the importance of
duplicating those social relationships most easily defined as personal and
human wherever they are found in the society. Since the family provides
the initial and most fundamental socializing experience for most members of society, it serves as a major anchor point in the presentation to
follow.

ASSUMPTIONS.   Several basic assumptions have guided this commentary
on adaptation possibilities:

1. Families and household groups represent strong centers of humanizing influence in this society and they are likely to remain so for an
indefinite period of time.

2. The demand for health-care services, especially for primary services,
is now well ahead of the supply, a discrepancy that is likely to continue
for several decades. There is widespread agreement on this general assumption.[5] In addition to aggregate shortages, there are serious problems
of geographic maldistribution that intensify public awareness and generate political activity to correct the situation. This means that we will
probably have to reshape public expectations concerning more realistic
forms and amounts of service at the same time strong efforts are made
to expand service capacity and increase productivity.

3. Health services are labor intensive and are likely to remain so for

many years. Very few activities in the health-care field lend themselves to substitution of machines for people. This is especially true for the interface between the patient and the health-care system.

4. With the mounting demand for service, a condition of chronic overload is developing in many medical offices, clinics, and hospitals. Health-care personnel who work continuously in situations of very heavy work loads are likely to become callous, indifferent, and impersonal in their interaction with clients.

5. Many improvements in the delivery of services that are being developed in the name of increased efficiency are likely to be perceived by clients as detractions from personalized care. Frequently we find a conflict between making changes for greater economic efficiency and trying to effect more personalized forms of client service. Despite this general trend, it may be possible to find ways to improve both the efficiency and the humanity of the system at the same time.

6. Many trends monitored for decades are likely to show major changes in patterning during the next 10 years.[6] Significant changes in the financing of medical care and the control of costs are now underway. The training of large numbers of family physicians and new types of physician assistants will increase the availability of high quality ambulatory services. Government agencies and university medical centers will assume greater responsibility for correcting the geographic maldistribution in medical care.

In the following examination of means to facilitate adaptation to more humanizing patterns, each major health-care setting, including the home, is studied in detail.[7] The home and family situation used as a reference point is considered to be fairly typical for the majority of the 50 million families in this society, but it does not reflect alternate patterns found among specific minority groups.

HOME, HOUSEHOLD, AND RESIDENCE. Nearly all people spend most of their lifetime at home. In fact, it is reasonable to estimate that most people spend 50 percent of their waking time in or near their place of residence. Biological and psychosocial requirements of human existence generate a daily round of activity that utilizes the residence as a base of operations. For young people who are "between families," the college dormitory or the shared apartment serves as a transitional substitute for a more permanent residence.

The home also represents the first site of health care if we extend our definitional boundary to include ethnomedical practices as part of the health-care system. When a person is entering an episode of illness or has suffered an injury, he or she returns home and stays home exempt from the routine activities at school, work, or play. Most of the restricted activity days registered in official health statistics are spent at home and the same is true for bed-disability days.[8]

Ill persons return to their homes to gain privacy and to ease the stress and anxiety associated with the first stage of an episode of illness. In this setting, patients usually feel that they have greater control over events that may aggravate the distress associated with their illness. At home patients can usually receive compassionate attention and important support services during the recuperative process. A variety of ethnomedical diagnostic and treatment procedures may be initiated here as well. In the great majority of illness episodes, spontaneous remission occurs, and the "patient" returns to the regular round of activities within a few days.

Given the natural advantages of the home as a recuperative setting, is it possible to deliver various health-care services to the patient's residence? It is apparent from cursory inspection that the diagnostic and treatment procedures most frequently conducted in a physician's office could be done in a patient's home. Physical examinations could be conducted with full privacy for the patient. Blood and urine samples could be collected for transport to a clinical laboratory. Prescriptions could be written and drugs delivered by messenger. Even electrocardiograms and simple X-rays could be taken with assistance from a mobile van parked outside the home. Education about behavior modification related to health (smoking, drinking, eating, exercising) could be provided quite effectively in the home, with members of the family listening and asking questions. Other preventive services could be delivered to improve the capability of members of the household, to prevent illness or injury, and to promote general well-being. The great majority of primary care problems could be effectively handled in the home setting.

By selecting the patient's home as a significant place for the delivery of professional services, we increase the probability that the manner of delivery of such services will be personal and humanitarian. The territorial qualities of the behavior setting will evoke a generic set of cultural expectations in both parties, and these situational determinants will tend to override the imprinting effect of professional socialization so easily activated in office or hospital settings.

When health-care personnel enter a home, they are likely to behave in a personal and humane way because most persons who enter a home are defined as "guests." Courtesy, friendliness, tact, and sensitivity to the needs of others are routinely expected in such situations. The act of travel to the place of residence has already indicated to the client that the professional person cares about the client's welfare. Normal expectations about the duration of a "visit" will require the provider to stay a reasonable length of time—a duration that is likely to give a sense of satisfaction to the patient. The visitor may be invited to use the toilet facilities and to share some refreshments. Thus, the delivery of a medical service within the patient's home nicely meshes with the more general pattern of gift exchange in the community at large.

This analysis suggests that serious efforts be made to shift services now provided in professional offices, clinics, and hospitals to home delivery. Newspapers, mail, milk, and appliance repairs are now delivered to the home. People are transported in and out of the home on a daily basis. It seems both possible and desirable to bring health services to the same location.

The basic arguments against home delivery are (1) inconvenience to the physician or nurse, (2) lack of access to equipment and supplies available in the office or hospital, and (3) poor utilization of the time of health professionals because of the need for travel. If we are serious about the proposal for the expansion of home health-care services, then we must cope with these objections.

I propose that nurses and physician assistants make the house visits, not physicians. Personnel with this level of training could handle most situations, and when faced with a serious medical condition could consult by telephone with a physician before taking action. If physician assistants and nurse practitioners were assigned to regular geographic districts, like the visiting nurses and public health nurses, then an economical route could be charted for the visits to be made in a given day. Patients would remain in a comfortable setting awaiting their appointment at home.

The normal procedures of interview, physical examination, and prescription of treatment could be handled by a physician assistant. Blood and urine samples could be collected. With the information available by observation during a home visit, the physician assistant could chart a realistic regimen that would have high probability of being followed by the patient with help from other family members. Prompt telephone consultation with a physician would be readily available. Prompt initiation of treatment procedures, including medication, would also be possible. And the patient would suffer a minimum amount of distress, inconvenience, and expenditure of time.

Although physician assistant services could be provided by men or women, the role might have special appeal to women. It represents a natural role extension for the profession of nursing, and it combines easily with the generic role for women in our society with reference to caring for children and the home. Mature women with nurse's training and with 15 to 25 years of experience in raising children would make excellent candidates for this type of work. If provided with specialized training, flexible hours of work, a service district near their home, and good supervision by a practicing physician, these nurse practitioners could make a major contribution in helping to expand the service capacity in primary care and family practice. These practitioners would work for private physicians, neighborhood health centers, public school systems, large business organizations, or municipal health departments. Charges would be made for their services in the home, and they would receive wages and expenses for their work.

The function of the telephone in the provision of health care in the home deserves a special note here. Many people have commented on the importance of the telephone in medical care. Telephones are found in nearly every home. They are used by physicians and other health personnel frequently during the working day, and provide a highly flexible extension of verbal communication capability.

The initial request for medical attention usually comes in over the telephone. The dialogue between the patient or the patient's agent and an agent of the physician generally starts the consultation process. Usually the major objective of this communication is to decide the time of an appointment to see the physician, but many other types of information can be transacted over the telephone. The patient's agent can report presenting complaints in detail and follow simple instructions to obtain additional data on the patient's condition. The physician's agent can give advice about danger signs or simple treatment procedures. Physicians and nurse practitioners are in a position to know the daily "weather map" of mild infectious diseases found within the community population. Thus, at the time of the telephone inquiry, they can usually make a good prognosis for the individual person who is beginning to experience an episode of illness.

Both the range and quality of the services provided over the telephone are related to several factors—how well the parties to the conversation know each other, the level of medical knowledge and experience of the doctor's agent, the level of anxiety in the patient and the patient's agent, and the level of concern among responsible professionals about the probability of malpractice litigation. When strangers talk over the telephone, there are serious limitations on how much they can learn from one another and how much trust they can develop in the relationship. The situation is quite different when two people know each other as a result of face-to-face interactions on a number of occasions. If nurse practitioners frequently visited patients in their homes and handled most of the telephone conversations with patients, the level of knowledge and trust would be adequate for the task. In the typical situation today, the patient or the patient's agent talks to an anonymous secretary in the doctor's office. The identity of the secretary as a person is seldom known to the caller, and the secretary is not expected to have any medical knowledge or professional expertise. It is only when the physician makes a return call to a familiar patient that conditions of prior knowledge, medical expertise, and trust are available.

Under the present rules of "telephone practice" nearly all of the initiative lies in the hands of the patient or the patient's agent. This makes sense for the initial request for service but becomes more difficult to explain once the service responsibility becomes operative during the later stages of the episode of the illness. After an office visit has taken place, there may be clinical laboratory results to report. A return call asking about the current level of suffering would be greatly appreciated. People who care about your welfare usually take some initiative in making further inquiries to see if the distress has lessened. If the condition has not improved, then they may offer further assistance or suggestions. An investment in follow-up telephone contacts could convey a sense of personal concern and allow the "helper" to assess the appropriate time for termination of service responsibility. With more telephone contact, situations of patient dissatisfaction and "change of doctor" would come more easily to the attention of professionals.

If nurse practitioners and physicians increase the amount of professional service they deliver via telephone, then it will be necessary to charge the patient or insurance carrier for telephone calls on a regular basis. This is an infrequent practice at the present time. Such charges could be automatically calculated by frequency and duration of telephone conversations. The accounting equipment is already in operation for direct-dial, long-distance telephone service.

The home visit, supplemented by secondary communication, offers many advantages to the effective practitioner of comprehensive, family, or social medicine. Direct observation of the patient in the home greatly enriches contextual information. Since many contemporary medical problems require patient education and behavior modification, the home setting gives an opportunity to plan and implement treatment strategies that are both more realistic and more likely to succeed than strategies outlined in an office or clinic setting.

PROFESSIONAL OFFICES.   It is estimated that in 1970 there were 214,000 doctor's offices and 83,000 dental offices in the United States.[9] In addition, there were approximately 1,200 mental health clinics engaged in office practice. And there are small numbers of neighborhood health centers, clinics, and dispensaries not included in these statistics that could be reasonably categorized as office settings as well. Medical groups, often called "medical clinics," are included in the generic category of "doctor's offices." Today these medical groups account for only a small fraction of the total offices, but their number is increasing.

It is further estimated that 184,000 physicians and 97,500 dentists were heavily engaged in office practice, and that they received 900 million patient visits in 1969.[10] This is a conservative estimate because the visits to mental health clinics, neighborhood health centers, and similar office facilities have not been added to this total. Yet, the volume of service is large especially when compared with the 31 million admissions to hospitals in 1969.[11]

The office setting usually provides a reception area, a waiting room, one or more examining rooms, and an office for the doctor or dentist.

Some settings have additional space for clinical laboratory testing, typing medical records, conducting diagnostic X-ray procedures, or performing minor surgery. A pharmacy is seldom available as part of the office. The key personnel are a secretary who serves as secretary-receptionist, and a doctor or dentist. Technicians, nurses, and clinical personnel are also employed in some offices.

The professional office is home base for the physician or dentist. This domain is under the doctor's exclusive control.[12] The doctor is the employer and direct supervisor of the secretary, technician, and office nurse. The office operates as a small private business with all of the financial requirements and opportunities usually associated with such a small-scale service organization. It is important to realize that the doctor does not directly own or lease many of the essential components of the health-care services that he or she is responsible for providing. Many of the diagnostic services frequently required are only available at the outpatient department of a hospital. Pharmaceutical prescription services are only available at the retail drugstore. The professional often subcontracts support services: bookkeeping, telephone answering, medical records transcription, clinical laboratory testing, and housekeeping services.

Are there ways in which patient experiences with the office practice of medicine could be modified to yield a greater degree of patient satisfaction? Let us consider this question in some detail. The first stage of interaction is called the "reception process." Many of the reception behaviors that are so well developed in fine restaurants and hotels could be practiced in professional offices. Patients could be greeted just inside the door, rather than from behind a desk or counter. Small, decentralized waiting areas with convenient and secure storage for outdoor clothing could be provided. Well-marked rest rooms could be made available near the entrance. Free refreshments could be offered. The receptionist could greet the visitor by name and give an estimate of the duration of the waiting period. If the wait is to be more than 5 or 10 minutes, an explanation for the delay could be volunteered.

The duration of waiting time is very important to most patients. Often they are in pain and feeling anxious. The trip to the office may have added to their discomfort and anxiety. Their place in line assumes greater salience as they enter a full waiting room. If the patient does not have to wait more than a few minutes in a public area before gaining the privacy of a consultation room, further positive satisfaction is achieved. Both the initial waiting and the total processing time are important to patients. They are usually viewed as basic indicators of sensitivity and responsiveness on the part of health professionals as they move to meet patients who request their help. Unfortunately, delays and "running behind schedule" are a chronic condition in most ambulatory health-care facilities.

But the critical encounter is with the health personnel who directly deliver the medical services expected. The nurse and the doctor must give full attention to the patient. Despite the reality of the presence of other clients and other personnel, individual patients want total and uninterrupted attention. Furthermore, they want a sense of unlimited time availability to solve their problems. When clients receive less than 10 minutes of uninterrupted private conversation with the physician, they feel that they are being treated in an impersonal manner.* In addition, patients usually need tactile interaction with the physician in the form of the procedures of physical examination. The generic importance of touching as a means for "gentling" persons who are upset or for conveying a sense of concern has been documented by Ashley Montagu.[13] We can assume that the diagnostic procedures that bring a physician and a nurse into physical contact with patients contribute a significant component to the message systems that communicate caring concern and healing intent.

The patient also expects the professional caretaker to remember him as a person, and not just as a "container" for a specific disease process that generated the need for the last office visit or the last entry in the medical record. In spite of the realities of a large volume of contacts with many different patients during each working day, physicians are expected to remember enough detail about each individual to be able to make an inquiry or comment that indicates a memory of the patient as an individual.

This expectation of the patient is tied directly to a fundamental requirement in the provision of health care of high quality. Each client

---

* This tentative hypothesis about a minimum threshold effect is based on two unpublished documents written in January 1969 by J. Samuel Chase and William R. Craig, members of the Harvard Medical School Class of 1971. One paper, "Time and Motion Study of General Practice," reports their observational data of 693 office visits with eight general practitioners in Oregon. The other paper, "The Physician's Use of Time," gives a review of the literature as of that date.

represents a fairly unique combination of allergic sensitivity, unhealthy living habits, disease history, social role responsibilities, and income. Physicians and nurses need a considerable data base on each patient to do an effective and efficient job of providing care at acceptable levels of quality and cost. The availability of good medical records can assist this process of knowledge in depth at the time of the patient visit. The newer form of record called the "problem-oriented medical record" is especially useful in this regard.

At the conclusion of the patient visit, the physician describes the symptoms and warning signs that should be monitored by the patient, suggests how the sick role should be played for the next few days, recommends changes in behavioral habits that will have a beneficial effect, and often perscribes some medication. Patients are generally advised to make an appointment for a follow-up visit. They are always told to call back if unexpected events occur or if "things get worse." At this point clients are normally left to find their own way back to the entrance door.

A careful analysis of the natural history of the patient visit suggests that there are several critical pressure points in maintaining a personalized level of service. Perhaps the most important issue is the amount of work scheduled to be done in a given period of time. Part of the work can be scheduled in the form of appointments, but emergency requests for service interrupt and interfere with the scheduled sequence. Further uncertainties arise in the match between patient problems and the blocks of time assigned in advance; some problems simply will not fit within the arranged time block. And in the long run, extended visits do not balance off with an equal number of shorter visits. Since additional professional staff are seldom in reserve, this situation creates longer and longer waiting times for patients.

The work overload generates stress in the entire set of interpersonal relationships within the office setting. People become irritable, abrupt, and contentious with one another. The doctor tries to shorten the time spent with each patient to an absolute minimum and begins to cut corners in the normal routine—not taking time to read the medical record before talking with the patient, or cutting out the physical examination. The doctor may allow interruptions when speaking with the patient, and may make errors in recording charges so the patient is billed for the wrong set of services. The cloak of tolerance and understanding gets extended by small increments until it reaches the limits of elasticity and finally tears. The physician and nurse suddenly realize that they have lost their sense of friendliness, sense of humor, and sense of compassion for other persons.

Everyone is placed in a serious position of conflict in this medical situation because they automatically accept two general cultural rules: "If you have any concern about your health, call a doctor"; and "Only a physician or dentist can provide diagnostic and treatment services." This means that only licensed physicians and dentists can work at the interface between the entire health-care system and the public. But these ancient cultural rules do not make sense in terms of the realities of the epidemiological profile of requests for service.[14] The overwhelming majority of these requests do not require a level of medical expertise beyond that found in the training of nurses, medical corpsmen, pharmacist mates, or physician assistants. Indeed, these personnel could do most of the professional work required in primary or family medical practice.

With the volume of requests for service mounting each day in the 300,000 offices across the nation, it seems reasonable to expand the number of health-care personnel working in and out of these locations. This can be done by short-term, "conversion training" of nurses and other occupational groups with health-care experience.[15] Such training programs are now available for "physician associates" and "physician assistants" under a number of different names. They represent a new form of continuing education for adults with considerable work experience. They open up new jobs and career opportunities for nurses returning to work and for veterans returning to the civilian work force. Since these programs require simultaneous working and learning under physician preceptorship, there is almost immediate expansion of the personnel available in the office practice of medicine. As physicians make their daily rounds of office, hospital, nursing home, and household, they add one or more nurse practitioners to expand their service capability. This process does not require a major reorganization of solo office practices into multispecialty group practices or the development of new types of health insurance.

Despite the current sensitivity associated with commenting on the role of women in the United States today, I venture to state that women have a natural advantage over men in dealing with sick people. This is particularly true if the interpersonal service requires a high component of *caring* communication rather than *curing* procedures. And this is the major component of service requirements in the field of primary care and family practice.

In addition it is important to remember that for most families the central figure in the practice of ethnomedicine is the wife and mother, who is often part-time "health-care practitioner" conducting most of the negotiations between the patient in the family and the health-service providers in the community. Some of these women who have had training as nurses could be trained to be nurse practitioners or physicians associates. Working "woman to woman" they are very likely to be able to negotiate and resolve many of the health-care needs that arise from day to day in residential locations. For those office practices that are organized as medical groups, neighborhood health centers, or mental health clinics, the pattern of using nonphysician personnel to provide direct professional services is already partially recognized as an operational norm.

Under present arrangements, it is very difficult for patient dissatisfactions to be expressed to physicians and dentists. Given the psychological realities of fear and anxiety experienced by the client during an episode of illness, there is little likelihood of complaint because of fear of retaliation from the professional provider. The expression of complaints is diverted into conversations with relatives and friends. Resistance comes in the form of tardiness in paying medical bills or repetitious patterns in changing doctors when this is a viable possibility. After the crisis is past, clients assume that complaints might jeopardize their future needs for medical service in a more serious emergency situation.

The availability of consumer boards with either advisory or executive responsibilities could provide a valuable channel for the transmission of dissatisfactions. Public groups defined as "trustees" for the collective interests of consumers and providers could buffer the relationships and tensions generated between frustrated clients and professionals working under stress. In this sense, a more formal organization might assist in humanizing services rather than leading to a greater degree of depersonalization.[16]

If consumers are given direct managerial responsibility as they often are in the operation of mental health clinics, or advisory responsibilities as they often are in neighborhood health centers, then we have another avenue through which the public concern for humanizing health care can be mobilized. It does not seem unreasonable for medical groups and

health maintenance organizations to adopt similar authority arrangements. Boards of trustees representing the community interest are an
accepted management structure for the operation of the majority of the
hospitals in this country. It would seem reasonable for medical groups
and district medical societies to take the initiative in establishing similar
groups to represent consumer interests and concerns. Perhaps some of the
public dissatisfaction now being registered through political legislative
action could be rechanneled to connect directly with service units managed by physicians and administrators at the community level.

Humanizing health care based in professional offices requires a strong
concern for accessibility and availability. Offices and health centers should
be located close to residential populations. Such service centers should be
convenient in terms of major transportation routes and parking facilities.
A reasonable cluster of equipment, supplies, and health personnel should
be available in any given primary care facility. Most clients do not feel
their needs are adequately met by a sequence of referrals with separate
waiting lines and transportation events. They expect comprehensive
packages of service in health care just as they usually find them in other
service facilities in the business community. Many clients feel that health
services are similar to the protective services provided by police and fire
departments.

In addition to geographic convenience, there is a strong concern for
temporal convenience. The schedule of service hours according to day
of the week and time of day is important to clients. Unlike the need for
food, gasoline, or educational services, the need for health care does not
always coincide with normal hours of business within the community.
Standby medical and dental services are necessary around the clock just
as are the protective services of police and firefighters and the organizations that provide essential utilities (telephone, electricity, water, and
furnace repair). In present practice, most professional offices close down
at night and on weekends. The telephones either are unanswered or are
shifted to an answering service. Suddenly there is a tremendous reduction
in the number of service centers with medically trained personnel on
duty. This creates a cascading of requests for service into the hospital
facilities on nights, weekends, and holidays.

There could be a better "fall-back" position for these office service
locations. Groups of doctors in community hospitals or district medical
societies could develop geographically-based rotation systems for on-duty

personnel in office sites. They could also assist the development of centralized and consolidated telephone answering coverage for all health-care personnel working in a given geographic area. The communications and transportation capability of police departments suggests a natural tie-in for off-duty health services in the community. The standby health facility might be a small room in the nearest fire or police station. Pharmacists as well as physician assistants (MEDEX and nurse practitioners) could take their turn along with physicians and dentists in staffing such facilities when offices are closed. Officials in municipal government and members of boards of trustees for hospitals and other health-care facilities could play a strong role in encouraging these improvements in service.

Departments of health might awaken to the realization that they have an obvious mandate to assist in the development of coordinated and comprehensive preventive and curative services for residential populations. School departments could press for comprehensive pediatric and mental health services to be made available in school facilities. It is time for the medical profession to show some initiative in opening up channels of communication and cooperative discourse at the level of the local community.[17] Many role players and interest groups would welcome an invitation to conduct open discussions about improving and humanizing health care in residential communities.

THE PHARMACY. The pharmacy in the local retail drugstore is not usually classified as a health-care setting, but good reasons exist for its inclusion. There are 129,000 licensed pharmacists in the country. Most of them work in 51,746 drugstores and 5,313 hospital pharmacies.[18] The volume of professional service they provide as measured by sale of prescription and nonprescription drugs is considerable. Pharmacists provided over 2 billion prescriptions in 1970; 1.2 billion of these were dispensed in retail drugstores. This means that the number of contacts per year between patients and pharmacists is probably close to four times the level of patient-physician contacts. With the current methods of manufacturing and packaging of pharmaceuticals, most pharmacists are overtrained for what they do. How could we enhance and humanize their encounters with clients?

The typical work setting for the pharmacist is a retail store with a variety of products on sale. Prescription drugs are embedded in counter displays of candy, perfume, photographic supplies, magazines, and greeting cards. There is no office for private consultation between client and pharmacist. Many clients find it stressful to select and purchase certain health-care supplies when they are in public view. If office privacy were available, clients could learn about side effects of drugs, compare costs of identical drugs manufactured with different trade names, and receive valuable consultation on ethnomedical practices of drug use in the home.

The traditional independence of physicians and pharmacists and their interprofessional conflict often work against the interests of the client. In many states, physicians are legally forbidden to dispense drugs in their offices unless they employ a pharmacist. The geographic separation of physician and pharmacist creates a transportation inconvenience for clients leaving the office with a prescription order. The presence of pharmacists and physicians in the same facility would improve for both groups the process of continuing education about new drugs and side effects. The availability of a pharmacist would help the physician cope with a steady stream of drug salesmen. Regular communication between physicians and pharmacists regarding generic and trade-name drugs and wholesale and retail prices would probably work to the benefit of the consumer.

Client concern about being exploited in the purchase and use of drugs and biologicals is strong. Consumers sense an almost impossible combination of interest groups aligned against their interests. Doctors are highly vulnerable to unreasonable influence from drug detailers who promote drugs that produce high profits for a specific manufacturer. Doctors write prescriptions without knowing the actual cost of the drug to their patients. Pharmacists are combination health-care professionals and small-business people. As long as they must manage a small retail store and be able to show no loss and some profit for the year, they will be tempted to increased their profit margin in the sale of perfumes and drugs to offset losses in the sale of other products. A reinforcement of the viewpoint that the pharmacist is a significant member of the group of people who provide health care might reduce the element of commercialism and exploitation now present in the sale of drugs to the American public.

Most pharmacists perform well in providing geographic decentralization, service hours in the evening and on weekends, emergency contact by telephone, and home delivery without charge. If their role as health-care consultants could be expanded for clients, physicians, dentists, and nurses, the result would be quickly appreciated by all consumers of pharmaceutical materials.

OUTPATIENT SERVICES AT HOSPITALS. The depersonalized health care available in hospital outpatient departments throughout the country is well known and documented. According to statistics compiled by the American Hospital Association, there were 181 million outpatient visits in 1972 (6,000 out of 7,000 hospitals reporting).[19] Only 45 million of these visits were classified as "medical emergencies" in the AHA statistics. The remainder were classified as "clinic" or "specialty referral." In terms of our analysis, it is necessary to subdivide "outpatient visits" into four major categories: (1) medical emergencies, (2) referrals for diagnostic tests, (3) referrals for specialty consultation, and (4) primary care services.

Medical emergencies are relatively easy to define, for example, traumatic injury, poisoning, attempted suicide, and cardiac arrest. Referrals for diagnostic tests are generated by physicians who do not have specialized diagnostic equipment and technicians in their own office facility. Since the community or teaching hospital often provides a convenient "office setting" for medical and surgical specialists, patients referred to specialists frequently come to the hospital for their office consultation. Primary care services are defined as those encounters between patients and physicians that are nearly identical with the encounters that occur in the offices of primary care physicians in the community.

In terms of necessary facilities, outpatient visits can be divided into two categories: medical emergencies and all others. Emergency medicine necessitates specialized areas that allow the rapid movement of patients and medical personnel. It also requires ready access to X-ray and operating rooms. All other forms of "outpatient visit" require the same set up that is found in the office practice of medicine and dentistry. The point needs to be made because most outpatient departments are organized with a large waiting room, a cluster of examination cubicles, and a very visible cashier's cage. To the degree that hospitals begin to differentiate clearly between "emergency medicine" and "ambulatory medicine" the necessary renovation of facilities and reorganization of work can proceed in a rational way.

In the interest of humanizing ambulatory health care, there are often good reasons to discourage most nonemergency outpatient visits to hospitals. Outpatient departments in large city hospitals could be dismantled and replaced by a decentralized set of health centers or doctors' offices in residential neighborhoods. A shift from the operation of one large outpatient department attached to a hospital to a set of small neighborhood health centers or doctors' offices would encourage the development of more personalized services. Fewer strangers are present in an office or health center practice. The traditional and unequal competition between inpatient services and ambulatory services within the hospital can be reduced by geographic and by organizational separation. Many urban-based hospitals are now following this course.

But even in those situations where ambulatory services remain in the hospital building, many improvements can be made to humanize care. Waiting rooms can be decentralized; furnishings and interior decorations can mimic the residential living room; an appointment system can be installed; full-time medical, dental, and nursing staff can be employed; nurse clinicians or practitioners can be utilized; waiting times can be reduced; credit billing can replace cash payment; convenient parking can be provided; family practitioners can be given office space. Features mentioned in the section on office practice could also be used to improve outpatient services at a hospital. Changes of this kind have already been made in a large number of hospitals.

The forces that shaped the traditional outpatient department are no longer the dominant pressures today. Many outpatient departments were organized to train student physicians and to provide free medical services to patients from low-income families. A special form of gift relationship was developed. The patient unable to pay for medical care was willing to help student physicians acquire their clinical training by going to outpatient departments in teaching hospitals. A form of second-class ambulatory medicine was fostered in this situation. Few licensed physicians were present on a full-time basis to provide direct service or to oversee student physicians. The continuous rotation of students and part-time preceptors created a form of territorial "no man's land" in the OPD.

Now things are different. There is health insurance coverage of various kinds for low-income families. Poor people expect to receive medical services of the type available to middle-class families who visit doctors' offices. At the same time, medical educators now recognize that ambulatory medicine has been neglected in clinical training. Student physicians are beginning to rotate through office and health center practices as a legitimate part of their training. The serious shortage of family physicians is apparent to everyone. Physicians in private practice and in academic medicine are generating a strong interest in prepaid group practices, health maintenance organizations, neighborhood health centers, emergency medicine, physician assistants, problem-oriented medical records, use of computers in medical practice, and a host of related developments. Some physicians are even interested in consumer participation in the management of health-care organizations.

All of these processes are likely to have a strong influence on the provision of outpatient services at hospitals. Insofar as physicians and dentists in private practice do not provide adequate care for low-income families or do not provide adequate standby coverage in their offices during evenings and weekends, there will be a mounting wave of requests for services based in hospital facilities.

The community or teaching hospital can respond in either of two ways. It can construct additional ambulatory service facilities adjacent to the hospital, or it can find ways to improve the performance of the other service units in the community at large. The rationale for centralized expansion of hospital facilities is persuasive, but I question whether the public interest is best served by such a policy. Inconvenience and depersonalization for the client always increase after a certain scale of operation is reached in one building. We can sense these things intuitively even when we do not have rigorous empirical evidence to pinpoint the threshold when dehumanization begins.

Given our American cultural assumption that the bigger something becomes the better it must be, I assume that most hospitals will expand if their neighbors allow it and if they can keep their charges for outpatient services competitive with office or health center practices. There is some evidence that outpatient costs and charges are indeed rising faster than the cost and charge for similar services in office practice. If such a differential does emerge, we might have powerful evidence to recommend the decentralized community strategy that seems warranted on grounds of more humanized service.

HOSPITALS. There are approximately 7,000 hospitals in this country, housing a total of 1.6 million beds. They receive 32 million admissions each year and have an average daily occupancy of 1.3 million persons.[20]

The number of beds and the number of facilities seem to be holding fairly constant in recent years. With the tremendous inflation of construction and operating costs, one might expect this condition of stability to continue for the next decade.

The incredible increase in hospial costs and the growing public dissatisfaction with services received by many hospitalized patients have led to mounting concern about the utilization of hospital services. The standard length of stay for various treatment procedures is being shortened. Some diagnostic procedures previously done on an inpatient basis are now being provided as ambulatory services. A search for unnecessary surgery is getting underway and may further reduce admissions. Patients normally cared for in hospitals are now being transferred to nursing homes and extended-care facilities. Some people have been so bold as to suggest that most babies could be delievered at home and that many terminally ill patients could be allowed to die at home. As hospital insurance coverage expands to pay for more and more ambulatory services, the pressure toward hospitalization for diagnostic studies or a "good rest" is likely to be ameliorated. As the cost increases, the consumer or the consumer's insurance carrier is more likely to challenge the physician's recommendation that the patient be hospitalized for a specific episode of illness.

A public policy could be adopted to reduce hospitalization to an absolute minimum while developing alternative capabilities to handle the service transfers involved. Preventive services and home medical services could be created and could generate a form of "back pressure" against the present tide that leads to more and more hospitalization. When hospitalization is likely to be depersonalizing, then such a policy position could be further reinforced. Those interested in humanitarian concerns and those interested in economic imperatives might join ranks on this issue. And it is not difficult to imagine such an alliance if one can believe the results of Titmuss' study of blood donor systems.[21] According to his comparative research, gift systems work better than commercial ones in terms of standard economic criteria. Because of its implications for the various exchange systems operating in the field of health services, this landmark investigation deserves careful study.

Given the continued need for hospitals, however, many things could be done to humanize their care of patients. In maternity services, fathers could be allowed to remain with their wives during most or all of the delivery process. A mother might be encouraged to keep her infant in her room rather than in a distant nursery, to hold and cuddle her baby, and to feed the infant by breast rather than by bottle. Siblings could be allowed to visit both mother and newborn infant. Plenty of folk experience as well as some scientific evidence show that a shift to these practices in the hospital would enhance the health and well-being of both mother and baby.

When children must be hospitalized, the physical facilities and hospital policies could support the presence of the mother or another member of the family to live-in with the child.[22] Strings of single rooms along a corridor could be replaced by clusters of rooms grouped around a common living room or patio. Space could be set aside as a playroom and be staffed by nursery school teachers or day-care personnel. Small kitchenettes could be provided to allow mothers and nursing staff to serve snacks and meals specifically tailored to each child's food preferences and needs.

The admission process could be modified to allow patients and their escorts to be ushered directly from the front door to the assigned room. The interviewing process needed to gain administrative data and to initiate the medical record could be conducted in the patient's room after the patient has taken up residence. Patients could be allowed to wear their own clothing. Recreational areas and food service areas could be provided so that patients would not have to remain in their bedrooms at all times. Visiting hours could be expanded and made more flexible to match the specific needs of individual patients and the convenience of visitors. Patients could be provided with their own appointment books so that they would know the schedule of events requiring their participation at bedside or in a specific diagnostic or treatment site within the hospital.

Health education programs could be broadcast on the television set. Self-instruction modules about common health hazards or about the condition that caused hospitalization could be offered each patient. A telephone could be available at bedside to facilitate communication with family and friends, with the attending physician, or with service centers in the hospital. Public address and intercom systems should be replaced by visible signal systems and telephones. All hospital personnel should be instructed to refer to patients by name and not to use slang expressions such as "the gall bladder in Room 34." Hours of waking, bathing, and eating could be adjusted on an individual basis. Many patients could be instructed to monitor their own illness and to record signs and symptoms.

Changes such as these would alter the emotional climate of the hospital.

As patients are discharged from the hospital, they should be asked to write candid observations, reactions, and suggestions in an anonymous questionnaire. The collected comments could then be compiled, duplicated, and distributed to all hospital personnel who interact with patients. Where necessary, the membership of the hospital's board of trustees could be changed to achieve broader representation from client groups that use the hospital. A standing committee on complaints and suggestions could be created with the authority to invesigate patient grievances and negotiate changes in staff behavior and attitudes. To foster a sense of direct representation, families who regularly use the hospital could be encouraged to get to know one or more members of the board of trustees. Because trustees are traditionally middle class, a rigorous expansion and recruitment program would be required to insure that the board's makeup reflected the population of the community.

Patients could also have their own personal medical record that approximated the hospital record in terms of essential facts and important medical interpretations and predictions. A key to continuity of care in a highly mobile society with pluralistic health-care services is a single, cumulative medical record that is the property of the person who has the most at stake in terms of personal health and well-being. In moving from one health-care provider to the next, the patient could carry the authoritative record. Ideally, it would contain entries for each service received from the event of birth onward.

Such a record could be used as a significant vehicle for the continuing, personal health education of the subject. It would provide a strong sense of identity, participation, independence, and control for the person entering into a new relationship with a health-care professional. The existence of this kind of personal record would reduce the redundancy in interviewing, sensitivity testing, diagnostic X-rays, and a variety of other reiterative health-care processing procedures. As the record grew in bulk, sections of it could be easily converted to microfilm. A duplicate record could be made and kept in a safety deposit box in the bank.

Many objections can be raised to this proposal. Again there is a major issue of public policy to be faced. We can move in the direction of computer data banks that contain medical data on many thousands of individuals, or we can move in the direction of placing crucial information about a person's health in the person's own possession. At this stage of our knowledge about the use of computerized data banks, we know that such systems do not provide acceptable levels of control over error, strong guarantees for protection against unauthorized use by government agencies or other interest groups, or convenient and complete review by the person whose records are kept in the system. Here again, in an effort to humanize health care we must give more information and legitimate authority to the client to offset the present imbalance in favor of health professionals.

In concluding this section on hospitals, I must offer a warning about the trend toward larger facilities. I believe we know very little about the optimal size range for organizations that provide human services. We have the suggestive study by Barker and his associates on the optimal size of high schools, but I know of no similar research in the field of hospital studies.[23] Given the tendency of economists to talk about "economies of scale," the public concern among government planning agencies about redundancies in capital equipment, the abundance of physicians with specialties that require the use of equipment in hospitals, and the current attitude of hospital architects, we see many interest groups aligned on the side of "growing big means getting better."

There is a fascinating paradox in the debates between those who recommend closing all hospital maternity services with fewer than 2,500 deliveries per year and those who recommend that all deliveries should take place in the home with a midwife in attendance. I suggest that policy-oriented studies with interdisciplinary representation be initiated to help clarify the central issue of what service load is in the best interest of the consumer-client and the general welfare of society.

CONCLUSION. In a social environment that generates a signal of urgency about the delivery of health services, there are many people hard at work trying to suggest or implement improvements. Most of these efforts are directed toward reducing costs, improving the equity of the distribution of basic services, and maintaining an acceptable level of quality. Attempts to rationalize the patterns of service are well underway. Specialists in the fields of management, economics, and law are being asked for their ideas. In all of this activity and political negotiation, we must remember the central requirement in the provision of health services: the demonstrable act of one professionally trained person offering help in a compassionate manner to a suffering human being. Mayerhoff has captured the focal message of this interpersonal transaction in the following words:

> To care for another person, in the most significant sense, is to help him grow and actualize himself . . . Caring is the antithesis of simply using the other person to satisfy one's own needs.
>
> The meaning of caring I want to suggest is not to be confused with such meanings as wishing well, liking, comforting and maintaining, or simply having an interest in what happens to another. Also, it is not an isolated feeling or a momentary relationship, nor is it simply a matter of wanting to care for some person.
>
> Caring, as helping another grow and actualize himself, is a process, a way of relating to someone that involves development, in the same way that friendship can only emerge in time through mutual trust and a deepening and qualitative transformation of the relationship.
>
> In the context of a man's life, caring has a way of ordering his other values and activities around it. When this ordering is comprehensive, because of the inclusiveness of his carings, there is a basic stability in his life; he is "in place" in the world, instead of being out of place. . . .
>
> Through caring for certain others, by serving them through caring, a man lives the meaning of his own life.[24]*

That is the central issue for our consideration. We ought not to act with timidity in our exploration of both realistic and idealistic potentialities for change in the health-care field.

NOTES

1. M. Mayerhoff. *On Caring*. New York: Harper & Row, 1971.
2. A. Etzioni. *The Active Society*. New York: The Free Press, Collier-Macmillan, 1968.
3. B. Commoner. *The Closing Circle*. New York: Bantam Book and Knopf Editions, 1971. J. K. Galbraith. "Economics and the Quality of Life." In *A Contemporary Guide to Economics, Peace, and Laughter*, edited by A. D. Williams. Boston: Houghton-Mifflin, 1971, pp. 1-25. R. Bauer, ed. *Social Indicators*. Cambridge: MIT Press, 1967.
4. W. H. Goodenough. *Cooperation in Change*. New York: Russell Sage Foundation, 1963.
5. R. Fein. *The Doctor Shortage*. Washington, D.C.: The Brookings Institution, 1967.

6. D. Michael. *The Unprepared Society*. New York: Harper & Row, 1967.

7. W. F. Maloney, J. Pollack, and H. H. Field. *To Facilitate Health: A Proposal to Establish Health Facilities*. American Institute of Architects: Task Force on a Health Facilities Laboratory. Boston: Tufts Medical School, November 1971.

8. *The American Almanac, 1972*. New York: Grosset & Dunlap, 1971, p. 76.

9. *Ibid.*

10. Maloney, et al. *Op. cit.*, pp. 38, 41.

11. American Hospital Association. *Guide to the Health Care Field*. Chicago: AHA, 1973.

12. E. Freidson. *Profession of Medicine*. New York: Dodd, Mead, 1970.

13. A. Montagu. *Touching: The Human Significance of the Skin*. New York: Columbia University Press, 1971.

14. P. B. Storey, J. W. Williamson, and C. H. Castle. *Continuing Education: A New Emphasis*. Chicago: American Medical Association, 1968.

15. C. E. Lewis and B. A. Resnick. "Nurse Clinics and Progressive Patient Care." *N Engl J Med*, vol. 277, December 1967, pp. 1236-1241. P. Andrews, A. Yankauer, and J. Connelly. "Changing the Patterns of Ambulatory Pediatric Caretaking: An Action-Oriented Training Program for Nurses." *Am J Public Health*, vol. 60, May 1970, pp. 870-879.

16. Personal communication from Rashi Fein.

17. E. Freidson. *Professional Dominance*. New York: Atherton, 1970.

18. Maloney et al. *Op. cit.*, p. 45.

19. American Hospital Association. *Guidebook*. Chicago: AHA, 1971.

20. J. S. Chase and W. R. Craig. *AHA: Guide to the Health Care Field*, January 1969 (unpublished).

21. R. M. Titmuss. *The Gift Relationship*. New York: Random House, 1971. (Vintage Book Edition, 1972.)

22. M. B. Kreidberg et al. *Problems of Pediatric Hospital Design*. Boston: Tufts-New England Medical Center, 1965.

23. R. G. Barker and P. V. Gump. *Big School, Small School: High School Size and Student Behavior*. Stanford: Stanford University Press, 1964.

24. M. Mayerhoff. *Op. cit.*, pp. 1-2.

CHAPTER ELEVEN

ALTERING ROLE RELATIONSHIPS

Commentary on Donald Kennedy's Model for Change

ELLIOT STUDT, D.S.W.

I am a social worker with extensive practice and research experience in corrections—prisons, probation, and parole. My major focus has been on the use of organizational change to "humanize" the delivery of service, and I am currently pursuing this interest through the comparative analysis of various types of service systems, some of which are medical. Because of my particular area of competence, I would like to discuss Dr. Kennedy's paper, not in terms of his substantive recommendations, but as an example of how to think about organizational change as a primary means to improve the delivery of services.

Dr. Kennedy's first step is to identify within the totality of medical services a series of task sequences by which the practice of medicine is currently organized for dealing with different kinds of medical problems and patient popultaions. As he analyzed what must be accomplished by each such functional process, he proposes alternative patterns for relating people and places to tasks. He envisions that these alternatives (processes of adaptation) might solve pressing work problems, such as chronic overload, while at the same time improving the client's experience of personalized care. In these "thought experiments" he rearranges the elements of task performance to make it more probable that human

215

concerns will be attended to in the course of providing the necessary technological services. Many of the changes he proposes involve modifying present roles for various kinds of medical personnel, or introducing new roles, or both. Implied throughout are corresponding role changes for patients.

The usefulness of such mind play with alternative patterns for relating people to tasks is all too frequently overlooked in planning for change. The usual issues seem to concern achieving technological excellence— through appropriate intake policy, specialized staff, advanced equipment, and adequate space. This focus is based on an unstated assumption that desired human relationships will be assured once the proper skills and accoutrements are provided. Unfortunately we are beginning to learn that organizational reality does not uphold this assumption. On the contrary, many research findings show that when the goal of change is to elicit the exercise of human compassion and creativity in the provision of service, the most direct and economical means for achieving such a goal is to change the way people are related to one another in the organization.

In the studies of diverse service systems that my students and I have been conducting, we have frequently traced the source of dehumanizing behavior on the part of staff to role anomalies arising from the way authority is distributed throughout the organization. These role problems seem to be particularly intense when a specialized expert assumes the top authority across the board over a variety of personnel with different kinds of competence. Evidence suggests that this type of role problem may also be operating in the organization of medical services.

It seems to me that the role of physicians is described primarily in terms of those medical situations in which their authority and expertise must be relatively absolute. Such situations present the most serious and difficult challenges to the particular kind of competence of physicians, leaving their role partners especially dependent on their guidance. Patients are in serious danger and are limited in their ability to judge for themselves, while the subordinate staff members are required to follow the physician's instructions implicitly. This set of role relationships is frequently generalized to other medical situations so that physicians are cast as top experts regardless of the tasks to be accomplished or the kinds of competence required for problem solving in the particular situation.

Our studies of service systems indicate that wherever the role of an expert is generalized to mean top decision maker in all operations throughout the organization, there are also strong tendencies toward routinization and segmentation among staff groups. This results in depersonalization and dehumanization expressed in relationships among subordinate staff members as well as in interactions between the employed personnel and recipients of service.

The process of defining all the doctor's roles in terms of the most serious and demanding task is similar to what happens in defining the authority of a prison superintendent and the role relationships that operate throughout the institution. The superintendent, or warden, in a prison is unilaterally responsible for "security," which means both preventing the escape of dangerous persons into the free community and protecting persons within the institution, both inmates and staff, from personal harm. Accordingly, in the prison the warden exercises absolute authority in matters of security, and all subordinate roles are designed to insure control over those inmates who are most potentially dangerous and most prone to escape.

Since any event in prison may have implications for security, the special authority of the warden is generalized to cover almost every type of decision making. The corresponding roles for both inmates and subordinate staff are therefore constricted, and all human contacts are suffused by concern about danger or escape. The prison example implies a lower level of intellectual and scientific competence in the authority structure than is true for the medical hierarchy. But it serves to illustrate the insidious effect of a hierarchical authority structure on the way lower echelon persons, including patients, are perceived and dealt with.

Three kinds of relationships in medical services require reexamination if we are to design roles that better support respect for human dignity and concern for the individual.

DOCTOR-PATIENT RELATIONSHIPS. It has been suggested that equality in the doctor-patient role relationship is one way of supporting more humanized provision of services. This formulation leaves me uneasy, particularly when I think as a patient. When I go to get help, I—and probably most patients—want the doctor to be far superior to me in diagnosing and prescribing. I have no desire to become the doctor's equal in that kind of competence. On the other hand, patients do have two kinds of "expertise" on which the doctor must depend if health is to be restored. In the first place, patients know more than anyone else, including the physician, about how the illness affects their functioning and what they experience under treatment. In addition, patients do the basic work of getting well; otherwise, the goal of medical service will not be achieved. Unless patients are mobilized biologically and psychologically to use the service they receive toward the improvement of their condition, they can nullify the doctor's efforts.

It seems to me that the attempt to modify doctor-patient relationships should move in the direction of idenifying the critical contributions of both roles to the process of achieving health. This will establish reciprocal, rather than equal, roles for each. Employment of medical personnel by consumer groups is one possible mechanism by which reciprocal roles between doctors and patients might be established in the economic area and encouraged in other aspects of the relationship.

THE PHYSICIAN'S RELATIONSHIPS WITH OTHER MEDICAL PERSONNEL. A similar principle can be applied in examining the role relations between doctors and personnel who work under a doctor's direction. In the present system, doctors are always the top definers of roles for the aides, the nurses, the social workers, and others. Inevitably, they see the work of these others primarily in terms of the way it affects their own work, often with too little regard for those aspects about which the others know far more than they know, such as which special techniques are appropriate to which task; what conditions might make it difficult to follow prescribed procedures; which activities are subtly demeaning while others carry rewards; and how the design of relationships among the various roles introduces conflict and disjunction into the flow of work.

Too often in medical settings, as in other service systems, people in subordinate positions work with a sense of frustrated creativity and depersonalization, feelings that inevitably affect the way they deal with patients. A work-group plan, in which the doctor and team members pool their various kinds of competence and knowledge and together design work patterns for group tasks, is one important mechanism for breaking down the monolithic authority structure of the medical setting and encouraging each person to perform at top capacity in achieving "our task." A primary means for changing people's attitudes toward themselves and others is to engage them significantly in remaking their own realities. In most cases, the resulting increase in self-respect, loyalty to the job, and work enjoyment leads to warmer, more sensitive relationships with coworkers and with patients.[1]

I can most easily illustrate this point by reporting one small "miracle" of attitude change in a "difficult" worker that occurred in a prison demonstration program of which I was director. In this program, a staff of 11 persons, including custody officers, counselors, researchers, and secretaries, were responsible as a work group for the care of, and services to, 130 randomly chosen young adult male felons, all of whom lived in a single housing unit. One custody officer, nicknamed Vince, was assigned to our staff to manage the evening watch. It was known throughout the institution that he was supposed to act in our project as the official spy for the custody division and as a curb on our "newfangled" ideas.

Vince was a stocky, gravelly voiced, retired marine sergeant. As I observed his domineering performance with inmates in the weeks before the project began, I anticipated difficulties for him and for others as we attempted to establish new relationships among staff and inmates. We did not try to turn Vince into a therapist, but we were committed to involving the custody officers in the problem-solving processes that we hoped would characterize all relationships on the unit. Therefore, we had regular work-group meetings in which Vince, along with the other officers, was involved. We invited his ideas, many of which proved to be valuable, and we discussed with him how the activities of other personnel affected his work.

A year later, when we conducted an inmate system survey, comparing the demonstration unit with others in the institution, Vince was reported by the inmates to be the custody officer they most often sought out for informal discussion. Almost uniformly the inmates in the survey spoke of Vince with respect and affection. Long after the project terminated a former inmate asked me for news of Vince, saying "I sure loved that old guy." Vince's former behavior had been shaped by the system that isolated him from his coworkers and rewarded his dictatorial approach to inmates. He changed when, in a different role system, he was treated as a person with potentialities in a pool of human resources and was invited to share responsibility for managing the use of these resources. He still performed the "dirty" job of custody, but the new role relationship allowed his natural warmth and kindliness to be expressed on the job (even though his voice remained loud and gravelly). The many contributions he made to the project were essential to its modicum of success.[2]

This story suggests that one of the best available tools for humanizing the way medical personnel relate to patients is to humanize relationships among coworkers. Although certain kinds of worker conformity can be secured through rules established by a remote superior, it is well known that no human being ever follows the rules èxactly and that rule conformity alone cannot insure humane behavior. A better way to achieve informed responsibility for the necessities of the task and warm sensitivity in human relationships is to provide an organizational setting that encourages each person to perform at that person's highest actual capacity.

THE DOCTOR AS ADMINISTRATOR.   I would like to suggest one other aspect of role design in the medical system that should be examined when planning for more humanized services. It concerns the doctor as administrator and the kind of skills needed to design effective role relationships in a large service agency. Let us divert our attention for a moment to airline pilots. It has been suggested that they must be highly expert in the job of piloting a plane; they are not also expected to assume responsibility for running the airline company and managing all other types of personnel necessary to make the pilot's expertise effective. Is it feasible to expect doctors to become, and remain, expert in the skills of doctoring, while at the same time developing the quite different skills required to design role systems that evoke and support humanized relationships?

If we want to produce administrators who can understand the special contributions of each type of competence to the medical service and design the total system as a set of mutually supportive roles, then perhaps we need a different type of educational process for them than for physicians who treat patients. This issue is only one example of the continuing debate about the relative importance of specialized substantive knowledge for managerial effectiveness. The question must be settled by each field of practice in terms of its own necessities. It remains, however, an important issue to be examined whenever one is planning for organizational change.

The process of organizational change that I have been describing is not as well understood as it should be, and pertinent literature is sparse.[3] We are well aware that demonstration programs frequently fail or disappear into the bureaucratic jungle. I would like to make four suggestions that, if implemented, might prevent some potential failures and, at the very least, insure that we increase knowledge about the change process even when particular programs fail.

1. Too often we introduce changes without knowing enough about the total system into which we are introducing a foreign body. An intriguing idea may be proposed in the literature or a consultant may report that some high-prestige institution has had glowing success with a new program, and we graft the new idea or program onto an established agency that operates on different assumptions.

Before we implement a new program, we should study the system in which it must survive, to answer such questions as: What forces in the system support change? What are the anticipated resistances? At what point can innovation be introduced most economically? What changes must be made before others are attempted? What commitments need to be secured before the innovation is introduced? Prior to designing a plan for change, one should describe and analyze the organizational environment within which the new program must operate, giving special attention to the action dynamics that characterize that system. Because we so frequently skip this preliminary analysis and planning, we often fail to demonstrate more effective services, and we also do unintended harm to the staff members and patients who are the subjects of our experimentation.

2. After an adequate analysis of the ongoing system has been made, it is wise to design a series of small experimental changes prior to attempting a major revision that affects the entire organization. In a small change program it is possible to observe unintended consequences as they appear and to modify the design accordingly while it is still tentative. Then, when more comprehensive changes are to be introduced, the planners will have the advantage of knowing how the system as a whole reacts to change and where problems are apt to occur. This information is usually available after intervention has been introduced, but not before.

3. The research associated with each of the changes in a service organization should not be just evaluative. In all innovative programs research on the processes of change per se should accompany the study of out-

comes. This will help us understand how change should and should not be introduced into service organizations and thereby help us avoid costly demonstration program failures.

4. We also need in the published literature more reports of the failures in attempted change programs. Too often unsuccessful ventures are hidden in the bureaucratic maze to save face as well as to protect future funding opportunities. However, if we are to make the failures worth something, in spite of their financial and human costs, we must subject such experiences to rigorous analytic autopsies and publish the results. We must also persuade funding bodies to support high-risk projects on the basis that, even if failure occurs, useful knowledge about the causes of failure will have been achieved. Only with this kind of knowledge will we be able to develop the expertise that will enable us to use organizational change as a professional tool in humanizing services.

To me, these remarks are not far afield from Dr. Kennedy's ideas. He is talking about using organizational change to modify attitudes and to improve the human quality of services. My plea is for a wider dissemination of this kind of knowledge and skill and for increasing scientific rigor in its practice.

NOTES

1. This organizational approach, identified as the human resources model, is discussed in "Human Relations or Human Resources?" by Raymond E. Miles (*Harv Bus Rev*, vol. 43, July-August 1965, pp. 149-156.)

2. The complete report of this demonstration program is found in *C-Unit: Search for Community In Prison* by Elliot Studt, Sheldon L. Messinger, and Thomas P. Wilson. (New York: Russell Sage Foundation, 1968.)

3. A recent book by Seymour B. Sarason, *The Creation of Settings and Future Societies* (San Francisco: Jossey-Bass, 1972) provides an important analysis of the process of organizational innovation, summarizing what is already known and projecting what needs to be known.

CHAPTER TWELVE

INCREASING CHOICE WITHIN LIMITS:

Commentary on Donald Kennedy's Model for Change

ELIOT FREIDSON, PH.D.

A number of issues deserve attention in Kennedy's paper, but I shall touch only a few. First, I think we ought to face the fact that some kinds of "dehumanization" are, in fact, desirable and positively liberating. There are many occasions in the use of everyday medical care when people want convenience and simplicity much more than solicitous human contact. If one is dying for a candy bar or some bubble gum, an automatic vendor is far preferable to a garrulous old salesman in a friendly neighborhood candy-gum-newspaper-magazine store.

Most people who drop into a drugstore and matter of factly buy aspirin for their headache, lozenges for their cough, suppositories for their piles, and douching powder for their vaginitis do not need humanized medical care. Perhaps it would be well, wherever possible, to present thoroughly mechanized care for such people, or for such disorders, so as to keep these things from cluttering up the appointment lists on which only the *worried* (sick or well) should really be. Perhaps it would be well to let people who want to do so manage more of their own care and save our efforts for those who truly need a human service from a professional.

In this sense, I argue that to release the resources needed for real humanized care, it might be well to deliberately dehumanize all amenable care for all amenable people. The first thing that could be done would be to minimize the necessity of any professional contact whatsoever. For example, why should it not be possible to provide officially approved versions of Merck Manuals, limited of course, in the drugs and symptoms covered? Why cannot medical people sit down and seriously think about expanding the diagnoses and drugs lay people can manage by themselves without the trouble of a visit to a bored practitioner who examines conditions and provides prescriptions so routine that they were probably not taught in medical school in the first place?

This would be beneficial, of course, only if what laymen could prescribe for themselves were limited. To control and limit the process, it could be constituted more in the manner of a bureaucratically formal self-prescription of which a record is kept than in the manner of a casual, over-the-counter purchase. Or the process could simulate a walk-in subway photomatic. One might punch in answers about history and symptoms in response to a computer's questions, have one's vital signs read, perhaps even have lab tests and X rays taken, and receive a self-portrait and fortune in the form of a diagnosis and prescription. The latter could drop out of the machine already formulated and packaged, like Raisinets or Milk Duds. Naturally, the computer would be programmed so that for some patrons there would be no prescription, only a referral to a human physician; for others, there would be only a placebo.

I am obviously suggesting more mechanization, but I believe that when people deliberately and consciously use machines because they are convenient and desirable, mechanization is not dehumanization. Where machinery is hidden behind fleshlike plastic and the pretense made that it is human, there is dehumanization. An even worse situation occurs when real, live human beings are trained to act like friendly robots. The latter transformation constitutes the profitable stock-in-trade of such recreation industries as Disneyland, mass restaurants, and the airlines. This type of mechanization is the true dehumanization, the dehumanization to be unmasked and resisted, because the "solution" involves calculated manipulation of people precisely on those occasions when they hunger for human contact and not machines.

For people who do need and want human support, the most important way of really providing it, and not providing plasticized machinery or mechanized human beings, is to do so in people's own homes, as Kennedy suggests. Health institutions should be avoided wherever possible. However, I differ with him in his apparent assumption that fully humanized treatment will be obtained from professional workers even when they are obliged to suffer the "indignity" of making house calls. Fully humanized treatment is likely only when those caring for the person also care for the person.

The limitations of professional and paraprofessional care must never be forgotten. Much attention is being paid these days to the development of new kinds of workers, more humble than the doctor, who will be able to bear much of the burden now borne entirely by the doctor, and at the same time might do so in the spirit of caring. Clearly, in the case of those conditions that patients cannot manage for themselves, some sort of increase in the number and kind of medical personnel is necessary.

It is very popular, indeed very fashionable, to talk about paramedical personnel taking over many of the doctor's jobs. I think, however, that health manpower planners are being naive in considering this to be a real solution. On the basis of "demonstration" experience with people who are brand new, who have never done the job before, who are freshly trained and enthusiastic, and above all, who are not yet organized as true occupations, they are planning for the future. The planners are not logical because they are comparing apples with pears. A new form of work, without tradition or identity, is not yet a true social enterprise. In time, however, it becomes a social enterprise, and in the course of doing so, changes itself. There is no reason to believe that new health workers are going to remain the same as they were when their occupation was being constituted. But this is what planners seem to assume.

There are processes of occupational self-identification, professionalization, and even unionization that have led drearily and uniformly to the stage of no longer wanting to do dirty work. The worker wants to become more and more professional, cultivate more and more distance from the client, practice job mobility. As Everett Hughes pointed out in his study of nursing,[1] the natural history of the so-called helping occupations in this country has very consistently been one in which low-status occupations were invented and trained for the performance of tasks that higher-status occupations no longer wished to perform. In time, those new, low-status occupations develop identification with their job, proceed to initiate organization, and then seek to drop the dirty work themselves, shoving it off to somebody else below them in order to "upgrade" themselves.

I do not think it inevitably happens that way, but in our own historical and national environment, with its virus of professionalism, with mobility through greater dignity, higher rewards, cleaner work, more intellectual work, and pleasant patients to deal with, it seems to be a "normal" process. Take nurses, who, of course, have been upgrading themselves every 20 or 30 years. In the past 80 years of "professional nursing" we have had the development of practical nurses to take over the dirty work that nurses did not want as they were being upgraded. Then nurses' aides were developed to take over the dirty work the practical nurses did not want, and so on, ad infinitum. And some nurses have left the bedside in order to be coordinators of care, while others seek to become practitioners. There is no reason to assume in this present era that this process will not continue to operate among physician's assistants, nurse-practitioners, and the like.

We must build into our conception of the development of these new kinds of health workers some way of coping with this self-defeating process. There is no reason to believe that it is not going to affect these new workers when they are trained and established. When they get their hands on patients and decide they are really doing a doctor's work, they are likely to decide that they should have the prerogatives of doctors, and they will struggle for some of the rewards, including cleaner work, and the right to be less humble and accessible. The first mode of dealing with the problem is, as I have already said, to maximize the possibility that lay people can care for themselves, and that they can be cared for by those who care for them.

Inevitably, however, there will be some people who will have to be dealt with by professional health workers in professionally controlled institutions. This creates the problem of routinization, no matter who the worker is. Regardless of good intentions, the fact is that day after day after day health workers see people who present problems that they do not see as idiosyncratic, but rather as an example of a general diagnostic and/or management class. It is virtually impossible to do otherwise. Though good manners may preclude addressing Mr. Jones as "the gall bladder in Bed A," patients inevitably become gall bladders. Dehumanizing categorizations are largely unavoidable. What are avoidable are bad manners and, so far as I am concerned, they are best corrected by dependence on the patient's good will.

The patient must have power. Medical pavilions are not half so notorious for the extraordinarily high technical quality of care they give as they are for the amenities, physical and psychosocial. And it seems no accident that wealth and power characterize the patients of medical pavilions: the amenities are precisely what go with wealth and power. History teaches us that extreme dependence on the patient and the patient's power can lead to care becoming simply a reflex of lay conceptions of what is needed. This, of course, destroys the whole point of a professional or expert service, and makes the expert a mere servant. If there really is expert knowledge, it deserves some independence; if there is not, then consultation is absurd. Obviously the power of the patient should be limited, but some kind of dependence on patient good will must be built into the system of health care. Kennedy's ideas of complaint services, evaluation questionnaires, and the rest are appropriate suggestions for developing such dependence.

Consumer participation is also appropriate. But when it comes to this matter, part of the problem in an area like health care is that people's involvement is far more episodic then their participation in such things as educational services. They are not involved day in and day out except for special cases of illness. A classic study of tuberculosis patients by Julius Roth[2] shows how much leverage patients could gain over the staff in their hospital. But they could do so in that context because they all had tuberculosis, which did not leave many of them comatose or bedridden, and they were all there for relatively long periods of time. They could thus develop the kinds of resources that could exert organized social control over the system of the hospital.

Ordinary, everyday health-care patients are involved mostly with episodic illness. He needs a herniorrhaphy or she is pregnant; they go in, they get fixed up, and they leave. I am not sure that such limited involvement is a very sound foundation for truly effective consumer participation. It is far more likely that given a formal system of patient participation, rather special kinds of people would come to serve as consumer representatives. They would professionalize the job and would in some sense sell out or be coopted. The danger of this is great for any consumer participation scheme, but it is particularly great in the case of something like medical care, in which consumers are not deeply or continuously involved.

Finally, I might point out that the adversary relationship created by consumer participation in the governance of health institutions is not the only way of countering dehumanization of care. It can also be avoided by mobilizing special motivation on the part of the providers—the health-care workers themselves. In some way, they must become somewhat less mechanically oriented. They must break out of their characteristic commitment to critical study and refinement of physical and manipulative *technique* while ignoring or taking for granted their relationship with the other people with whom they work, and with those on whom they practice their technique. The tendency to value technique in and of itself, without concern for the goals of human service and caring which justify the development and application of technique to human beings, must be tempered markedly. This is unlikely to occur through the mere increase of countervailing power. It is far more likely to occur through the institution of new forms of organization of the health workers themselves, and a head-on confrontation with traditional notions of collegial etiquette that prevent the very possibility of realizing the ideals of professionalism.

NOTES

1. E. C. Hughes, H. M. Hughes, and I. Deutscher. *Twenty Thousand Nurses Tell Their Story*. Philadelphia: Lippincott, 1958.
2. J. A. Roth. *Timetables: Structuring the Passage of Time in Hospital Treatment and Other Careers*. Indianapolis: Bobbs-Merrill, 1963.

PART FIVE

AN OVERVIEW

CHAPTER THIRTEEN

COMMENTS ON DEHUMANIZATION: CAVEATS, DILEMMAS, AND REMEDIES

JAN HOWARD, PH.D., AND CAROLE C. TYLER

The symposium on Humanizing Health Care, which served as a catalyst for this book, involved a diverse and vibrant group of health professionals. Many delivered formal papers that became the nuclei of articles included here. Others voiced their views orally in the cross discussion that followed each set of papers. In reviewing tapes from the conference, we were impressed by the richness of debate and the wealth of ideas expressed. Instead of presenting the remarks in chronological order, we selected the most cogent comments—those that made us pause to consider broader implications of conceptual schemes, research approaches, and innovative modes of care. To be parsimonious and still retain the flavor of the original argument, we paraphrased thoughts and organized them around specific questions that were raised time and again throughout the conference.

THE DILEMMA OF AMORALITY VERSUS MORALITY. For those attending the symposium the issue of humanizing health care was extremely impor-

Carole C. Tyler, R.N., M.S., and M.A., is a doctoral candidate in sociology at the University of California in San Francisco.

tant. This was not coincidental, since a deliberate effort was made to invite "heads with hearts" and "hearts with heads." Given their orientation, participants were somewhat startled by data from Charles Lewis that showed that a sample of respondents in Los Angeles rated humanization of care relatively low on a scale of priorities.

> Out of a group of several hundred, no one placed what we are talking about now (seeing the same doctor and nurse and being treated like human beings) above seven in a list of ten. Twenty-four hour availability of care and life-saving intervention were rated one and two. Our sample included people from various backgrounds, age groups, and settings—people who have the problems most of us say exist.[1]

The first reaction to this finding was to attack the research orientation. One person noted that dehumanization in the abstract may differ greatly from dehumanization in concrete terms and that findings depend on the nature of the question asked. He argued further that patients are very concerned about communication with their doctors regarding therapeutic regimens and that this is part of the humanization process. Others suggested that the Los Angeles respondents did not know their own best interests. Thus, Robert Cooke pointed out that continuity of care helps insure therapeutic compliance whether patients appreciate it or not.[2]

After this initial response, the conference confronted the fundamental question posed by these data. Who should decide what is good for patients? Patients themselves? Health professionals? Policy makers? A group of outsiders such as behavioral scientists? The patient perspective was defended by Rashi Fein, who was wary of the tendency of researchers to impose their values on others.

> Patients may want something very different from what we believe is best. Our priorities may not be their priorities. Our "trade offs" may not be theirs. Investigators must consider what patients want, what components of care enter into their definitions of humanization and dehumanization. In spite of complexities involved in asking questions about dehumanization, we should not be dissuaded from inquiry. Surely it is important how the question is asked, but it is also important not to reject asking it of patients.

The gist of this posture was unequivocally challenged by Eliot Freidson. He forthrightly argued that "we have an obligation to consider what patients *should* want, not just to decide what they do want." His logic follows:

Any system you set up influences human beings. It can create little Mickey Mouse automations as Disneyland does. It can create brainwashed people as our contemporary television does. And we can say, "Well, that's what they want; we asked them in a survey." We can plasticize it, make it personalized, provide it at least cost; we can use all the devices of our contemporary culture. But by giving them what they want, we are producing them at the same time.

The other approach, which is elitist I agree, is to consider what a fuller, richer life could be and what services might conceivably lead to different responses in a different kind of world. I don't think we can approach it passively because by giving them what they want, on the basis of having no experience with anything else, we continue to maintain them exactly the way they are. We have to face our own feelings and our own conceptions of what human beings can be, as opposed to what they are. I don't think we can avoid that dilemma. We have to assert some kind of moral conception of our own. Otherwise we are implicitly asserting a different kind of moral conception.

The moral dilemma portrayed by Freidson was not resolved by the conference. It reappeared in somewhat different form during the discussion of racism and change, summarized under "Geiger's Framework" below.

APPROPRIATE BOUNDARIES OF MEDICAL SYSTEMS. Generally speaking, medical systems are viewed as humanizing institutions. Thus, some humanists want to expand the boundaries of medicine to include as many people and problems as possible. Three arguments for caution were voiced at the symposium.

Jeanne Benoliel criticized medical institutions because she believes that they are sickness oriented and that rewards go to treatment of the sick rather than preventive care. She felt this was implicitly dehumanizing for those professionals who work in the broader field of health care and for patients who are perceived and treated in terms of their pathology.

A physician and lawyer by training, Dr. Perpich* had misgivings about other facets of medical systems. He questioned the modern view that drug addiction, alcoholism, mental retardation, and psychological disorders are not criminal justice problems but societal problems and, more importantly, health problems. Impressed by Thomas Szasz's[3] writings, Perpich suggested that defining all of this in terms of natural illness is itself dehumanizing.

> When I worked in prisons, many prisoners told me, "I don't want you to send me to your criminal division and label my problem medical illness or psychiatric illness because in a way that makes me less than a man. At least I own my own body; I'm a prisoner and I have an identity. If I go to the psychiatric system I'm a patient, and I'm in there forever. I have none of the due process rights that a prisoner has."

One rationale for expanding the definition of health problems to embrace certain crimes is that our society is possibly more disposed to allocate resources to medical systems than to systems concerned with criminal justice. And, perhaps, it is easier to humanize medical care than the care of prisoners.

The boundary dilemma was also mentioned by Philip Lee† in addressing the issue of drug use and abuse. He maintained that the pharmaceutical industry and the medical profession have redefined a whole series of problems as medical and treat them with drugs. For every conceivable complaint from headaches to examination anxiety, there is a drug for an answer. According to Lee, "this interferes with human interaction and humanistic approaches to problems. The most obvious example is with narcotic addiction where we choose to substitute one form of addiction for another. Heroin was the answer for morphine and now methadone is the answer for heroin."

REMEDIES FOR DEHUMANIZATION: PITFALLS, SIDE EFFECTS, AND COUNTERTHERAPY. In each of the four major papers, the authors suggested vari-

---

* Mental Health Career Development fellow, NIMH; law clerk for David Bazelon, Chief Judge, U.S. District Court of Appeals, Washington, D.C.; staff member, Senate Health Subcommittee.
† Currently director of Health Policy Program and Professor of Social Medicine, University of California at San Francisco; formerly Assistant Secretary for Health and Scientific Affairs, DHEW, and Chancellor of UCSF.

ous ways of personalizing care. During the discussion more proposals were made. Because of their diverse backgrounds and experiences, participants in the conference could point to a number of pitfalls in translating abstract models into reality. Occasionally, too, they prescribed antidotes for problems they foresaw.

Geiger's Framework. Jack Geiger's paper provoked a heated debate concerning better and worse approaches to eliminating institutionalized racism in our society. Philip Lee felt that Geiger had soft-pedaled the possibility of change from within institutions through affirmative action programs and new admission policies in professional schools. "Even if you don't deal directly with the care process, if you change the climate and the people who are involved, more humanized behavior will follow."

This approach was too benign for Dr. Geiger. He strongly argued that possibilities for combating racism are greatest where outside forces apply pressure for change. Even with regard to affirmative action programs, he believed that pressure from the federal government and local constituencies were a more important impetus for change than voluntary efforts from within. Based on his own experience, he accused universities and medical schools of exploiting affirmative action: "Their interest tends to stop when the overhead stops or as soon as pressures get to the point where internal structural changes are called for."

In essence, Geiger looked to organizational constituencies that could exercise power through some sort of threat.

> I think more has been done by people who are in a position to boycott, picket, set fire to, throw rocks at, cut off the funds of, or otherwise influence medical schools and universities than has been done by the action of the university itself in hiring more minority people.

Price Cobbs took vocal issue with this position on two grounds: insiders have a moral responsibility to be agents of change, and passing the buck to outsiders further victimizes victims.

> All too often when we say the system has to be changed from the outside, most of the people from inside are saying it. Yet none of us are opting out of the system. We keep paying our mortgages; taking vacations; trying to get our kids into college. I think it's a copout for me or anyone in the system

not to declare: "I guess if it's going to change, I'll have to try to change it from the inside." If there's another group out there that may be somewhat divergent from me, maybe I can get some input from them and vice versa, but I can't look for any primary source of change other than myself or starting with myself.

The tenor of Cobb's argument caused Jack Geiger to retreat somewhat from his earlier position. He concluded that there are actually three alternatives. One is for professionals alone or others within the system to say to those being victimized: "We will do it for you. We'll initiate change from the inside." The second option is for the victims to do it all from the outside. The third approach depends on advocacy and says in effect: "We will form alliances between insiders and outsiders. We can do it together, negotiating where possible and taking account of our respective responsibilities."

In his paper Professor Geiger identified the "tyranny of technology" as a dehumanizing influence in health care. During the discussion he carried his thinking further by criticizing the tendency to substitute machines for people. The machines may pretend they are in personal communication with us, as is true for answering devices and computer programs that interview people;[4] but plastic communication often heightens the patient's sense of isolation. Rashi Fein offered a counteridea in suggesting that technology can be a friend rather than a foe of humanization. He turned to the airline industry to show that the computer can be made a "liberating force."

> On Eastern Airlines shuttle, you're herded like sheep—no computer is used. You just come and get on the plane. And it's miserable. American Airlines, because they use a computer, has a reservation system. You come up and get your ticket. You're greeted by name and treated like a human being. The computer has enabled American to do something Eastern has chosen not to do, but they don't have a computer.

Dr. Geiger had strongly endorsed the proposition that health care is a right rather than a marketplace commodity. One means of implementing this ideology is to substitute national health insurance for fee for service. From an economist's perspective, Professor Fein stressed the importance of structuring the exchange relationship between consumer and provider in a manner that gives the consumer real power even when there is no financial transaction involved at the time that care is rendered. Without such structuring, he anticipated that the shift from a fee-for-service model to government payment or capitation might increase depersonalization by removing the power of the consumer implicit in fee for service.

> If we take certain constructs we have been advocating such as consumer participation and ability to go elsewhere, they often accompany fee for service. Now if this isn't doing the job, and I would not claim it is, consider how much worse we might be if we move, as I hope we will, to a national health insurance program in which there is no financial transaction between the patient and physician. I'm not saying that national health insurance must carry this high cost, but it might. Effective substitutes for the financial transaction are needed—substitutes that give the consumer power to withhold "purchase."

As a solution, Fein proposed that incentives be built into the system to encourage achievement of humanistic goals that providers and patients might agree upon.

> Let's say 90 percent of mothers shall have prenatal care by the third month, and there's a bonus to the group if they in fact achieve that. The same could apply to personalization of care. If you don't structure things, there's every reason to believe that the method of payment might make things even worse than they are now.

Howard's Model.   Jan Howard's conceptual scheme was criticized from two points of view. Irving Janis took issue with several dimensions of her model on the grounds of a potential conflict between research findings and the impetus to bring about change based on moral principles. He argued that freedom of choice, equality of status, and shared decision making are dangerous things to start tampering with.

> I have found that those surgical patients who become most disturbed emotionally are physicians and nurses who are treated exactly this way. Their practitioners will turn to them and say: "Doctor, you know as much about this as I do: What do you think we ought to do? Should we operate, or shouldn't we?" Equality of status and involvement in decision making sound wonderful—but these people were miserably upset. So I see empirical issues here that call for consideration before we try automatically to apply any of these concepts.

Another potential pitfall was anticipated by Dr. Howard in her discussion of empathy and affect, but it was elaborated on at the conference. Her contention that these are crucial dimensions of humanized care was underscored by Anselm Strauss with data from his studies of acute-care units. He noted that in the Burn Unit the therapy process itself intensifies pain to the absolute maximum, so an entire team is mobilized to shorten the time it takes to go through that pain. Yet members of the team rarely talk to patients about their suffering. It's taboo.[5] "All my researcher has to do is come close to a patient and give what we call 'presence,' and the patient bursts forth with comments about pain." Thus, the Burn Unit is superbly organized to minimize pain, but depersonalization results from the reluctance of personnel to become emotionally involved with patients.

An expression of concern for the patient in this situation would be interpreted by Strauss and Howard as humanizing behavior, but it was seen by Jeanne Benoliel as possibly dehumanizing for the health worker. Speaking from the vantage point of a nurse, she stressed the human cost of trying to relate to very sick patients. "When you're on a surgical ward, every patient is very personally focused on himself. If you walk in and show interest, everyone unloads on you. That's why its hard to stay with it. It takes so much energy to stay involved."

Leventhal's Model.   Howard Leventhal provided an information-processing model to serve as a guideline for personalizing care. The model was well received but invoked pleas for caution from the audience. Their first question concerned the amount and type of information patients should be told about their cases. Two problems were posed: limits on patients' ability to understand and negative effects of threatening information.

Dr. Cooke was especially pessimistic about the capacity of laypersons to comprehend elementary medical facts such as genetic probabilities of one in four. One cause of this difficulty was identified by Dr. Janis: physicians try to instruct patients at a time when they are in no position to receive and assimilate new information. For example, Ley and Spelman[6] found that their patient sample remembered 86 percent of the doctor's statements about their diagnoses, but they remembered only 43 percent of the doctor's instructions. According to Janis, this highly significant difference suggests that when the diagnosis is absorbed, emotional processes are set in motion that prevent other kinds of information from being assimilated. A further source of "noise" is the inability of health workers to understand their own abstractions. This obviously interferes with clarity of expression.

Assuming the patient *is* able to comprehend the facts communicated, what is the professional's role in sharing threatening information? The dilemma was succinctly stated by Dr. Cooke:

> I'm worried about the problem of the patient's knowing when he or she can't do anything about it, as is true for Huntington's Chorea. You may have a child who at 12 has serious deterioration of the central nervous system. You make a diagnosis. We can now make the diagnosis on his newborn sib, age one week; and you say to the family: "I can tell you with 100 percent certainty this child is going to be just like your older child and be deteriorating and dead in 5, 6, 7, 8, 10 years."
>
> In genetic disease we're opening up a fantastic number of biochemical determinations that tell you what's going to happen a few years from now. What we need to know is what this kind of knowledge does to the patient and his family. I get very different opinions from different people. But no facts.

There was general agreement that practitioners in this situation have a moral responsibility to help the patient cope with the knowledge at hand, but the "how" was in doubt. Albert Jonsen* proposed that ministers might be trained to facilitate communication with patients about taboo or threatening subjects and that clinical-pastoral education programs[7] should direct attention to this problem: "Patients may react negatively to the presence of conspicuously religious figures, but they could play a very important role, particularly since they rotate through different medical services."

Several members of the conference identified a further dilemma concerning communication with patients. In many situations, various therapeutic options are available, all of which are acceptable to health professionals. The patient needs to know the range of choices and weigh their pros and cons. Who should provide this information? Physicians? Other patients? Outsiders?

* Adjunct Associate Professor of Bioethics, Health Policy Program, School of Medicine, University of California at San Francisco.

Fritz Redlich* had misgivings about professionals as sole sources of information for patients because their action bias at times prevents objectivity.

In the case of a serious illness (like partial thrombosis of the retinal vein) which requires drastic procedures, the ill person is advised by his opthomologist of alternative approaches to therapy. The patient inquires about his prognosis and possible consequences of the various procedures and finally asks: "What should I do?" The surgeon, the opthomologist, is inclined to say: "Let's do such and such a procedure (laser treatment, for instance)."

In general, any kind of therapist is more inclined to be active because that's his job, his profession, his living. And he has also seen some bad consequences when other options are chosen. However, if a patient asks: "How many bad cases have you seen? What are the statistics?" he doesn't usually get this information even if it exists. So what can the patient do? He can ask for consultants, but they are chosen by the therapist.

A better solution might call for the intrusion of outsiders to supply facts, as is true for the purchase of commodities. Data come from other consumers, from published research, and so forth. Redlich observed that in medicine, we do not even have that: "We have an extraordinarily obscure situation which is highly protected by a guild. If we are going to humanize medicine, we have to change this situation. Otherwise, the patient is treated in a dehumanizing way even if no cruelty is involved." Eliot Freidson proposed that a directory on the order of *Consumer Reports* would be useful. It could describe and list options, probabilities, expert opinions, and physicians who tend toward one or another approach such as the Lamaze method of delivery.

The group also suggested that patients who have experienced certain procedures could be helpful in providing information to other patients— more helpful than medical personnel in describing the realities of the experience and how it affected their lives.

Besides questions concerning the content of information to be communicated and who should provide it, Howard Leventhal's model invoked still another question from the audience. This concerned possible boomerang effects of institutionalizing humane tasks such as those of a paramedical instructor. Professor Freidson wondered how the para-

*Professor of Psychiatry and director of Behavioral Sciences Study Center, Yale University.

medic's task might be transformed by workers in the course of routinization, as they moved from the freshness of interactions in the laboratory
to more stable relationships in the outside world:

> What if you take the results of these experiments described by Dr. Leven-
> thal, apply the knowledge in social policy—carving out time in the descrip-
> tion of paramedical tasks—and they proceed to perform these tasks rou-
> tinely, day in, day out? How will they perform these jobs once they become
> routine; and how will that influence the effectiveness of the process itself?
> Assuming Leventhal's findings could be put ponderously as a scientific law,
> the problem is translating that into routine human activities in an
> organization.

Dr. Freidson's plea for caution gained support from other members of
the conference. One person cited data from innovative mental health
programs suggesting a point at which they cannot sustain the same kind
of energy and enthusiasm; so the patients fall back.[8] Further evidence
was offered by David Hayes-Bautista* from his experience as director of
a free clinic. He observed that free clinics start out very human because
they self-select the people that staff them. But patient volume leads to
work fatigue and a burned-out feeling among professionals. Tom Scheff†
argued that boredom is a crucial factor in the dynamics of routinization.
When a health worker keeps doing the same thing with a patient or
what feels like the same thing, it starts to show. That shuts the patient
off, which exacerbates the situation because "you get more bored dealing
with shut-off people." The cycle escalates until there is no contact at all.
Both parties behave like robots.

Although routinization is a severe problem, several participants proposed methods of countering, or at least neutralizing, its impact. From
Jan Howard's perspective, the antidote lies in the reward structure. "I
find anything routinizing (even talking to students) if it interferes with
my research, which is what universities really consider important. But
I can dot i's and cross t's all day if I know I'll be rewarded by the
system."

A different approach was taken by Irving Janis in considering the
problem of fatigue among psychological experimenters. To counteract
the feeling of staleness that occurs when only a few psychologists have

---

* Ph.D. in sociology; director of Clínica de La Raza, Oakland, California.
† Professor of Sociology, University of California at Santa Barbara.

to deal consecutively with a large number of subjects, Janis's team has adopted the following procedure. The main recommendations (regarding a dietary regimen, for example) are recorded on tape in the voice of the experimenter. This gives continuity without the need to repeat the same instructions time and time again. Further communication is more open-ended. With respect to the interactional process being studied (the effect of positive versus neutral social reinforcement, for example), the investigator as well as the subject can make some personal revelations.

> The morale of the investigator stands up beautifully. The problem of habituation and degradation of procedures goes on at a much lower rate. So my idea is that standardized information can be given in packaged form once you have established the proper type of relationship, and interactions would be of a kind that keep interest alive.

A similar technique was endorsed by Norma Raynes* on the basis of her field experience. Conducting hundreds of interviews can be very alienating. So Dr. Raynes starts talking to respondents about herself— her problems, what she was doing yesterday, and so on. The interviews take longer, but they are far less boring for everyone involved. "In essence, this approach recognizes the existence of human beings on both sides."

Use of volunteers and quasi-volunteers is still another way of countering the cycle of routinization. Julius Roth† suggested that if writing a job description destroys innovation, one remedy is to try to avoid turning tasks into jobs. Some responsibilities can be left in the hands of the patient, members of the patient's family, and friends. Health professionals might find models in religious institutions where work is seen as a calling rather than a job. Other possible prototypes are free clinics, VISTA, and the Peace Corps.

In Tom Scheff's opinion, affect can play a crucial role in mitigating boredom. He maintained that people who do not become routinized in their tasks are those who have learned to handle emotional tension. They can be warm to other people because they have someone who is warm to them. Scheff speculated that the humanitarians in religious institutions undoubtedly have at least one person who keeps them going by provid-

* Director of Sociological Research Unit, Eunice Kennedy Schriver Center for Mental Retardation, Waltham, Mass.
† Professor of Sociology, University of California at Davis.

ing emotional support. He felt that mechanisms for affective support and the discharge of emotional distress might be made an integral part of health-care organizations—through cocounseling,[9] for example.

Kennedy's Model. Donald Kennedy's focal theme was decentralization of services, with particular emphasis on the home as a setting for health-care delivery. His argument raised two fundamental questions among listeners. The first concerned its middle-class bias and the second, the public's willingness to accept decentralized care. Rashi Fein feared that using the home as a locus for service might tend to reinforce two systems of care—"one for those who have homes they aren't ashamed to invite physicians into and one for other people." Fein also wondered how residential mobility among particular groups of workers might affect the possibility of humanized care at home.

The second caveat was articulated by Jack Geiger in describing decentralized care in a Mississippi OEO project. Geiger helped develop a program for making hospital beds out of plantation shacks because not enough beds were available in hospitals.

We discovered that we could put together a package that we loaded on a pickup truck, consisting of 100 gallons of clean water, a portable hospital bed, a portable chemical commode, a portable water heater, and a nurse-aide. And we took care of people with coronaries and pneumonia in a shack.

The big question posed by this experience is whether an urban nuclear industrial family would be as willing to accept "inpatient" home care as were the rural extended sharecropper families of Mississippi. As Dr. Geiger noted: "In settings of great deprivation this represents an advance. It may not work among populations with very different ideas about what medical care comprises." A similar caveat applies to the People's Republic of China where there is local control over the ward, hospital, commune, and brigade. Accountability is maintained in the presence of an overriding social ethic. One should not assume, however, that practices among people who have suffered many years of deprivation can be successfully transplanted to American soil.

Fragmentation of care was mentioned as a possible consequence of decentralization, and some members of the conference addressed this issue. The most significant suggestion came from Tom Scheff who described treatment systems for so-called "network problems." He referred specifically to two types of network approaches, one involving practitioners and the other laypersons. For illustrative purposes he cited *Away With All Pests*[10] in which a meeting is described in a Chinese hospital. The entire network of people participating in the patient's care are present: nurses, doctors, orderlies, the hospital administrator, and a representative of the patient. During the meeting those in charge of the case engage in self-criticism. If they forget their errors, others remind them. The discussion continues until mutually satisfying solutions are arrived at. The approach puts each specialist in proper perspective within the whole, makes all present accountable for their own actions, and gives a sense of unity to the care process.

Another network model was implemented by Ross Speck,[11] a Philadelphia psychiatrist, for crisis intervention. He believes that when people are psychologically disturbed or mentally ill, their situation becomes more critical if they have no supportive social network around them or if their network falls away. Such persons are resourceless and defenseless. So Dr. Speck assembles or reassembles the network. He tries to find the people in his patient's life who are relevant resources and sources of information; then he gets them all together. The meeting may include from 3 to 45 people. Professor Scheff would apply this perspective to all kinds of chronic illness in which there are feelings of helplessness and despair. "Even if services are decentralized, you can still assemble groups of relevant people, let them confront each other, exchange information, become emotionally motivated, and get a sense of an ongoing meaningful system of human values."

Creating A New Profession of Humanists. In addition to considering the pros and cons of ideas expressed in the four focal papers, those attending the symposium advanced other suggestions for humanizing care. One tack was to propose changes in the practice of care and those who practice it. Thus, Irving Janis recommended the creation of a new profession that would work to understand the patient's fears, facilitate the flow of communication, and increase motivational power. He recognized that psychiatrists and social workers could play these roles but felt their training was not entirely appropriate.

Janis's suggestion provoked negative reactions from certain listeners.

One person felt it would exacerbate fragmentation: "Now you go for diagnosis; now you go for therapy; now you go for niceness—three different waiting rooms." Others speculated that the new profession of humanists would have low paramedical status. "Human work" might be perceived as scut work to be avoided or tolerated until one could advance to a higher level in the pecking order. It was also feared that paramedical assistants might try to gain prestige by emulating the worst attributes of physicians. And the virus of professionalism was seen as an anathema to innovation. There seems to be a tendency for new professions to emerge prepackaged with instant boards of directors, codes of ethics, and newsletters, but with little genuine interest in rendering a service to society. Janis acknowledged these problems but thought they could be solved if the new professional roles were properly defined and supported by institutional norms.

Revamping Professional Education. An alternative to creating a new profession of humanists is to alter the orientation of existing health professions. This would necessitate change in the educational process because professional training in large health-science centers tends to perpetuate dehumanization. As Warren Richards* described the situation: "There's a lack of sensitivity on the part of our medical aristocracy (professors in medical schools, professors in hospitals) that becomes an inbred genetic thing because the residents copy their professors, the interns copy the residents, and medical students copy the interns."

The best approach to change was not at all clear. Professor Cooke was hopeful that education could raise the level of moral development among health professionals by exposing them to moral dilemmas, and teaching basic principles of justice. "Students have to learn to give up rights as they acquire greater responsibilities and capabilities." Others were wary of the value of abstract principles and rules. Howard Leventhal argued that humanization has to be made an integral part of the health professional's job and that we need a set of tools as rational and concrete as the tools for treating a sore.

If we can get to that level, then we can teach medical students how you

* Associate Professor of Pediatrics, University of Southern California; Director of Ambulatory Services and head, Division of Allergy, Children's Hospital, Los Angeles.

handle these particular things in this setting. I agree we're very far from that, and it's not the whole bag, but once you have this trapping of some theory and research you can institutionalize specific practices and make clear to the student that "It's part of your job, buddy."

Thus, the student learns to give patients information on the sensory feel of a procedure because he has been trained in the theory and research that says it is part of treatment. The student asks the patient his interpretation of an instruction, because asking is programmed by the knowledge that the patient's comprehension and retention is necessary for compliance to medical care. The student's behavior becomes an expression of a detailed theory of practice.

Leventhal's perspective drew a sharp retort from Rashi Fein, who strongly contended that no one in the health system today is going to be saying: "Buddy, it's your job," unless it is the consumer. If there is no premium on being nice, medical students will quickly forget humanistic values.

I'm not advancing a concept of original sin, but I'm not optimistic that people are inherently going to be pleasant to other people. If solo practitioners are nice or respectful or whatever, it's because there is a premium— the client can go elsewhere. It's not merely because this is the way they were taught to be.

Dr. Fein then suggested that we need to structure the environment in which health professionals practice so they are forced to treat patients as human beings. In the process they may even learn to value this approach.

One thought along this line was advanced by Jack Geiger from his Columbia Point experience. Students in the health professions could be assigned to patient-teachers with the stipulation that they could treat patients only if they continued to be acceptable to those involved. "There's a lot to learn from the consumer, and this would counter the idea that patients are only guinea pigs."

Expanding the Role of Consumers. Generally speaking, participants in the symposium were not optimistic about the possibility of changing attitudes and actions of the professional segment of health-care systems. Therefore, it seemed appropriate to consider ways of enlarging the responsibility of consumers as caretakers. This perspective was consistent with Jan Howard's conception of humanized care as involving equality of status, shared decision making, and freedom of action. It also coincided with emerging ideologies of consumer power and women's liberation, exemplified in Ellen Frankfort's *Vaginal Politics*.[12]

The idea of consumers as providers is hardly new. At a White House conference in 1965, Secretary of State Rusk speculated that 90 percent of medical care in the United States is provided by mothers.[13] In deciding when members of their families seek care and under what circumstances they will accept or reject advice, mothers are essentially captains of the health team.

Obviously, most consumers are laypersons who cannot easily be converted into medical experts. They are supposed to defer to physicians or designated others with proper credentials. But some members of the symposium had grave misgivings about professional expertise and its dysfunctional by-products. They recognized a tendency to exaggerate the value of this expertise, both inside and outside of health-care systems, and to underestimate the potential ability of laypersons. Thus, Julius Krevans* noted that as Dean of the Medical School, he is a symbol of inhumanity to all the other health professions. One reason is that people define roles and competence in relation to a false assumption: that the physician can operate anywhere on the long line of things necessary for the patient's care, from opening the door of the office to taking out a piece of the frontal lobe. Everyone else has a part of that line short of what the physician has, which leads to feelings of frustration, inferiority, and jealousy. The assumption of physician expertise extends outside regions in which his or her competence could in any way be genuine—to PTA meetings, for example. This further alienates segments of society.

From the standpoint of consumer participation in the care process, a more important consideration is the physician's limited expertise in dealing with a number of chronic and acute illnesses for which there is either no treatment of choice, or one that is relatively ineffective, protracted, and costly. These diseases include alcoholism, drug addiction, and mental disorders for which formal and informal lay groups have served as successful therapists.

An informed consumer population is one means of exerting control

* Dean of the Medical School, University of California at San Francisco.

over professionals and increasing the overall quality of health care. Evidence suggests that, once they have the facts at hand, consumers respond rationally to information. According to Philip Lee, the use of oral contraceptives was significantly reduced when women became aware of their dangers.[14] Thus, some members of the conference believed that information regarding adverse effects of drugs should be more readily available to the public through widespread distribution of appropriate Merck-type manuals and the *Physicians' Desk Reference.*

Others looked with disfavor on use of drugs as the primary mode of self-care. Dr. Lee stressed the need for alternatives and foresaw the emergence of nontraditional therapeutic approaches. He noted that transcendental meditation has produced dramatic reductions in drug usage among people who have been habituated or addicted to amphetamines, barbiturates, and a number of other medications.[15] Self-care could also include nutrition and exercise.

For the most part, the conference endorsed the idea of greater consumer participation in health care, but they raised a number of cautions. An important reservation was expressed by Dr. Geiger who feared that the value of professional expertise was underestimated. He agreed that the vast majority of illnesses are self-limiting and that GP's or mothers can handle 85 percent of the problems brought to the attention of medical systems. But this begs the question of determining whether or not a particular problem belongs in that category. It is only retrospectively that laymen can distinguish these illnesses from the 15 percent that require expert consultation. According to Geiger, "That doesn't help us prospectively when we first feel sick. We have to remember that all of that expert knowledge and machinery is there for a purpose."

The prospect of widespread self-medication brought further criticism. People would be treating themselves unnecessarily and magnifying the danger of iatrogenic injury. Many felt that wholesale distribution of Merck manuals would exacerbate the tendency to seek technological solutions to problems in human relations, and there is no guarantee that the average consumer could begin to understand Merck verbiage and its implications. The same criticism applies to patients having copies of their own medical records.[16] They would have difficulty interpreting them even if they wanted to, and charts might well be lost along the way.

In this vein, Jack Geiger advocated that self-care be distinguished from self-diagnosis and treatment.

What we ought to be talking about is not self-diagnosis and self-treatment but the acquisition of knowledge and information by people about themselves, their bodies, and disease. It's important that women know how their bodies work, what kind of examination they should get from their physician, what the cervix is, even what it looks like. That's different, however, from doing pelvic examinations and diagnoses oneself.

Professor Geiger also warned the audience not to overestimate the desire of laypersons to learn about health, or the possibility of getting this kind of information out or into people.

I think all of us connected with health, whether we are social scientists or physicians, are more interested in health, bodies, and illness than are other people. It's not clear to me, I wish there were some data, that women were all that interested in their bodies until it became an ideological issue. Much of health education has failed over this kind of problem.

A provocative footnote to the discussion of self-care and physician expertise was provided by Charles Lewis. He had just completed a comparative study of pavilion care and ward care in the same institution. Patients on the elitist floor (the pavilion) were matched by diagnosis with ward patients, and nurses were assigned to the two floors on a reasonably random basis. Quality assessments showed that the ward patients, who were treated by house staff, were actually receiving better care than patients in the pavilion, even though pavilion patients paid more and were treated by a variety of specialists.[17] Lewis concluded that there is a certain danger in being elitist—in having too many consultants, too many drug reactions, and being too much in charge of one's own care.

The only response from the audience concerned the options available to the elite. They are facing voluntary dangers. If they become dissatisfied with the treatment they receive, they can choose an alternative mode of care. Indigent patients have no such options. They face dangers involuntarily.

It is clear from the foregoing discussion that those attending the conference did not blindly endorse proposed antidotes for dehumanization in health care. They subjected each remedy to critical scrutiny. Some were generally wary of the prospect of change and what it might leave in its wake. Influenced by his training as a biologist, Julius Krevans questioned whether change per se is always good: "In social change I am not persuaded that there isn't at least some carry over from biology; so we ought to evaluate the situation to see whether the proposed solution is going to benefit society or be a detriment."

A second argument for caution was advanced by Marie Callender.* She was primarily concerned with technological change and its consequences for health care: "Are we doing in health care some of the same kinds of things we have done in other industries, providing an environmental or ecological base which in the long run may be more detrimental to the individual or society than if we did not produce that kind of technology?"

Professor Fein foresaw problems in allocating scarce resources and advised the group not to go overboard in trying to humanize care. There may be trade offs. He noted that many people have adjusted at no great cost to depersonalization in a variety of settings, such as transportation, and that selective change is called for:

> In certain parts of the medical system personalized care may be vital for our well-being. In other parts the energy devoted to getting it may be misspent. So let's examine the institutional settings and tasks carefully. Let's not make the system respond in all its facets to the fact that we want it to respond to the life-and-death situation, which isn't what all of medicine is about.

Another plea for restraint was voiced by Norma Raynes who was especially dubious of change induced from the outside. "I've seen change agents from the outside become the new victimizers. They appear as angels and crusaders, but they are really pursuing their own damned interests." Dr. Raynes was also leery of the bandwagon phenomenon which she found more characteristic of the United States than England. "The impulse to change and change fast is OK when we're talking about what to wear. It's very different when it's human lives."

According to Charles Lewis, innovative movements in health care tend to be cyclical. If one were to study the natural history of innovations dealing with quality of care and dehumanization (for example, home-care programs and comprehensive-care units), one would probably find that they have a three- to five-year life at most. Lewis hypothesized that deviant true believers provide the initial impact for these programs,

* Formerly Special Assistant for Nursing Home Affairs, Department of Health, Education, and Welfare.

expend their energy, and generate vigorous antibodies because their efforts are counter to the main value priorities of the institution. So these tend to be self-executing kinds of experiments that reoccur later when a new crop of true believers reinvents them.

IMPLEMENTING PROPOSALS FOR CHANGE ON A POLICY LEVEL. Assuming one wished to alter existing systems of care to make them more humanistic, how might policy makers be approached? This question captured the interest of Joseph Perpich and other members of the symposium who had policy orientations. Perpich suggested that decision makers are primarily influenced by dollars and cents and, therefore, the best way of convincing them to reform current practices is to show that humanism can have economic benefits. Data from the Egbert study,[18] which was quoted by Irving Janis, seemed particularly pertinent.

Egbert found that giving surgical patients preoperative psychological preparation reduced the time of their confinement. They left the hospital 2.7 days earlier than the control group and required less narcotics. Janis observed that on a strict cost-accounting basis, this kind of treatment has an enormous payoff. However, he cautioned the group not to assume that humanization of care will always pay economic dividends. Further research has shown that patients react differently to the same procedure;[19] and personalized approaches to treatment can be very expensive, depending on the professional group involved. All things considered, Janis believed that humanizing care will increase its cost. But research can help us determine for whom a given type of treatment is most effective and give us a rational basis for measuring the full range of benefits and costs.

Not everyone accepted the notion that policy makers are only persuaded by monetary considerations. Some felt that consumer power could effect major changes in the delivery process. If that power were properly organized and directed, decision makers would be forced to allocate resources to humanize care even if they had to divert funds from other activities. It was also noted that the dollars-and-cents approach overlooks the human cost of dehumanization and that cost/benefit analyses are too instrumental in their orientation. Personalized care can be viewed as an end in itself, not simply a means to other ends such as shorter periods of confinement. To adequately assess direct and indirect effects of various approaches to care, one should focus on long-term as well as short-term consequences.

A crucial factor affecting the possibility of humanizing health systems was identified by Marie Callender. In a new, significant trend, decision making and accountability are being transferred from traditional providers to absentee industrialists who deliver care as a subsidiary activity. Hospitals, long-term care institutions, and medical practices are being absorbed into larger corporate structures such as insurance companies, hotel chains, and fast food enterprises. The accountability of the provider is to a fiscal manager, which is somewhat divorced from the provision of care and which has a proprietary interest rather than a service profit interest.

Dr. Callender estimated that 80 to 90 percent of nursing homes are controlled and owned by proprietary "persons,"[20] and 60 to 70 percent of the beds in these proprietaries are controlled by interstate corporations engaged in absentee ownership.[21] Thus, health professionals who usually conceive of themselves as insiders may, in fact, be the outsiders. "We are not only dealing with patients in that kind of system, but we as providers are caught up in it, too." Dr. Callender expressed extreme pessimism regarding the ability of health workers to control these institutions, because power lies in the hands of a distant agent with organizational leverage over employees.

> I'm not suggesting that proprietarism is totally bad, but I think it adds a dimension to care that is not easily controlled by health professionals. Up to now, we've been talking in terms of a model which is a little too ivory-tower insular and a little too antiquated for the realities we are going to have to deal with.

A surprising response to the prospect of industrial control over the health field came from Elliott C. Roberts, Commissioner of Hospital for the City of Detroit. He speculated that, as in private industry, a business orientation among hospitals might indirectly facilitate humanism by providing an element of competition.

> These institutions are dependent on those who come to them and who will come back if they get what they're paying for. Profit-oriented businessmen and administrators have to please their customers. Too many hospitals have had a captive audience for far too long.

ISSUES AND QUESTIONS CONCERNING CONCEPTUALIZATION AND RESEARCH. In her presentation, Jan Howard proposed an eight-dimensional scheme for conceptualizing humanistic care. Charles Lewis had responded with a single-faceted definition in terms of self-image. The audience was then faced with two conceptual blueprints, one relatively simple and the other quite complex. They found simplicity appealing but were skeptical of its relevance to real-life situations. David Mechanic ventured that people can suffer frustration and humiliation in medical settings without any measurable impact on self-image. He suggested that perhaps the only commonality in the various portrayals of dehumanization was its negative impact on people; research necessitates a more sensitive definition.

> We keep referring to different levels of phenomena. As we get to research we can't operate on a level of generality. We have to cut the concept up in different ways, to take a piece at a time and ask questions about it.

Another approach to the dilemma of simplicity versus complexity is to emphasize a particular dimension of a conceptual network. Thus, Jack Geiger championed the view that *power* is the most important factor in humanization or dehumanization of care and that members of the conference were retreating from this issue. Power was also a crucial variable in Albert Jonsen's conceptual scheme. He contended that patients are fearful; the sicker they are, the more frightened they are. And they are put in situations where they are faced by very powerful people.

> Being a patient is like going to church. You are put into a strange situation where special rituals are being performed; where there are specialists up front who know all the secrets; and where fear and reverence are supposed to be the primary emotional attitudes. But in religion, people who don't like dehumanization can quit. You can't leave the health-care system so easily.

The only way to humanize medical care, according to Dr. Jonsen, is to find some way for patients to respond to power with a power of their own.

Tom Scheff visualized the patient-provider relationship in somewhat different terms. He singled out *affect* as the critical concept, not power. Thus, in a humanized interaction, there is mutually acknowledged and mutually intelligible expression of emotion.

I think the way people identify others as human beings like themselves and feel that they, too, are identified as human beings is by expression of emotion—especially fear, anger, embarrassment, disgust, humiliation, grief, and boredom.

Medical settings are unusual in two ways: the intensity of these emotions is overwhelming from the patient's side; and you have two people, one of whom is feeling all these things, and the other is more or less immune. So in medical settings you have less reciprocity and acknowledgment from the other person involved. This gives rise to feelings of dehumanization among patients.

A second theoretical question concerned the universal applicability of particular models for humanizing care, such as that set forth by Howard Leventhal. People in different social locations vary so much in their actions, attitudes, and expectations that it may be impossible to apply a given model across the board. Modifications might be necessary to insure compatibility between the theoretical design and the specific population being studied. The relevance of Kluckhohn and Murray's[22] paradigm was mentioned: in certain respects we are like all other people; in other respects we are like some others; and in still other respects we are unique. It was noted that medical clinicians have understood this for years. They constantly have to keep these three categories in mind, shifting back and forth among them.

Another fundamental issue was posed by paradoxes in the way the group conceptualized patients and practitioners and planned the task of research. Some wondered whether the dialogue and research posture of the conference were themselves dehumanizing. Thus, Julius Krevans strongly criticized the tendency of discussants to personalize objects, institutions, and organizations.

I have never seen a human hospital or a human group-practice or a human anything that is not alive and human. I have a James Barrie concept of what is causing the loss of humanity. Everytime somebody calls a physician or nurse a "provider," an angel dies; and everytime somebody calls a patient a "consumer," an angel dies. When all the angels are dead we will have a totally inhuman system. We ought to be cautious of the effect of language on concept and concept on process and remind ourselves that humanity is interaction between human beings, not between institutions.

Dr. Geiger immediately challenged Krevans's viewpoint, suggesting that the dyad of sick patient/physician must be accompanied by negotiation between groups of consumers and groups of providers on the basis of equality and accountability. He argued that this is a major source of positive change: "I disagree that everytime that happens an angel dies. I think it's an equally tenable position that it would be a lot better if the angels had a union."

With respect to research into the ways health systems affect people, several participants speculated that the intrusion of social scientists might serve to aggravate rather than ameliorate dehumanization if they superimpose their rationality on spontaneous interactions between patients and personnel. Paradoxically, the value of research regarding humanization of care may be directly related to the degree of intrusion into existing processes and practices. For example, if one wants to understand why some systems (possibly religious institutions for the mentally retarded) are more humanistic than others, one confronts the problem of self-selection. As Jack Geiger observed:

It is not at all clear that a humane physician in one setting would be humane in another because health workers select themselves into different settings. Furthermore, patients have preconceptions about existing systems that influence perceptions of what they find there. The same behavior (e.g., a 30-minute wait) in two different places may look very different to the same patient.

The solution to the selection problem would be to have the same patients and professionals function seriatum in two different environments, but a controlled experiment of this kind is difficult to design and implement. And it would, of course, be open to criticism on grounds of dehumanization through manipulation.

During the course of the conference it became abundantly clear that most of the questions that concerned the group could not be answered to their satisfaction, because little research has been conducted relevant to humanization and dehumanization of care. Few facts are available regarding the consequences of various approaches to treatment, the causes of existing practices, or possibilities for making health care more humanistic. To carry us beyond the tenuous realm of speculation, systematic research on a variety of fronts is called for.

The discussion that followed Charles Lewis's presentation concerning research issues revealed the diverse perspectives of scholars from different disciplines. In selecting areas for study, investigators tend to be guided by their own theoretical and pragmatic priorities. Thus, in planning the section on research we felt it imperative to tap the thoughts of more than one analyst. The next set of chapters provides a look at research issues from the point of view of a physician, a medical anthropologist, two medical sociologists, and an architect-planner. As a logical extension of ideas expressed above, the papers illustrate in no uncertain terms that the problem and task of humanizing care mean different things to different people, and thereby inspire qualitatively different blueprints for research and action.

NOTES

1. Unpublished data.
2. M. H. Becker, R. H. Drachman, and J. P. Kirscht. "A New Approach to Explaining Sick Role Behavior in Low Income Populations." *Am J Public Health*, vol. 164, March 1974, pp. 205-216.
3. T. S. Szasz. *The Myth of Mental Illness*. New York: Harper & Row, 1961.
4. W. V. Slack et al. "Patient-Computer Dialogue." *N Engl J Med*, vol. 286, June 15, 1972, pp. 1304-1309.
5. S. Fagerhaugh. "Pain Expression and Control on a Burn Care Unit." *Nurs Outlook*, vol. 22, October 1974, pp. 645-650.
6. P. Ley and M. S. Spelman. "Communications in an Out-Patient Setting." *Br J Soc Clin Psychol*, vol. 4, June 1965, pp. 114-116.
7. E. E. Thornton. *Professional Education for Ministry: History of Clinical Pastoral Education*. Nashville, Tenn.: Abbington Press, 1970.
8. D. Mechanic. "Issues in the Sociology of Organizations and the Administration of Mental Health Services." In *Politics, Medicine and Social Science*. New York: John Wiley & Sons, 1974,pp. 203-223. J. Wing and G. Brown. *Institutionalism and Schizophrenia: A Comparative Study of Three Mental Hospitals, 1960-1968*. Cambridge: Cambridge University Press, 1970.
9. T. Scheff. "Re-evaluation Counseling: Social Implications." *J Hum Psychol*, vol. 12, Spring 1972, pp. 58-71.
10. J. Horne. *Away With All Pests*. New York: Monthly Review Press, 1971.
11. R. Speck and C. Attneaue. "Network Therapy." In *The Book of Family Therapy*, edited by A. Ferber, M. Mendelsohn, and A. Napier. New York: Science House, 1972, pp. 637-665.
12. E. Frankfort. *Vaginal Politics*. New York: Bantam, 1973.
13. D. Rusk. "Address." White House Conference on Health, November 4, 1965.
14. M. Silverman and P. Lee. *Pills, Profits, and Politics*. Berkeley: University of California Press, 1974.
15. B. Brown. *New Mind, New Body: Biofeedback: New Directions for the Mind*. New York: Harper & Row, 1974.

16. Cf. p. "248" of this book.

17. Unpublished data.

18. L. D. Egbert et al. "Reduction of Post Operative Pain by Encouragement and Instruction of Patients." *N Engl J Med*, vol. 270, April 16, 1964, pp. 825-827.

19. I. L. Janis. *Stress and Frustration*. New York: Harcourt Brace Jovanovich, 1971.

20. U.S. Health Facilities Survey, 1960. National Center for Health Statistics, Department of Health, Education, and Welfare.

21. Unpublished data from Subcommittee on Longterm Care, Committee on Aging, Chicago, 1971. M. A. Mendelson. *Tender Loving Greed*. New York: Random House (Knopf), 1974.

22. C. Kluckhohn and H. Murray. "Personality Formation: The Determinants." In *Personality in Nature, Society, and Culture*. New York: Knopf, 1953, pp. 53-55.

PART SIX

RESEARCH
ISSUES

This part differs from the others in two major respects. It focuses primarily on research, and it offers the insights of five people who see the issues from coordinate but distinct towers of observation.

Charles Lewis combines the experience of a doctor of medicine and a doctor of science. He is presently Professor of Medicine and Public Health and head of the Division of Ambulatory and Community Medicine in the School of Medicine, University of California at Los Angeles. Over the past 10 years he has helped design a number of innovative programs in ambulatory care, emphasizing the utilization of varied forms of manpower. He has also been interested in multidisciplinary approaches to care at undergraduate and postgraduate levels. Dr. Lewis's publications are too numerous to list in full. Recent contributions include: "Acceptance of Physician's Assistants," *J Am Hosp Assoc*, vol. 45, June 1971, pp. 62-64; "Experiments in the Delivery of Health Care and Their Impact on Medical Schools," *Arch Intern Med*, vol. 127, February 1971, pp. 312-314; "Information for Planning and Evaluating the Education for Health Manpower," *Med Care*, vol. 11, March-April 1973, pp. 81-86;

"The Quandary of Quality: Incompetence Among the Excellent," *Am J Occup Ther*, vol. 27, March 1973, pp. 59-63.

Professor Clifford R. Barnett holds a dual appointment in the Departments of Anthropology and Pediatrics at Stanford University. For many years he has served as Director of the Program in Medicine and the Behavioral Sciences at Stanford. Dr. Barnett has a long history of research in epidemiology and the provision of health care across cultural barriers. Of late he has focused on the organization of health care for neonates, interactions between mothers and infants, and on physician-patient communication. His concern for humanizing health care demonstrates sensitivity to the multiple needs of professionals and patients. Publications include: (with D. Rabin), "Collaborative Study by Physicians and Anthropologists: Congenital Hip Disease," in *The People's Health*, edited by J. Adair and K. Deuschle, New York: Appleton-Century-Crofts, 1970, pp. 128-139; (with others) "The Effects of Denial of Early Mother-Infant Interaction on Maternal Self-Confidence," *J Pers Soc Psychol*, vol. 26, June 1973, pp. 369-378; (with others) "Mother-Infant Interaction: Effects of Early Deprivation, Prior Experience and Sex of Infant," *Biological and Environmental Determinants of Early Development*, The Association for Research in Nervous and Mental Disease, vol. 51, 1973, pp. 154-175.

Anselm Strauss is a professor of sociology, and former head of the Graduate Program in Sociology at the University of California, San Francisco. He also teaches in the School of Nursing on this campus. Before joining the UCSF faculty he directed social science research at Michael Reese Hospital in Chicago, and taught in the Department of Sociology at the University of Chicago. He has been involved for some years in research and teaching, much of it in the area of health and illness. Among the books he has authored or coauthored are: (with others) *Psychiatric Ideologies and Institutions*, New York: Free Press, 1964; (with B. Glaser) *Awareness of Dying*, Chicago: Aldine, 1965; (with B. Glaser) *Time for Dying*, Chicago: Aldine, 1967; and in press, with Mosby Company, a book on the social and psychological aspects of living with chronic illness.

Sol Levine currently holds three positions at Boston University. He is a University Professor, a professor of sociology in the College of Liberal Arts, and a professor of community medicine in the School of Medicine. He was formerly professor and chairman of the Department of Behavioral

Sciences and the director of the Center for Urban Affairs at Johns Hopkins University. As a medical sociologist Dr. Levine has written many articles and explored a number of themes including social consequences of medical science, life stress and coronary artery disease, new careers in health care, and change in community health organizations. Since 1972 Professor Levine has published several articles with Sydney Croog on responses to severe illness, and served as editor (with H. Freeman and L. Reeder) of the *Handbook of Medical Sociology* (Englewood Cliffs, N.J.: Prentice Hall, 1971, rev. ed.), in which he was also coauthor of two papers. In 1970 with Norman A. Scotch he edited *Social Stress* (Chicago: Aldine). *Social Policy and Changing Organizations* (New York: Random House) is in preparation.

Roslyn Lindheim is a professor of architecture at the College of Environmental Design, University of California, Berkeley, and is chairman of the Committee on New Ideas, Chancellor's Advisory Committee on Health and Medical Sciences. She is a member of the Institute of Medicine, National Academy of Sciences. Since 1970, Professor Lindheim has served as director of a special program of study on the interrelationship of social, psychological, and economic factors and the physical environment, sponsored by the National Institute of Mental Health. As an architect, consultant, and researcher, she has been primarily interested in the relationships between health care and the institutions that deliver it. Recent publications include: (with H. Glazer and C. Coffin) *Changing Hospital Environments for Children*, Boston: Harvard University Press, 1972; *Uncoupling the Diagnostic Radiology System*, Chicago: American Hospital Association, 1971; "Introduction" at the 1973 conference of the Gerontological Society on Housing and Environment for the Elderly; "Environments for the Elderly: Future Oriented Design for Living," *J Archit Educ*, vol. XXVII, June 1974, pp. 7-10. Forthcoming is *The Hospitalization of Space*, London: Calder and Boyars.

CHAPTER FOURTEEN

A PHYSICIAN'S PERSPECTIVE

CHARLES E. LEWIS, M.D.

The procedures to be followed in conducting research into the dehumanization of patient care are no different from those observed in the study of any topic. There are reasons, methods, results, and conclusions. In more "basic" research (that which does not directly involve social issues), the summary may be framed in a matter-of-fact way: "thus enzyme X has been demonstrated to be essential for the conversion of . . ." However, in studies of variables that are confounded with or measured in terms of "good-bad" or "right-wrong," the conclusions frequently include prescriptions for the immediate initiation or cessation of something that the investigator believes is needed or unneeded.

In this kind of research it is essential to avoid the pretext that the conclusions, as well as questions asked, are value free. If the researchers are truly concerned with "objective inquiry," they should declare their relevant values in advance. An investigator may hold strong opinions and values—most of us do—and these may actually enhance the quality of our work. However, there is a difference between a biased individual and a biased experiment, and the "results" should not be commingled with our "discussion." If research findings are to be credible and generalizable, then the hypotheses, designs, and instruments used must not result in self-fulfilling prophecies.

The images of cruelty and indifference that are provoked by the topic "dehumanization" invite impassioned rhetoric far more than objective inquiry. Yet, many questions in this area deserve dispassionate research. From my perspective as a physician, the following questions seem particularly cogent.

How Do You Define Dehumanization or Humanization of Care? To avoid a mere listing of problems, I suggest that depersonalization or dehumanization be defined as a reduction in self-esteem or loss of self-image or dignity. Assuming, then, that dehumanization is something that happens to human beings, evidence of the process might best be obtained from observation and testing of a particular experimental subject. For measurement purposes, the investigator could employ a variety of attitudinal scales related to self-esteem and self-concept, could monitor physiologic parameters, or assess the excretion rates of certain body metabolites that reflect "stress." It should also be possible to conduct experiments measuring the reverse of dehumanization; that is, situations in which an individual's self-esteem or sense of positive image is enhanced or increased. While some might enjoy the anger that is aroused by a discussion of a dehumanizing experience, perhaps we should take a more positive view of the research question, asking, for example: "What do we know about 'natural' treatments that seem to produce humanization?"

Several years ago, in assessing the performance of nurses trained for coronary care units, we took graduate students from a drama department and programmed them to play out scenarios designed to test the nurses' ability to deal with certain social-psychological situations that might occur in this type of care setting. The actors were placed in beds and wired with appropriate monitoring equipment. Then the interactions between nurses and actors were viodeotaped. We observed how different nurses dealt with their "final examination," how they managed a hysterical wife who threw herself on her husband's bed or a business partner arguing with his infarcted colleague over the future of their "big deal." We subsequently interviewed the actors with regard to their impressions of each of the nurses. Our own observations of the quality of the interventions were highly correlated with the subjective impressions of the professional actors, based solely on the degree to which *they* felt comforted, reassured, and cared for.

WHAT IS THE EPIDEMIOLOGY OF DEHUMANIZATION?   To whom, where, and when does it occur? Following the epidemiologic model, one might speculate about certain high-risk situations. What host (patient) factors predispose to this phenomenon? What are the characteristics of agents (providers) who reduce or enhance an individual's sense of dignity or self-esteem? What environmental variables lead to interactions of host and agent that result in positive or negative experiences? One might hypothesize that surgical patients more often sustain "loss of identity" than do those on a medical service, that this more often occurs on in-patient services than in physicians' offices, and in larger rather than smaller organizational entities. One might also predict that "loss of identity" is a function of the sociocultural distance between doctor and patient. Given a set of even "tentative hypotheses" it might be possible to make observations and examine the extent to which depersonalization or dehumanization is found in certain settings and on certain occasions more often than others.

WHAT IS THE NATURAL HISTORY OF DEHUMANIZATION?   It is doubtful if this phenomenon occurs only as a result of interactions with health pro-fessionals, or only in the health-care system. One might suspect that lowered self-esteem begins early in childhood and that, like many proc-esses, it is completely reversible *only* in its earliest stages. Does deper-sonalization among different age groups have differing long-term effects? Are these effects cumulative? Does "healing" occur? How effective is repersonalization therapy?

Just as Dr. Leventhal sees depersonalization as a normal process in the perception of illness by patients, a certain degree of depersonalization of patients may be essential for the psychological well-being of providers. It may not always be a pathologic entity. One of the most important hypotheses that needs testing is the following: "A positive self-concept in the provider is a prerequisite for humane care" (translated as follows: "I cannot meet your needs very long, unless I am meeting my own."). Does dehumanization of providers precede or predispose to dehumaniza-tion of patients? If such a sequence of events could be established, then perhaps we need to focus our attention on the selection and education of health professional students as a means of "prevention," rather than focusing on "treatment" or rehabilitation. Furthermore, if research findings document a relation between provider and consumer dehumanization, then major reorganizations in the health-care system need to be accomplished in ways that do not result in *further* depersonalization of the process of care.

OTHER RESEARCH QUESTIONS. What organizational structures facilitate behaviors that increase the individual's self-esteem or dignity? What are the types of transactions that accomplish these desired results? What is the relation of "humane" interactions to dependency needs and behaviors? Under certain conditions "doing good" or making people "feel better" may be confounded with transactions that foster dependency of patients on providers. Such therapy would seem to be akin to treating a cough due to carcinoma of the lung with a proprietary cough syrup. The patient may feel better, at least temporarily, but . . .

What is the relationship, if any, between humane care and the quality of *technical* care provided? Behaviors that may cause the patient to "like" the doctor may not reflect the physician's technical competence. When quality is evaluated objectively by professional standards, it is not related to patient satisfaction with the treatment received,[1] and it probably is not associated with enhanced self-esteem. The relationship between humane treatment and technical quality may well depend on the seriousness of the illness and possible outcomes of a humanizing transaction. Under some circumstances, care that is depersonalized, because it involves a minimal transfer of information, may achieve the best results in terms of another view of humanization (survival of the patient), as long as the quality of care is technically superb.

How can we change behaviors of providers to achieve more "humane care"? One hypothesis drawn from learning theory suggests that this will be accomplished best when desired behaviors are reinforced at the time of learning, rather than by attempts to extinguish negative behaviors. That is, medical or nursing students who demonstrate "humane care" should be commended by their "chief," who should model the kinds of interactions desired for the learner. When negative behaviors are observed, it may also be necessary to demonstrate alternative kinds of actions, and to reward (with positive reinforcement) those behaviors by providers that increase the dignity of human beings.

What is the effect on humanization of informing the consumer about the health-care process? The amount of information exchanged between participants may not be an appropriate proxy for the kinds of behaviors that affect humanization-dehumanization. Is there a way to involve the participation of individuals in their own care that achieves the desired results, that is, an increase in self-esteem and positive self-image? We are currently experimenting with an approach that involves children between the ages of 6 and 12 in the decision-making process with regard to their own health services. We believe that it is critical at this stage to enhance the patient's ability to make decisions and to reinforce the desired behaviors positively. Further, we feel that these interactions *do* increase the child's sense or self-esteem and provide a sense of internal control over his or her own destiny.

In summary, a variety of questions beg answers. Relevant research will not be easy. The results will have their greatest impact if studies are conducted as objectively as possible. Physicians are not necessarily "all bad." We are selected primarily to be puzzle solvers in a complex field of molecular biology. I suspect that the aggregate evidence indicates we do this reasonably well. Once upon a time, we lacked the tools to solve these puzzles—in fact, we did not even know some of the problems existed. During that phase of medicine, the physician's primary instrument of healing was himself or herself, and most doctors used "it" extremely well. There is some evidence, as Marshall McLuhan[2] has suggested, that our new technology has tended to "amputate" or replace those original skills that still represent the most effective treatment modality for dehumanization. However, I see no reason why competence in an affective domain cannot at the same time be associated with competence in a cognitive one.

If physicians are to "hear" the message, it is necessary to speak to them in terms they can appreciate and understand. To learn how to deal with patients more effectively—more humanistically—they must realize the value of designing intervention strategies that improve the patient's self-esteem, and they must see and comprehend experimental evidence that indicates that certain types of transactions are more useful in accomplishing this goal than others. Those academicians who are interested in meeting the needs of human beings (other than themselves) and avoiding dehumanization in care might spend more time designing and conducting research and less time engaging in rhetoric that reduces the signal/noise ratio.

NOTES

1. Columbia University: School of Public Health and Administrative Medicine. *The Quantity, Quality and Costs of Medical and Hospital Care Secured by a Sample of Teamsters Families in the New York Area.* New York: Columbia University Press, 1961, p. 6.

2. M. McLuhan. *Understanding Media, the Extensions of Man.* 1st ed. New York: New American Library, 1964.

CHAPTER FIFTEEN

AN ANTHROPOLOGIST'S PERSPECTIVE

CLIFFORD R. BARNETT, PH.D.

A number of the contributors to this volume have called for a better definition of humanization through research. This is not surprising, since the presentations cover a range of "needs" from better communication between physician and patient, through the need for more representatives of minority groups in the medical establishment, to direct consumer control over the health delivery system (sometimes described as a means to humanization and sometimes viewed as a form of it). "Humanization" and "dehumanization" are labels that may be useful in rallying popular support for changes in certain medical-care practices, but they are hardly useful for designing research. Indeed, everyone who has used or alluded to research has had to redefine "humanization" so that it could be operationalized through a protocol demanding specific observations or measured through the use of research instruments.

This is not a call for an idle academic exercise, since there are significant basic questions to be answered if we are to approach the many facets of humanization in a knowledgeable way. The emotional impact of certain medical situations understandably motivates us to take or demand immediate action, even though the grounds for such action are poorly drawn. How can we not respond in an emotional way to the following example (received as a response to a question on a mail survey that our research group sent to intensive care nurseries throughout the United States)?

In May of 1965, we had a baby expire from a heart condition, who had been with us for 3 months (since birth). At no time did we consider the feelings of the parents, although not a day went by that both parents did not come to the nursery to see their baby from the outside window. When the baby died, the mother asked to hold him. This she did, sitting, rocking and crying. She made the statement that this was the first time she had touched it. From that time until now, all mothers of prematures are allowed to scrub, gown and stick their hands in the incubator to touch their babies, regardless of the baby's condition.

I think most readers would agree that this nursery adopted a very humanistic procedure in allowing mothers some contact with their infants during the immediate postpartum period. But if we move from an empathic or propagandistic stance to a research position with regard to this case, we must ask some critical questions. Was there sufficient evidence that it would be better for mothers if they were allowed to enter the intensive care nursery? What was known about the impact this would have on the infant and the organization of care in the nursery?

One approach to the latter question would be to examine why parents were kept out of nurseries. Initially, this practice was designed to decrease the risk of infection to the infant. Thus, parents of low birth-weight babies in intensive care nurseries were permitted only to observe from a viewing window, as described in the poignant example cited above. This separation period could last from several weeks to several months. In the 50 or so years since the establishment of hospital nurseries for premature infants, there have been many technical innovations (disposable syringes and other items, positive pressurization, new antiseptic solutions) for preventing infection, as well as new drugs for treating infections when they occur. Nevertheless, the entry of mothers into intensive care nurseries was an untested practice in the United States in 1965 when the cited nursery (along with a number of others) adopted the practice for humanistic reasons. It was not until the end of 1969 and early 1970 that studies appeared regarding the safety of admitting mothers to these nurseries.[1]

The research group of which I was a part carried out a pilot study to determine whether infection risk increased with the presence of mothers. The investigation was done as necessary preparation for testing a set of specific hypotheses directed toward humanization. In the central study we used an experimental group (mothers in the nursery) and a control group (mothers kept out of the nursery). We asked whether the separation of a mother from her infant in the immediate postpartum period affected how she felt about herself and about her baby, and whether her separation affected her maternal behavior when the baby was discharged to her care. In brief, a question about the humanization of care became a basic research question about the impact of separation on the maternal-infant relationship. The form of the findings bear mention here.

We found that separation from her infant in the immediate postpartum period had a clear negative impact on the primiparous mother but little effect on the multiparous mother.[2] Whether primiparous or multiparous, however, women who initially had low self-confidence in their ability as mothers remained low or dropped even lower in self-confidence as a result of the separation. On the other hand, women with low, initial self-confidence gained in assurance when they maintained contact with their infants in the intensive care nursery. Our findings thus defined a group "at risk" as a result of separation.

All mothers in the experimental group were given the choice of entering the nursery when they felt ready for contact with their babies. All entered eventually, but clearly some felt "ready" to do so before others. Thus, we are not suggesting that all mothers must enter the intensive care nursery, thereby substituting one rigid system (all mothers in) for another (all mothers out). We are opting for individual choice.

When humanization of care questions are framed and researched in this manner, dealing with specific populations in clearly delineated circumstances, we will avoid completely the standardization issue raised earlier by Eliot Freidson. In his commentary on Donald Kennedy's presentation, Freidson suggested that some patients (at least some of the time) might prefer to have their medical history taken via a computer terminal and to be treated efficiently through a relationship that involves a minimum of human interaction. In my opinion, humanization research should specify the conditions under which specific populations prefer or are in need of certain types of care alternatives. If humanization is to mean anything, institutions designed to serve human needs must allow maximum choice and maximum alternatives to match the great variety of human desires. As an anthropologist who has been impressed by the diversity of human behavior and human-created institutions, I am most skeptical about single solutions to complex questions.

There is another advantage to raising researchable questions in terms of patient or consumer response within specific situations. This posture will prevent us from entangling ourselves in the problematic attempt to define panhuman needs in absolute terms. It may be true that all mothers have a panhuman need for physical contact with their infants shortly after birth, but it is far more feasible to document the differential response of mothers to contact or no contact. Further, the delineation of "high risk" groups in need of special attention or procedures means that resources (which are always scarce) can be allocated where they are needed, rather than indiscriminately. Such an approach is likely to have greater impact on the health-care system and prevent the development of monolithic organizational structures.

This is not to say that it is unimportant to be sensitive to untested assumptions about panhuman responses. These often are the underpinnings for the development and perpetuation of certain health-care practices. The initial response to our nursery study, for example, clearly indicated how procedures in British nurseries were based on certain assumptions about human nature. The *British Medical Journal* commented editorially about how unnecessary our study was, stating:

> It would be natural and normal for a mother of a premature baby to be helped to feel close to him . . . to maintain contact with him in hospital from the time of delivery to the time when she leaves for home where she will have to do everything for him—and to feel the great satisfaction that she has helped to save her child from the valley of death.[3]

For the anthropologist, appeals to what is "natural and normal," "common sense" or "what everybody knows" are markers for areas of the culture where key assumptions are being made. Another feature of common understandings is that commonly held contradictory understandings can often be found, each of which is "logical" in a given situation.

The location of such contradictions may provide fruitful areas for humanization research in medical care because contradictions in practice that are based on assumptions about human response often result from a lack of research findings. The old argument of whether "to tell" or "not to tell" the terminal patient is a case in point. We found in our nursery survey that some nurseries generally allowed mothers to enter except when the infant was critically ill or terminal. Others generally did *not* allow mothers to enter except when the infant was critical or terminal. Proponents for either position can make a good case.

One side has argued that if a mother has contact with a critically ill infant she will be more involved and attached, and thus will feel the loss more. Others argue that it is better for a mother to grieve for a real infant than for one who is so removed she can fantasize about it. Both sides can make their assumptions about the human response because as yet only one pilot study has been directed to the question of how contact affects the grieving process.[4] Studies such as these will provide a solid theoretical and empirical base for humanization, for they will also state the variety of response under differing conditions.

Dr. Lewis concludes that what is needed is less "rhetoric that reduces the signal/noise ratio" and more time devoted to "designing and conducting research." Although research may be better than rhetoric under certain conditions, its design and conduct are not necessarily divorced from propaganda or social action. Every anthropologist who has studied programs of directed cultural and social change has pointed out that such change is facilitated if the innovating agency can make appeals that agree with the values of the target population that hopefully will accept the innovation. Further, it has been suggested that if recipients participate in innovation programs, this will also facilitate acceptance of change. Certainly, scientific research is highly respected by members of the medical establishment, so any changes in the delivery of care would have a better chance of adoption if they were based on scientific research, especially if it involved the potential adopters.

Furthermore, research can and should include variables that may help "sell" the innovation. This is implicitly recognized in studies of the *cost* differential of using the allied health worker in contrast to the physician in providing certain kinds of services. Similarly, with reference to Dr. Leventhal's research, it is important to the physician to learn that patient compliance during endoscopic examination is increased if the patient is psychologically prepared beforehand. That finding has a better chance of leading to acceptance of the new preparation procedure than would the finding that the patient feels less anxiety and in general feels better about it.

Research carried out for propaganda purposes alone, however, does not seem very exciting. The dearth of good studies by social scientists on humanization of health care may reflect the general view that the problems are so applied in nature that they have limited theoretical scope. Instead of turning away, we must seek out the basic research questions that may underlie the immediate clinical question being posed.

Some areas of health-care humanization mentioned in this volume lie outside the domain of research at the present time. Once the finding is made, for example, that medical care of a certain quality (as measured objectively by outcome) is unevenly available to various groups in the population according to their social class, color, or area of residence, then additional research to document the unequal distribution is not going to change the situation. Various experiments can be carried out to test ways of overcoming inequality, but the essential issue has passed from research to the political arena.

In summary, there are a number of guidelines for developing productive research in the area of concern here. First, the very word "humanization" suggests assumptions about human nature. The goal of humanization in the health-care context has been to make the medical-care system come as close as possible to meeting human needs. However, as we have learned from psychology and other social sciences, the attempt to define needs (or instincts) is a blind research alley. We would do much better to think in terms of the responses of defined populations to specific situations. Once we pose the problem in this way we will be able to carry out empirical research because we will be studying how people with known characteristics respond to defined situations.

Second, a very useful way to discover significant problem areas for behavioral research in medicine is to seek out those places where health personnel are making assumptions about human responses to certain procedures. These areas often can be identified by observing the occurrence of conflicting practices or rationales among practitioners and institutions. Close examination of such situations will reveal that practitioners are flying by the seat of their clinical pants in the absence of any guidelines in the research literature.

Third, one result of research in these areas will be the delineation of response patterns that will differ according to the desires, expectations, and needs of the population studied. This should lead to recommendations for a variety of approaches in health delivery to meet the variety of responses in the population to be served. The question no longer is: "How can we humanize the system?" Rather, it is: "What is the best procedure for what kind of patient?" Once there is variety, informed choice becomes possible for the patient. We should not fall into the trap of prescribing a new monolithic system for the present one, no matter how "humanized" the new system may appear. A monolithic system (i.e., one without variety and choices) cannot be a humanized system.

Finally, in some areas of social change, research has been viewed as a substitute for social action or as a diversionary tactic to delay or prevent change. Within a subculture such as medicine, however, where research is highly valued, this need not be the case. By appealing to the values of the people in the subculture and involving them directly in the investigatory process, research can be a vehicle for change.

NOTES

1. C. P. S. William and T. K. Oliver. "Nursery Routines and Staphylococcal Colonization of the Newborn." *Pediatrics*, vol. 44, November 1969, pp. 640-646. C. R. Barnett et al. "Neonatal Separation: The Maternal Side of Interactional Deprivation." *Pediatrics*, vol. 45, February 1970, pp. 197-205.

2. M. Seashore et al. "The Effects of Denial of Early Mother-Infant Interaction on Maternal Self-Confidence." *J Pers Soc Psychol*, vol. 26, June 1973, pp. 369-378. A. Leifer et al. "Effects of Mother-Infant Separation on Maternal Attachment Behavior." *Child Dev*, vol. 43, December 1972, pp. 1230-1238.

3. Anonymous. "Mothers of Premature Babies." *Br Med J*, vol. 2, May 30, 1970, p. 556.

4. J. H. Kennel, H. Slyter, and M. H. Klaus. "The Mourning Reseponse of Parents to the Death of a Newborn Infant." *N Engl J Med*, vol. 283, August 13, 1970, pp. 334-339.

CHAPTER SIXTEEN

A SOCIOLOGIST'S PERSPECTIVE

ANSELM STRAUSS, PH.D.

In discussing dehumanization we have tended to emphasize four major themes: the impact of strict professionalism, the impact of modern technology, the increasing organizational size of health facilities, and the inequities in American life. Each was explored quite thoroughly. Yet that exploration, I think, does not adequately account for what goes on under the name of dehumanization.

It might even be maintained—at least in devil's advocate fashion—that our discussion has mostly examined only surface manifestations of something far more basic. I refer to the astonishing change in recent decades in the nature of disease (predominately chronic now rather than acute), and the implications of a substantial amount of chronic illness among the populations of the more economically developed nations. It is to that phenomenon, and its further relevance for the humanization-dehumanization issue, that I adress myself in this research note.* After discussing some of the implications of chronicity, I shall touch on research areas that need to be investigated.

"Chronic illness" tends to conjure up the illnesses of old age. It is true that the elderly suffer more than others from such illnesses, but the extent

* My approach is based on several years of interviewing and observation of the chronically ill together with Barney Glaser and our students. The research was supported in part by the Russell Sage Foundation.

of chronicity in the general population is suggested by some 1964 figures published by the Department of Health, Education, and Welfare. They indicated that approximately 46 percent of our population suffered from one or more chronic diseases, while one of every four was so afflicted that they had lost days away from work. A Social Security survey for 1968 suggests the amount of chronicity for younger people, although its author focuses on the age differential: "The rate of disability in the older population, aged 55-64, was more than three times that of the population aged 18-44, and about one and a half times that of the 45-55 age group."[1] In light of such figures, one may well ask why the contributors to this volume have referred only glancingly to the kinds of patients who have diseases like cancer, diabetes, heart disease, asthma, cystic fibrosis, arthritis—the patients who fill our hospitals and the corridors of our clinics.

Throughout our book, "the patient" appears in various guises: frustrated by the professionals, anxious about a disease, victimized by bureaucratic impersonality and the inequities inherent in American class and racial distinctions. Only occasionally does the patient appear as someone who has a specific illness, and usually then as an illustration of some specific point.

I should like to suggest that health professionals have not yet really grappled with the implications of widespread chronicity. Of course, they know that most patients are in hospitals because of a chronic illness—they are there to be diagnosed, treated, and sent home if possible with the disease partly reversed or at least temporarily arrested. Nevertheless, the professionals are oriented primarily toward disease systems and the handling of acute phases of chronicity. Why should they not be? After all, that is what medical technology is mainly about, and that is mainly what the training offered in medical schools is all about. (Nursing schools are moving toward a clearer understanding of "long-term" disease and what it might mean for nursing care.) Perhaps hospital-based physicians come to recognize what it really means to be incurably sick either when the patient is actually dying or when survival depends on the physician's management of delicate "home conditions" (as it does with kidney transplantation).

If we look squarely at how chronically ill persons manage their daily lives, we see that their main concern is not with the disease but with living as best they can despite the disease.[2] Translated into concrete images, this means they must learn how to minimize the effect on their lives of not only their symptoms but also their prescribed regimens. They may have to adjust to changes in the course of their disease, whether they have remissions or just worsen steadily. They may have increasingly to bear the retreat of their kin and their friends. Virtually all chronically ill persons have to manage their social relations so as to keep them as near to "normal" as possible. And, of course, many are confronted directly with the problem of paying for their treatments as well as managing in the face of lessened income.

To handle all such problems calls for an organization of effort that, more often than not, involves kin, friends, and even neighbors. To establish and maintain that organization requires various resources (financial, medical, familial) as well as various interactional and social skills. Health professionals are included in such arrangements—especially insofar as they involve regimens and the combating of medical crises—but they are not necessarily as crucial as they might think to the central issue of living with a chronic illness. Medicine may certainly contribute to survival and "being better," but it is just as surely secondary to what some patients aptly term "carrying on."

Hospitals get these patients for diagnosis or in the acute phases of their illnesses. Clinics and physicians' offices tend to get them in their recuperative phases or for routine chronic care. Nursing homes get them after hospitals discharge them, and often take them through to death. But, of course, most of the "living in face of chronicity" goes on at home where most illness behavior takes place, as Dr. Kennedy has insightfully emphasized.

Said another way, chronic patients have biographies that encompass not only their experiences with disease and its home management, but encounters with health-care personnel and their medical facilities and experiences with the changed social conditions brought about by their disease and its medical management. In the facilities, the personnel do not know very much about those other experiential biographies nor understand their bearing on the patient while under care.

An example or two may help to underline this point. Ulcerative colitis patients learn to monitor themselves very carefully, hour by hour. But when they become sick enough to come to the hospital, they cede all that personal responsibility and control to the hospital staff who do not generally have the least understanding of what it means to move from such an outside status to a hospitalized one. Often when the staff recognizes that a cronically ill patient has an illness biography—as when the patient seems to know a great deal about drugs—then that knowledge may only ruffle their professional feathers, which leads the patient to consider them annoyed, distant, "impersonal."

So we are back again to the issue of impersonality—dehumanization. According to views expressed in this book, dehumanization is related to the size and nature of the health facilities, and to the accompanying medical technology, professionalism, and social inequities. I believe that the very structure of the health facilities and the character of the medical technology are clearly associated with the predominant kinds of disease now being combated by health professionals. For instance, on many intensive care and cardiac units, an elaborate technology (comprised of machinery and skills) is used to monitor seriously ill cardiac patients minute by minute, and there is an organizational structure to match (notably the arrangement of space, the subtle management of time, the complicated organization of work, and the utilization of highly specialized staff).

As for professional training, it is related both to educators' conceptions of disease processes and to their views of how these processes are to be approached, treated, and managed. Understandably their conceptions are not linked closely with the patients' problems of living at home. What is more, they are just as understandably removed from concern with patients' problems of living while they are at the facility. Common professional jargon notes this by stating that the patient as a "total" or "whole person" is not really being treated. Those terms are applicable to treatment only if it is understood—it is not usually—that the whole person includes all those biographies noted earlier that patients bring to the hospital with them, generally unnoticed by the staff.

We must begin to think through the implications of illnesses that cannot, on the whole, be cured but only "managed" and that, in any event, must be lived with. One set of implications certainly pertains to how our facilities need to be reorganized to take into account the illness-health care-social biographies that precede, accompany, and persist beyond visits to the facilities. We must understand that organizational restructuring is necessary not merely for humanitarian or humanistic reasons, but quite literally to keep some people alive and certainly to give them better medical and nursing care. I even hazard to say that such care would be cheaper in the long run, keeping more chronically ill persons away from more facilities for more time; that is, this kind of reoriented care might contribute to a spacing out of the acute flare-ups that repeatedly bring the chronically ill into our professional domains.

The necessary reorganization of health facilities and health care surely should involve both the facilities and the conditions that patients confront at home. Consider, as an example, the difficulties experienced by cardiac patients. First, it is worth mentioning that cardiologists, being focused on survival and disease, have discovered that a great proportion of "cardiacs" die before actually reaching the hospital. Therefore, rescue care now begins in the ambulance. But when cardiac patients leave for home, they are typically not instructed in many things that may be necessary to prevent a relatively speedy relapse. They are given vague prescriptions—"take it easy," "don't overdo it," "find your own level of activity" —but they are on their own to operationalize those prescriptions. We will find, too, that as soon as such a patient meets other people, they will raise his level of anxiety by inquiring why he is or is not doing special exercises, or why he is still eating butter, or why he deviates from some other regimen they have heard about or are following themselves.

At home, also, marital difficulties may contribute to a relapse. That may be recognized by the physician; but generally the physician does and can do very little to ease the situation since our "health-care system" is not organized to help with such matters. It is not even organized, although it easily could be, to help with questions about sexual activity —questions that patients are unlikely to ask their physicians because of embarrassment or the feeling that they are not legitimate "medical" questions.

Other issues affecting cardiacs go far beyond what might be expected of health professionals and health-care organization; for instance, getting legislation that would require physical transformations in public buildings (ramps instead of steps) and on city streets (lower curb stones), as well as getting legislation or the necessary public pressure that would move insurance companies and employers to remedy a chief problem facing cardiacs: obtaining proper funding when they lose the capacity to work or cannot find employment because they are known to have had heart attacks. Undoubtedly, cardiacs would also appreciate any public pressure that would make employers more willing to hire or rehire them.

In short, helping cardiacs to manage better the problems that may bring relapses or contribute to quicker disintegration would require considerable new organization: new kinds of personnel, new kinds of tasks for current personnel, new legislation, and so on. As for the current health facilities, if we took seriously those multiple biographies of the cardiac, we would need considerable reorganization of tasks, training, and division of labor. The point is obvious if one thinks of giving more "humanized" terminal care—care that is more psychologically and socially oriented for patients who are dying.

Organizational restructuring is just as necessary for patients who are going to be discharged. A small illustration: the typical interaction around someone who has just had a myocardial infarction is characterized by intensive care and concern. However, as the patient moves further away from what the staff define as the time of greatest danger then, understandably, they give the patient less of their time and attention, turning instead to others who are more critically ill. But it is precisely then that the less endangered patient begins most to need some sort of psychological care—reassurance, or what have you. Frequently such patients are forced to go without that reassurance. Furthermore, everyone who passes by their beds is likely to define differently what "rest" consists of, and so although the patients are enjoined to rest, they receive divergent messages about whether they are obeying that injunction—not a situation calculated to allay their anxieties about potentially sudden fatality nor to increase the speed of their recovery.

Citizens of Great Britain or Scandinavia have great advantages when it comes to monetarily surviving their chronic illnesses or getting relatively equal care regardless of their social class, because their countries have more extensive and equitable insurance and health-care systems than ours has. Amazingly enough, however, these patients seem no better off than their American counterparts when it comes to the help they receive in handling their illnesses while at home and getting reasonably good psychological and social care while at the health facilities. To begin to make headway with such care, it is first necessary to recognize that chronic illness (and care, not cure) is the name of the illness game, at least in all the industrialized countries of the world. It is my contention that the increased humanization of health service is closely linked with that recognition.

Below is a brief set of suggestions about research areas relevant to the issue of "dehumanization" that would seem to need investigating.

1. My discussion so far is based on studies of sick people who had only a few of the possible chronic diseases. Since the major problems of living are bound to vary in accordance with salient properties of given diseases and their associated regimens, it is necessary that we study many additional—and different—kinds of chronic disease in relation to their impact on the sufferers' lives. This research ought to include cross-cutting variables such as sex, social class, marital status, life styles, and chronological age. On these matters, there is really a paucity of literature in general, let alone research.

2. The problems of "living with" chronic illness are not just the problems of the sick person but almost inevitably involve spouses, children, siblings, and close friends. With acute disease one might speak realistically of "the patient"; but with chronicity, the family context (or its significant absence) is realistically the frame of reference. So the networks of affected and of supporting others need to be studied intensively. It is there that we can get important information that will suggest how health personnel can be added to, or geared into, the lay networks.

3. Apropos of health personnel, it would be useful to have specific knowledge concerning the range of relationships currently extant between them and the chronically ill and their families. This focus ought to include interactions in home settings as well as hospitals and outpatient facilities. It ought also to include all health personnel, not merely "the doctor-patient relationship" (which tends to be discussed rather unrealistically as a one-to-one interaction). A major pragmatic question concerns the best means of improving these relationships. The answers depend on those to a prior question: What situations actually prevail today? This, of course, is the "dehumanization" area par excellence, or at least most obviously so.

4. Research should also explore some of the larger, public policy aspects of chronic illness. (Today those aspects are conceived almost totally in terms of geriatrics.) Some of the questions here pertain to the major perspectives on different chronic illnesses in relation to their effect on public action. Of further interest is the impact of new trends (Medicare, minority group rights, consumer movements) on the lives of the chronically ill. In this policy area, what is especially needed is applied research on what could be done to make less difficult (less dehumanized) the living of the ill. This means instituting actual programs and then evalu-

ating the results, including lobbying and legislative campaigns, legal action, work with trade unions, and education-information campaigns.

These are only a few of the potentially useful research areas. Any researcher or policy maker who is convinced of the genuine importance of the problem of chronicity (who does not merely assign it to the limbo of geriatrics) ought to be able to think of many additional and perhaps equally important areas for research.

NOTES

1. L. Haber. "Epidemiological Factors in Disability." In *Social Security Survey of the Disabled, 1966*. DHEW, Social Security Administration, Report no. 6, February 1969.
2. A. Strauss. *Chronic Disease and the Quality of Life*. St. Louis: Mosby, 1975.

CHAPTER SEVENTEEN

A SOCIOLOGIST'S PERSPECTIVE

SOL LEVINE, PH.D.

For many of us who have labored in the health field as teachers, research-ers, and administrators, the humanization of health services has been an underlying value, an organizing theme, and a guiding, broad, conceptual framework. My task here is to specify and formulate research questions relevant to humanizing care. One who assumes this role must, for awhile, shun metaphors and become circumspect and skeptical, for who has not been humbled by subjecting scintillating hypotheses to the naked and sobering exposure of empirical testing? Furthermore, the trumpeter's call to study X, Y, or Z may not be urgent or compelling for everyone. The research-oriented scholar has to be pragmatic and recognize that limits must be placed on the range of questions that can be explored fruitfully with a reasonable expenditure of time, money, and effort.

Thus, I raise a few brief questions about (1) the definition and impor-tance of the concept of humanization, (2) humanization as a dependent variable, (3) humanization as an independent variable, and (4) policy questions and change strategies.

DEFINITION AND IMPORTANCE OF HUMANIZATION.   What do we mean by humanization of health care? Is it roughly equivalent to patient satis-faction? Should we use a definition that permits us to judge a health system to be "dehumanized" even though patients may actually be happy with it? Has our health system, in fact, become more dehumanized, as many assert? How do we know? Despite the laudable elaboration of the concept of humanization by Dr. Howard and other contributors, from a research point of view there is still considerable need to define the concept operationally and, even more, to develop appropriate indicators. It is necessary to ascertain whether some of the indicators are redundant, measuring essentially the same phenomenon. We must also learn whether some of the dimensions of humanization are more highly prized than others. For example, if people could be assured that they were receiving excellent technical care, which is readily available and dispensed, with minimal pain and discomfort, would they be able to tolerate such unpleasant features as impersonality, a sterile and antiseptic environment, a lack of tender loving care, and other features usually regarded as evidence of the dehumanization of health care?

How salient and important, then, are different dimensions of humanization in the minds of patients? Are its components as meaningful and important to patients and to the general public as they are to the writers and academicians who have elaborated the concept? Whether we construct our own paper and pencil tests or observe real life situations in which health care is rendered, how much *reliability* is there in different people's ratings of the various dimensions of humanization?

These questions become even more interesting when we ask how salient and how important different aspects of humanized health care are for different segments of the population who vary by age, sex, social class, ethnicity, and type of illness. Would older people, who tend to be more bored, isolated, and physically vulnerable, show a greater preference for the kind of health professional who spends time with them, considers their individual needs, and dispenses tender loving care?

Are young, upwardly mobile, middle-class persons—people in a hurry —more likely to accept, indeed welcome, certain aspects of *impersonal* health care: speed, precision, and predictability? Are the less educated so overwhelmed by the mystique and uncertainty of the illness experience that they are especially appreciative when they receive benevolent and humane care? Or, has this group been so numbed by life experiences in general, and exposure to the service system in particular, that they are almost inured to the assaults and indignities of a dehumanized health-care system?

And is the type of illness, as well as its severity, related to variations in the preference for different aspects of humanized health care? While some writers make a very good case for the position that illness *per se* entails dehumanization, it would appear that some types of illness, as well as certain stages of the same illness, would make the patient yearn for more humanized care. It would be worth learning, for example, whether patients with an undiagnosed internal ailment are especially attuned to the need for humanized care, whereas those with more simple and routine problems may be less concerned with humanization. To what extent do the needs of the patient vary as we move from diagnosis to surgery to rehabilitation?

HUMANIZATION AS A DEPENDENT VARIABLE. What factors are presumed to promote humanistic care among health practitioners? In recent years, a number of deans and medical school faculty members have alleged that, more than brilliant minds, they are seeking candidates who "really care about people" and "want to take care of patients." What, in fact, is the relationship between such characteristics as the background, values, interests, and even the ideology of entering health science students and their subsequent behavior as health professionals? If a student scores high on altruism, is he or she more likely to manifest a sensitive and sympathetic orientation toward patients?

Some proponents of change seek to achieve a more humanized health system by utilizing the socializing climate and influence of the professional school. Others emphasize the overwhelming importance of the context in which one works or practices: the incentive system to which one is oriented, the organization of the health setting, and the attitudes and behavior of significant others within the health environment. How is the practice of care affected by each of these critical variables: the characteristics of the health professional, the socialization milieu of the educational institution, and the structure of the work environment? This question has important policy implications, but is most difficult to answer, for these three major factors contain a host of subvariables.

It is easy to overlook the crude but powerful role of the time factor and patient load to which Mechanic alludes in his Introduction. What is, in fact, the relation between the amount of uninterrupted time a health practitioner, or a health team, can spend with the patient, and other indices of humanization of care? Take the best health practitioner or health team one can imagine. Gradually increase patient load and monitor and document the changes that occur in the various humanization indicators. One need not be a Solomon to predict the general direction of findings, but the specific variations that emerge among different types of health practitioners may prove to be interesting, and also enlightening with respect to other questions:

1. Which health techniques and procedures can be streamlined and accelerated without accompanying feelings of dehumanization on the part of the patient?

2. How effective are varying arrangements and modes of allocating and deploying personnel as a means of meeting heavy patient loads? For example, do patients feel "dehumanized" if the nurse instead of the physician provides the health instruction? If the physician's assistant instead of the orthopedist applies the plaster cast? If the dental assistant instead of the dentist inserts the filling or inlay? How can these alternate modes of care be made compatible with patient needs and expectations? Is it true, as has been alleged, that humanized services to patients are positively associated with humanized relationships among health personnel?

It would also be useful to explore and study alternative modes of reimbursing health professionals to encourage them to spend more time with their patients, answer their questions, and provide appropriate health instruction. Nowadays, few internists have any incentive, aside from altruism or dedication, to devote more time to patients.

HUMANIZATION AS AN INDEPENDENT VARIABLE.   Hardly anyone can question the principle of humanized health care—for those who wish it, at least—but, aside from its intrinsic value and the satisfaction it gives patients, how is it related to other health goals we embrace? For example, does humanization of care reduce morbidity and mortality? Here, of course, relevant intervening variables would also be of interest. Patients who are exposed to a more humanized health experience may for that reason be more likely to engage in appropriate self-care and health promotion, to seek professional help when it is indicated, to raise and discuss problems and complaints with their therapists, and to comply with the medical regimens prescribed for them.

Leventhal's imaginative experiment suggests that when proper psychological orientation is given to patients, their distress may be reduced, and they are more likely to comply with recommended actions. Other research findings plus common experiences also indicate that different components of humanized health experiences have happy and salutary outcomes. But I believe it important to delineate and document carefully the relative contribution of each of the components of humanization to each of the desired outcomes and to designate the respective acts that are entailed in the humanizing process.

POLICY ISSUES AND CHANGE STRATEGIES. It has been suggested that to fulfill the various canons of humanization outlined in Dr. Howard's paper and to construct the kind of humane health-care system that is projected would be very time consuming and, hence, very costly. Clearly, responding to a patient as a dignified person instead of a passive object or thing would appear to take more time. But are all the steps toward more humanized care more time consuming and more costly? This is a matter for research. Are there alternative arrangements that could equally achieve humanistic goals but that would vary by time, cost, and modes of utilizing and deploying personnel? It may well be that a number of major features of humanization can be achieved with relatively little time and cost. Furthermore, even if there are considerable immediate costs, these may be minimal when the long-range beneficial consequences (such as avoidance of absenteeism and unnecessary hospitalization) are reckoned.

But what if the costs of creating a humanized health-care system do prove to be conspicuously high and, except for the fact that it is preferred by recipients, other reasonable benefits cannot be readily identified? Suppose we think of humanization as a continuum, with each additional increment requiring an additional expenditure of resources. Assuming that patients are assured that the technical quality of care will be rendered satisfactorily, how much will they be willing to pay for each additional improvement in the degree of humanization? Unpalatable as it may be to pose questions in these terms, it would be worth knowing how many Americans would choose the added increment of having the same personal physician who continually provides care, as opposed, for example, to having a full tank of gas for their cars or partial college tuition for their children.

Many of the issues discussed in this book raise the fundamental question of whether we can really be successful in effecting organizational change. But among the key obstacles to realizing proposed changes are the health organizations and the health professionals who enjoy considerable control over them. Can we be optimistic about the possibility of achieving these changes if professionals perceive them as threatening to their status, to their culture, to the prerogatives they enjoy, or to the resources they command? As long as any change is interpreted as threatening to professionals in power, it may be blocked, diverted, or rendered innocuous. For example, there is good reason to believe that the introduction of new careerists into the health system has been opposed because professionals with vested interests view these new workers as threats to their habits and cultures.

We know too that there are limits to the inroads that can be achieved on the organizational level without simultaneously achieving necessary changes in legislation on the state or national level. Here, also, new health careerists are a case in point. Can they become a permanent feature of the health organization system unless they are licensed by the state legislature and legitimized by relevant professional or accrediting bodies? Although a specific health organization may recognize the role and career pattern of new careerists, they will not become an institutionalized part of the health system unless appropriate measures are taken in the larger social environment.

Discussions of organizational change tend to be blurred or obscured because we often are vague in specifying and delineating some of the principal components of the dynamic phenomenon. It may be useful to conceptualize the change input in terms of the degree to which it represents a departure from the established habits and culture of health professionals. Some changes or innovations that are perceived as entailing no disruption or dislocation may be readily embraced by health professionals, while those that appear to be at variance with the culture of health professionals will be resisted.

The critical problem that confronts health administrators who are trying to humanize their organization system is how to construct ideal nonzero sum situations so that the projected changes are viewed as rewarding to everyone and, in fact, are. How do we establish a reward system for health personnel so that the kinds of changes we wish to inaugurate benefit the principal actors in the drama? It would appear worthwhile to explore this question as fully as possible, though we may actually find that some proposed improvements are only amenable to zero sum strategies.

It is also necessary for us to engage in the much needed exercise of critically examining and explicating the causal models underlying various change efforts and strategies for humanizing health systems. As we review previous efforts (or were they gestures?) at altering health institutions, they appear to have been dictated more by wishful thinking than by a clear model of planned social change. What mode of reasoning could have led us to believe that education and demonstration projects would effect important changes in the health system? Or that such endeavors as Regional Medical Programs and Comprehensive Health Planning (which were supported by so little leverage) could have any appreciable impact on the organization and delivery of health services? Or that planning bodies and coordinating agencies engaging in rationalistic exercises, but with no power to implement policy, would serve to reorganize the health system?

Of course, there are times when a relatively simple strategy such as merely conveying new information through research reports or demonstration projects, may be effective. But this tends to hold when there is a high degree of consensus among organizational participants, in the first place, or where the new information is consonant with existing practices or proclivities. What types of strategies are more effective when the organization is not characterized by consensus and when the desired change represents a departure from ongoing practices and orientations?

On the other side of the spectrum of approaches to change are those involving the use of power or coercion by significant population segments and forces that exert pressure on the organization.[1] Indeed, in some cases, these strategies may involve a threat to the integrity or survival of the organization. Toward the middle of the strategy spectrum is one to which I am strongly committed (though each approach has its unique function or advantage): the strategy of changing or restructuring the reward system.

Professionals and other organizational participants are as well motivated as other people, but there is a limit to which they can engage in the "right" behavior (e.g., humanistic behavior) unless such actions are consistent with the reward system in which they work. It does not help to cajole or plead with an internist to spend more time with a patient, when insurance companies do not acknowledge health education or psychological assurance as services to be reimbursed. The task before us, it would seem, is to create those conditions, those sets of rewards, that would make normal and natural the kind of behavior we are trying to promote.

Before we allocate major national resources in trying to produce a more humanized system of health care, we should have outlined in some detail a model of change that is based on empirical data. If we want to make our health system more humanized, we should be reasonably sure that our modes of intervention are really strategic. Should we focus on the would-be health professionals? The schools? The methods of reimbursement? The system of accountability? All of these? Why?

Few social objectives are more consonant with some of our most cherished values than is the humanization of health care. It would help us progress toward our goal if we could answer some key research questions and develop a strategy that is not based on impulse or fashion but on knowledge, experience, and a logical causal model of intervention.

NOTES

1. R. Chin and K. D. Benne. "General Strategies for Effecting Changes in Human Systems." In *The Planning of Change*, edited by W. G. Bennis, K. D. Benne, and R. Chin. New York: Holt, Rinehart and Winston, 1969, pp. 32-59.

CHAPTER EIGHTEEN

AN ARCHITECT'S PERSPECTIVE

ROSLYN LINDHEIM, A.I.A.

Buildings reflect the basic values of a society. It is possible to reconstruct from its architecture the nature of an institution and the priorities held by its decision makers. Architecture has been referred to as "frozen music." We might also call it "frozen ideology." The man-made environment mirrors our values without platitudes or rationalizations. These values show themselves in the relative size and scale of buildings, in the organization of spaces, in the relationship of parts to the whole, and in the location and interrelationship of the segments.

Similarly, values are reflected in the environments we provide for medical care. If we say that it is important to encourage early diagnosis, preventive medicine, and readily accessible ambulatory care, and then design giant centralized medical centers far from where people live and work, the facts contradict the words. If we talk about the need to personalize care and then design medical centers that are so large and impersonal they defy human scale, we are operating under a different set of priorities from those we profess.

No building complex in the city today is as large or as costly as the modern medical center. Its very size and monumental form symbolize power and the dominant role modern medicine plays in our lives. On a national scale, the health sector accounts for 7.6 percent of the gross national product. Hospitals are a major consumer of the health-care

293

dollar: more than 40 percent goes into their construction and operation.[1]

Since World War II technological medicine has come into its own. We are proud of the miracles of modern medicine—heart transplants, cobalt machines, kidney dialysis, intensive care units, coronary care—as well as of the new medical marvels to come. Laboratory and X ray have replaced the doctor's handbag as ordinary medical tools. The doctors themselves have clustered their offices around the technological hub of the hospital, forming larger and larger medical complexes.

Parallel with this increase in the role of technological medicine is the increase in medical domination over many functions of society previously controlled by the church, the state, the family, and the individual. The natural processes of birth and death are treated as illnesses and located in the hospital setting under the control of the physician. In many cases, fitness to work is certified by a medical examination; a psychiatric patient may be totally banished from society by a psychiatrist. Drug addiction and alcoholism are now labeled medical diseases, and treatment is in the hands of the medical profession. Doctors have taken over some of the functions of the religious clergy, such as rites of passage; and they use similar trappings: white coats, Latin terminology.

The dominant role of modern medicine in our society is partly maintained by professionalism. "In health above all, but also in law, education, welfare, and to a degree religion, the market is restricted to that which is licensed, certified, accredited, or otherwise officially approved, and control over the definition of services is held by those who control the *production* of services rather than those who consume them."[2] The buyer or patient is at the mercy of the medical institution or seller. This in itself is dehumanizing.

Thus medical dominance over much of our lives is possible because of our belief in the power of medical technology. Most patients, and most doctors, are convinced that industrial populations owe their high health standards to scientific medicine. They believe that such technology as currently exists is largely effective in coping with the tasks it faces and that it offers great promise for the future. The engineering approach to the improvement of health has become a dominant force in our lives, enforcing its own rules: professionalism, bureaucracy, and standardization.

A fundamental contradiction exists between technological medicine as it is practiced in modern medical centers and our ability to render personalized care to the individual. We have been trapped into becoming slaves of this technology rather than mastering it for our own benefit. Paradoxically, the achievements of modern technology have created their own Frankenstein. The therapeutic techniques developed to prolong life can cause incredible suffering by keeping people "alive" in name only, when there is no hope for their recovery. And many medical advances designed to cure illness actually cause illness.

To be effective, highly developed medical technology requires standardization, professionalism, and economy of operation. From the technological point of view, the less participation on the patient's part, the better. Yet we know intuitively that a most imporant and little-understood ingredient for patient recovery is patient participation and will to get better. This contradiction is reflected in design requirements for medical facilities. The need for sterile environments, efficient utilization of highly trained personnel, and meticulous coordination of people and machines conflicts with the human need for reassurance, sympathy, comfort, and contact with people who really care.

Doctors and administrators commonly specify that medical centers be centralized and efficient—and hopefully "homelike" as well. They assume that a humane environment can be achcieved by painting walls, carpeting floors, and arranging chairs in groups instead of rows. I take issue with the "cosmetic approach" to humanization. I do not want to minimize the value of superficial amenities, but it is like applying visual placebos to root out cancer.

It is possible for personalized medical care to take place in miserable settings, but it requires a tremendous expenditure of additional energy to overcome the environment. Conversely, impersonal medical care can occur in attractive new buildings. A building has no power to humanize or dehumanize care; it is a reinforcing system within which activities take place—in an easier, more pleasant, and more humane manner—or the reverse.

To develop viable alternatives, the term "design" must be interpreted to have a broader meaning than simply physical design. According to Webster, design is the "deliberate purposeful planning [of a] settled coherent program [for] selecting the means and contriving the elements, steps, and procedures [that] will adequately satisfy some need."[3] The humanization of the environment of the future will depend largely on who makes what "design" decisions now, to satisfy what needs.

A key question concerns where we want to put our resources—even our research resources. Do we want to put our money into the design of larger centralized medical centers, into smaller decentralized neighborhood centers, in people, in training—where? Decisions such as these will drastically affect the type of facility we build and will determine what we mean by humanized medical care.

The San Francisco Chronicle recently reported the projected construction of a 105 million dollar hospital to be built at Travis Air Force Base, California. This new structure is described as "an enormous new generation hospital . . . [that will] serve as a model and as an experiment into the 21st century."[4] It is my hope that before we build more of these giant medical centers we pose some alternatives. Research is needed to answer the following questions:

1. How can we demystify commonly held myths about medical technology and objectively appraise its costs and benefits?
2. What approaches will resolve the conflict between the requirements of technological medicine and the needs of human beings?
3. How might we develop alternative choices outside of the hospital for the natural processes of life—birth and death?

DEMYSTIFYING MYTHS AND APPRAISING COSTS AND BENEFITS.   Despite all its complex technology, the hospital as it is presently constituted is not a viable institution for the relief of human suffering. There are strong indications that many people who are there do not belong in the hospital, that many people cannot be cured by modern technology, and, in fact, that the technology itself can create illness. Moreover, our faith in technological medicine actually prevents us from focusing on those other aspects of health that might do far more than medicine to effect our well-being.

Florence Nightingale began her *Notes on Hospitals* with the following words:

> It may seem a strange principle to enunciate as the very first requirement in a Hospital that it should do the sick no harm. It is quite necessary, nevertheless, to lay down such a principle, because the actual mortality *in* hospitals, especially in those of large crowded cities, is very much higher than any calculation founded on the mortality of the same class of diseases among patients treated *out of* hospital would lead us to expect.[5]

Perhaps we must again enunciate the "no harm" principle as the first requirement in the total design of our health systems.

There is evidence that hospitals often do real harm. It has been shown that 20 percent of patients admitted to hospitals acquire a iatrogenic disease during their stay.[6] Most of these patients are victims of hospital mistakes in administering drugs or of adverse complications from diagnostic and therapeutic procedures. The wide array of articles on iatrogenic disease in *Index Medicus* for the years 1967 to 1973 is alarming.[7] Unnecessary surgery (hysterectomies, ovarectomies, tonsillectomies) is also a source of concern.

Although Americans spent an estimated $94 billion on health care in 1973,[8] there is substantial evidence that for many of them, particularly the poor and ghetto dwellers, the existing system is inefficient, unduly expensive, and plagued by unequal distribution and utilization of medical manpower. Furthermore, the system cannot adequately cope with institutional cost structures and user expectations in today's society.

We are spending a great deal of money and energy on the construction and maintenance of our giant medical centers, yet more and more people are questioning their validity. René Dubos writes that "the extent of health improvement that ensues from building ultramodern hospitals with up-to-date equipment, is probably trivial in comparison with the results that can be achieved at much lower cost by providing all infants and children with well-balanced food, sanitary conditions, and a stimulating environment."[9] It should also be noted that the enthusiasm associated with current developments in medical technology contrasts with the reality of decreasing returns to health for rapidly increasing efforts. In the past two decades, when scientific medicine is alleged to have blossomed, its effect on health has been minimal.

According to Charles Steward, "the high costs of medical treatment, combined with their low correlation with life expectancy, do suggest that treatment is a relatively poor investment."[10] In the United States, life expectancy at birth increased 20 years between 1900 and 1950, but since 1950 it has increased only 2 years more. We are bewitched by the myth of modern medicine—and now it appears that the reality of the situation is quite different from the myth.

I have raised the issues of iatrogenic diseases, the dangers of hospitalization, and some of the myths of modern medicine because it is assumed that people get "cured" in hospitals and by doctors. Many do, but there are risks in going to hospitals, risks in taking drugs, risks even in diagnostic procedures. Those who raise questions about the hazards of hospitals and pose alternative environments for care are labeled "romanticists." It is even more "romantic" to be unaware of some of the hazards of hospitals, drugs, and medicine. We urgently need research and clarity concerning the myth versus reality of modern technological medicine. Otherwise, we may misdirect our health resources into the wrong channels.

RESOLVING THE CONFLICT BETWEEN TECHNOLOGICAL MEDICINE AND HUMAN NEEDS. As an architect and consultant, I have been involved in the planning or design of many types of health facilities: a large county hospital, private hospitals including one for children, neighborhood health centers, medical office buildings including group practices, and private doctors' offices. I have worked with patients, doctors, nurses, technicians, and administrators who were truly concerned about humanizing facilities. Yet despite well-meaning efforts by everyone, all of these settings for the delivery of care reinforced dehumanized treatment to some degree.

Even those institutions that gave lip service to community participation and primary care did not develop the kinds of places that people could relate to in a human way. I believe that unconsciously all medical facilities are influenced by the hospital model, particularly by its narrowly interpreted criteria of economy, efficiency, and productivity. Doctors, nurses, technicians, and even patients accept—and do not question—the hospital model, because they respect the technological capability of the hospital. Yet the very logic of this model demands standardization of people and activities.

In his book *Asylums*,[11] Erving Goffman refers to certain establishments as total institutions, and notes that administration of the inhabitants in total institutions is geared to standardization of all of the individual's activities, from the most intimate to the most social ones. This standardization is not necessarily due to deliberate intent but is made necessary by the very real need for utilization of administrative time, energy, and resources.

The physical structure of the hospital, as well as of clinics and private offices, reinforces this standardization. By making everything the same— the nursing units, nursing stations, examination and treatment rooms, corridors—one bed becomes like another, and people cease to be individuals. Even attempts to bring a little variation to the rooms by differences in colors, sheets, spreads, and furniture are defeated by institutional dictates of laundry economy and uniformity of purchasing.

We know that patients need comfort and care, both as tools for curing and as supports when cure is impossible. Yet in the design process—more specifically, in the cost-cutting process—the first things to go are patient amenities. Priority is always given to architectural paradigms designed to render the hospital efficient and flexible. In most new hospitals entire floors devoted to mechanical and medical equipment are located between every two nursing floors. This new structural/mechanical remedy, called "interstitial space," is prescribed by hospital planners to achieve flexibility. It allows easy change in the mechanical system without disrupting the entire structure. But flexibility comes at a very high price. Mechanical services alone take up about 60 percent of the floor space and cost of hospitals.

When I was first involved in hospital design, we figured their cost at $20,000 per bed; rough estimates now range from $70,000 to $80,000 per bed.[12] In 1950, care in a large urban hospital cost a patient $15 per day; it has risen to $100 per day—$300 for intensive care. By 1980, according to estimates, the cost of a bed in a major urban hospital will rise to $1,000 per day.[13]

The high cost of medical technology has made space so expensive that it cannot be "wasted" on mothers, fathers, husbands, and friends. In a study of children in hospitals, we showed that many of them, particularly the younger ones, experienced ill effects from being hospitalized. In reacting to institutionalism, children manifest retardation, worsening medical conditions, reversal to infantile practices, and so forth, and often must be sent home to recover before they can be treated.[14] Children need their parents with them in order to get well. Similarly, women delivering babies need their husbands, and the sick, the lonely, and the old need family and friends.

In a highly mechanized environment where costs are so high, another way to save money is by using so-called "replaceable" personnel: orderlies, clean-up people, and practical nurses. By degrading their jobs, we exclude them from participation in the therapeutic environment, when in fact they may be the staff most able to relate to the patient in a humane way because of similar ethnic backgrounds or socioeconomic status.

The "thinging" phenomenon referred to by Jan Howard[15] is reflected in the design fo highly technological areas of the hospital, such as intensive care, coronary care, and recovery rooms. Until a few years ago when it was pronounced illegal, these areas had no windows—rationalized on the grounds that the patients were too far gone to notice, and efficiency was the first priority. No one mentioned the needs of the staff, the needs of family and friends, or the sensitivity of patients, even when they are extremely ill or semiconscious.

I have concentrated primarily on dehumanization as it affects bed patients. Ambulatory facilities, too, are dehumanizing, particularly for the urban poor. Until OEO neighborhood health centers and free clinics were established during the 1960s, which together account for a small percentage of all primary physician visits, the urban poor received their medicine in outpatient departments and emergency rooms of large city hospitals, built like fortresses. The images of long waiting lines, rows of chairs, dismal surroundings, and police officers everywhere have been well documented. It is no wonder that the poor go to these places only in times of crisis and believe, particularly if it is a teaching hospital, that they are being used as guinea pigs. Those who are frightened by the overbearing size and impersonal treatment become twice dehumanized— by the nature of the place and by their lack of choice as to where to seek treatment.

Despite these conditions, I have heard the academic staff in such hospitals talk proudly of the quality of care that their patients were receiving. It is only relatively recently that there has been medical recognition of the importance of a patient's emotional state to his or her physical recovery. It is necessary to carefully research the many factors that affect a patient's well-being. The same setting can have very different connotations to different people, depending on the age, bias, background, and perceptions of the user. There is no single best environment. Instead, we must research a variety of different environments to determine the best fits for the diverse needs of people. The notion of diverse solutions is in opposition to the trend toward universality of hospital and clinic design.

DEVELOPING CHOICES OUTSIDE THE HOSPITAL FOR THE NATURAL PROCESSES OF LIFE. The natural processes of life—birth and death—are treated as sicknesses in our society. We use expensive facilities to house these functions, which in most cases do not belong in the hospital but at home or in a homelike setting close to home. Having a baby is not an illness, and most pregnant women do not need to be looked on as patients in a hospital. The United States is one of the few countries in the world where most babies are born in sterile white delivery rooms, located in wings virtually interchangeable with their medical and surgical counterparts.

There is increasing reason to believe that today many aspects of medical obstetrical practices do not fit with the needs and expectations of significant numbers of individuals. Despite our advanced birth technology, many couples are deliberately bypassing or trying to change their relationship with the physician and other trained obstetrical personnel. "Natural childbirth" organizations are teaching women techniques that are often in conflict with the dependency-oriented practices of most obstetrical services. Fathers are insisting on being participants in all aspects of the labor and delivery process. An increasing number of women demand to return home immediately after delivery, with or without official sanction from the obstetrician or pediatrician. Further along the spectrum are the "hippie" communes where members often spurn the simplest medical amenities during childbirth. Ten years ago these and similar practices such as home delivery began to attract a small, rebellious, and alienated clientele. Today, their adherents are to be found in more impressive numbers.

Lower economic and minority groups are also alienated from mainstream medical systems, including obstetrical services. Prenatal care and ancillary training and service programs are poorly utilized by this group. There are deep-seated resistances to the place, form, and context of the care offered in prenatal clinics and labor and delivery rooms. Underuse of available facilities is due partially to their location, distant from the user's home, and to the hostile environment to be found there.

As a result, many women arrive at the hospital for the first time late in labor. That their health care suffers is clearly reflected in the high maternal and infant mortality and morbidity rates for this group. Research is needed on how to identify high-risk birth cases that can benefit from medical technology. Birth environments outside of hospitals should also be studied to determine their potential as settings for more humane care.

As with birth, so with death. It, too, is treated as an illness. Everybody dies—death is an integral part of life—but in the United States, half of us die in hospitals where death is treated impersonally as a routine matter. "Hegemony in the affairs of death has been transferred from the church to science and its representatives, the medical profession and the rationally organized hospital."[16] The very society that has so controlled death has made it more difficult to die with dignity. America's way of life insulates us from death and dying. In *The Psychology of Death*, Robert Kastenbaum and Ruth Aisenberg describe how illness and death are removed from household management and how even within hospital walls, the patient is not supposed to die in just any place at any time. It is deemed important that the survivors (other patients, staff, visitors) not be exposed to the phenomenon of death except under carefully specified circumstances. The staff is angry when death occurs in the wrong place.[17] The isolation of death from the natural processes of life has a drastic effect on the way we design our hospitals. The morgue is always located so the body can be sneaked away without being seen by patients or visitors. Isolation rooms—which are really dying rooms—hide death from the rest of the patients; yet they generally know where the room is, and what it is for.[18]

In his article "Death and Social Structure," Robert Blauner writes that "in premodern societies, many deaths take place amid the hubbub of life, in the central social territory of the tribe, clan, or other familial group."[19] Ivan Illich has written a brilliant article, "The Political Uses of Natural Death," in which he shows how the ritual nature of modern health procedures hides from doctors and patients the contradiction between the ideal of a natural death and the reality of the clinical death where most contemporary lives actually end.[20] Our vulnerability in the face of death, and its physical location away from where we live our lives, has stripped us of our ability to deal with it in a dignified manner, as a natural process of life.

The physical implications are difficult to formulate, but once again our homes must accommodate dying as a part of life. Death at home must be recognized, as well as death in other less technological and more humane places. If dying occurs in institutions outside the home that are only associated with the old and sick, then these institutions, including the hospital, will be viewed as death houses, no matter what their other functions might be.

CONCLUSION.   Much research is needed, particularly as we are on the threshold of a national health-care system. Will the highest priorities be given to cost effectiveness as seen by the insurance companies, or will the health needs of the people, with all their diversity, be met and resolved with their participation? Before we commit ourselves to one pattern of medical intervention, it is necessary to examine the whole system. By concentrating only on the technical mastery of disease we may lose sight of more fundamental questions affecting health, such as how to change our life styles and habits.

Paradoxically, although it is technically possible and economically necessary to decentralize medical care, this choice is not really feasible because of poor housing and poverty in people's homes, the reluctance of physicians to make house calls, and lack of available ambulant services. Thus, if we are to practice the humanization we preach, we cannot reduce the minimal health care facilities that are now available until other alternatives are implemented.

I have attempted to deal with some of the contradictions inherent in our medical system and reflected in most glaring form in our large urban medical centers. Beliefs in the power of medical technology versus the real consequences of this technology; the space priorities for machines versus the space needs of people; the natural processes of life—birth and death—versus their treatment as diseases; standardization of procedures versus the need for individualism; professional domination versus personal initiative. These contradictions—and many more—require the urgent attention of researchers from all disciplines. In working out the answers to these dilemmas, the foundation for more humane environments can be developed.

NOTES

1. A. R. Somers. *Health Care in Transition: Directions for the Future*. Chicago: Hospital Research and Educational Trust, 1971, p. 31.

2. E. Freidson. *Professional Dominance: The Social Structure of Medical Care*. New York: Atherton, 1970, p. 169.

3. *Webster's Third New International Dictionary*. Springfield: G. & C. Merriam, 1965.

4. N. Melnick. "$105 Million Hospital to be Built at Travis AFB." *The San Francisco Chronicle*, January 20, 1974, Sec. A, p. 3.

5. F. Nightingale. *Notes on Hospitals*. 3d ed. London: Longman Green, 1863, preface.

6. H. N. Beaty and R. G. Petersdorf. "Iatrogenic Factors in Infectious Disease." *Ann Intern Med*, vol. 65, October 1966, p. 641.

7. R. H. Moser, ed. *Diseases of Medical Progress: A Study of Iatrogenic Disease*. 3d ed. Springfield, Ill.: Charles C Thomas, 1969. J. C. Doyle. "Unnecessary Hyster-

ectomies." *JAMA*, vol. 151, January 31, 1953, pp. 360-365. J. C. Doyle. "Unnecessary Ovarectomies." *JAMA*, vol. 148, March 29, 1952, pp. 1105-1111.

8. B. S. Cooper, N. L. Worthington, and P. A. Piro. "National Health Expenditures, 1929-1973." *Soc Secur Bull*, vol. 37, February 1974, pp. 3-19, 48.

9. R. Dubos. "Man and His Environment: Biomedical Knowledge and Social Action." From a series of PAHO/WHO Scientific Lectures, presented September 29, 1965, published as *Scientific Publication No. 131*, Pan American Health Organization, March 1966, p. 10.

10. C. T. Stewart, Jr. "Allocation of Resources to Health." *J Hum Resour*, vol. 6, Winter 1971, pp. 103-122.

11. E. Goffman. *Asylums*. Garden City, N.Y.: Doubleday Anchor Books, 1961.

12. R. Kotelchuck. "How to Build a Hospital." *Health/PAC Bull*, vol. 41, May 1972, p. 3.

13. A. R. Somers. *Op. cit.*, p. 33.

14. R. Lindheim, H. Glazer, and C. Coffin. *Changing Hospital Environments for Children*. Cambridge: Harvard University Press, 1972.

15. See Jan Howard. "Humanization and Dehumanization of Health Care: A Conceptual View," in this book.

16. R. Blauner. "Death and Social Structure." In *Life Cycle and Achievement in America*, edited by R. L. Coser. New York: Harper Torchbooks, 1969.

17. R. Kastenbaum and R. Aisenberg. *The Psychology of Death*. New York: Springer, 1972.

18. Death in the modern hospital is the subject of sociological studies by Sudnow, who focuses on the handling of death and the dead in a county hospital catering to charity patients, and by Glaser and Strauss, who concentrate on the dying situation in a number of hospitals of varying status. D. N. Sudnow. "Passing On: The Social Organization of Dying in the County Hospital." Unpublished doctoral dissertation, University of California, Berkeley, 1965. B. G. Glaser and A. L. Strauss. "Temporal Aspects of Dying as a Non-Scheduled Status Passage." In *Middle Age and Aging: A Reader in Social Psychology*, edited by B. L. Neugarten. Chicago: University of Chicago Press, 1968.

19. R. Blauner. *Op. cit.*, p. 238.

20. I. Illich. *Alternative: Health Care*. Cuernavaca: Centro Intercultural de Documentacion, 1973. (APDO 479, Cuernavaca, Mexico.)

EPILOGUE

Humanizing Health Care Through National Health Insurance

PHILIP R. LEE, M.D.

National health insurance provides an excellent framework to consider many of the issues discussed in this book. The difficulty in determining what kind of national health insurance will best serve the country illustrates the problem of applying the concepts of humanization in terms of a practical public policy.

This problem was outlined by Professor Mechanic when he defined one of the purposes of the Symposium as:

> an attempt to develop more carefully the assumptions and ethical bases of medicine as a humane social institution, and to consider the implications of these assumptions and perspectives for policy as this nation looks toward national health insurance.

To consider the "assumptions and ethical bases of medicine as a humane social institution" within the context of national health insurance is difficult because the subject is so complex.

Philip R. Lee is director of the Health Policy Program and professor of social medicine at the University of California in San Francisco. He was formerly Assistant Secretary for Health and Scientific Affairs in the U.S. Department of Health, Education, and Welfare and later Chancellor of UCSF.

As an instrument of public policy, national health insurance has the
potential for articulating the goals of our health-care system. But are we
clear about those goals? Have we defined what our national effort is all
about? Will the nation, through national health insurance, attempt to
maintain the status quo, or will it attempt to make it possible for Americans to have a health-care system that is available to all, accessible to
all, where cost is not too high, and where service is provided in a humanized manner?

There has been growing recognition of the need for all people to be
covered by health insurance. There has been less recognition of health
care as a right. In the debate on national health insurance little attention
has been paid to the question of the right to health care or to such issues
as social justice and equity. It is precisely because these issues are so big
and difficult to grasp that they are often ignored.

It is my thesis in this epilogue that an adequate health-care system
would be based on a strong foundation of social justice and individual
rights, which would result in a resolution of the problems of access, availability, and reasonable cost. The basic foundation, once built, would
allow a clear focus on humanization of care. My premise is that health
care will never be truly humanized unless social justice and individual
rights are recognized and fulfilled.

Dr. Howard provides a clear analysis of the philosophical dimensions
of humanization in her article, "Humanization and Dehumanization of
Health Care: A Conceptual View." At the heart of humanization is our
image of man, how we value man and how we treat the individual. It
can be described most succinctly as recognition of the inherent worth of
the individual. Dehumanization, then, is unequal recognition of the
inherent worth of the individual.

The relationship of the philosophical concepts of justice and rights to
practical problems in the delivery of health care and in physician-patient
interactions is not always, nor even often, evident. This has been considered by Jonsen and Hellegers in relation to the moral problems of
medicine. In their view many of these problems are problems of justice.
In discussing justice, they note:

> The traditional definition of justice is "giving to each his due." The problem
> of justice is defining what is "due" to each. This is done, first by recognizing
> that the "each" of the definition is both everyman, with a basic humanness
> shared by all, and this single person, different in ability, merit and need

from all others. Justice thus requires an impartiality resting on the fundamental similarity of all persons and an equity which allows for different
treatment justified by different conditions of ability and merit.[1]

In other words, in relation to medicine, justice involves a just distribution of medical care.

Like justice, rights are key to any discussion of humanization. There
are two distinguishable meanings of "rights," and they are relevant to a
consideration of the right to health and the right to health care. The
right of an individual to health may be called a fundamental right. It
expresses the profound truth that a person's autonomy and freedom rest
upon his or her ability to function physically and psychologically. It
asserts that no other person can, with moral justification, deprive that
person of that ability. The fundamental right to health is justified by
inspecting the very nature of human beings. To the extent that "being
healthy" lies within human power, it is clear that being healthy is a
precondition for being free and autonomous.

The right to health care, on the other hand, is a "consequent or qualified right." It is directly implied by the fundamental right, and it is
implemented by individuals in institutions and practices only when such
is possible and reasonable and only when other rights are not thereby
infringed. The right to health care can be justified only after inspecting
the actual conditions of society and of medicine. A consequent or qualified right is justified when it becomes evident that the benefits and bur-
dens of a society are unfairly distributed. Unfair distribution means
distribution whereby some benefit, while others are deprived.

Where does humanization fit into this picture? It is important to recognize that it is possible to have a just system of health care—one in
which care is equitably distributed—and a system that considers individual rights, but in which at the same time the care is hurried, impersonal,
and dehumanized. Empathy cannot be legislated. It is also possible, however, to establish a health structure that has an adequate supply of services, that recognizes the worth of the individual, and that calls on people
to behave in a certain way. In short, by laying the foundation for the
individual to be seen as a person who has rights, who feels, who cares,
and who has intelligence, we can begin to realize humanized health care.

The problem then is to gain the acceptance of the idea that every
citizen has a right to *humanized* health care and to translate that concept
into specific policies. This should be the goal of national health insur-

ance. It is not an easy task. It will require that the costs be determined, that the sources of financing be identified, and that the means and manner of providing the services be delineated. It will require that ways be found to redress the present inequities in financing and delivery of health care, being careful to retain the essence of health care. It will require that other justified rights not be limited or impaired. And it is not easy to reconcile the problems of individual rights of physician and patient with the needs of society.

There are those who would argue that it is unreasonable or impossible to finance a comprehensive program of national health insurance for every citizen, particularly when many of the services provided, such as nursing home care, may bear little relationship to an individual's health. Debates rage on the equity of the various systems of financing that have been proposed as well as on the means of assuring access to and the provision of high quality care. If the goals can be clearly articulated and understood, the decisions can be made more wisely.

THE HISTORY OF FEDERAL SUPPORT FOR HEALTH-CARE PROGRAMS.   Federal support for health-care programs has long been justified on the premise that certain groups of individuals (the aged, the poor, the mentally ill) bear an unusually heavy burden of illness and do not, in fact, have access to the kind and quality of medical care required to meet their needs. A host of programs were established in an attempt to overcome the obstacles to access and to solve what was looked on as social injustice. They began in the 1920s with very small grants by the federal government to state public health departments for maternal and child health services. These programs were terminated temporarily in the late 1920s during the administration of President Hoover but were reestablished on a permanent basis with the enactment of the Social Security Act in 1935.

After gradual but steady expansion in the 1940s, 1950s, and 1960s there are now massive federal expenditures for several hundred different health programs, including those for the purchase of medical care by the aged, the poor, the permanently disabled, and individuals with end-stage renal disease who require kidney dialysis or transplantation.

Other groups felt to be in special need (native Americans, Alaska natives) or to merit special status because of their contributions (members of the armed forces, veterans with service-connected disabilities, merchant seamen) were provided medical care directly by the federal government.

In the past decade the federal government has adopted policies based on four different concepts: (1) the need of the individual (Medicaid for the poor), (2) merit or societal contributions (Medicare for Social Security beneficiaries and expanded medical care benefits for veterans), (3) similar treatment for similar cases (kidney dialysis and transplants for patients with end-stage renal disease), and (4) private health insurance as an appropriate means to meet the health-care needs of the majority of the people. None of these has emerged as the most dominant in terms of national health insurance. All are likely to be incorporated to some degree in the plan that is adopted.

Experience with these programs has made it clear that assuring equal financial access to medical care does not necessarily result in equal access. Racial, social, geographic, and other barriers remain. The Medicare experience, particularly, teaches us that a program that assures equal financial access will favor high-income persons, whites, and those living in areas with an abundance of physicians and other medical resources.

Equity of access to medical services requires not only the elimination of financial barriers for those in need, but the development or deployment of personnel and services to supplement any financing plan.

In public and private health insurance programs, the United States has followed a pattern that is significantly different from those of Canada, the United Kingdom, or most European countries. It has provided support through publicly financed programs for selected groups of beneficiaries (the aged, crippled children, the poor), whereas most other countries have made benefits (hospital care, physicians' services) equally available to the entire population. In Canada, for example, the approach has been to provide equal opportunity for all by eliminating financial barriers to those services that are available. Many say that the categorical and incremental approaches adopted in the United States will more quickly correct inequities in access and in the scope and quality of services made available to the poor and other people with greater need. But I believe the Canadian approach is more equitable and more rational.

Unlike the United Kingdom or Canada, a great deal of attention has been focused in the United States on the use of deductibles and co-insurance to deter overuse of services by patients. This approach is hard to reconcile with the fact that it is increasingly recognized that the physician is the one who determines utilization. The physician orders the tests, writes the prescriptions, arranges the hospitalization, carries out the surgery, and otherwise determines both utilization of services and the cost of care. The "consumer" has neither the expertise nor the ability to have much impact on this process.

NATIONAL HEALTH INSURANCE—GOALS AND ISSUES.   The debate on national health insurance has focused largely on specific legislative proposals. The emphasis has been on cost or political considerations, with little attention paid to such basic questions as:

1. What should be the relative emphasis on equity of access, scope of benefits, quality of care and cost control?
2. Should health care be regulated by the government or the private sector?

Other questions that relate to the planning of health services and the · behavior of physicians and other providers might also be considered because they concern possible paths of intervention in health care. But I focus on the two mentioned above.

Equity of Access.   Equity of access to health care and equity in the scope and quality of services available, in relation to the needs of the patient, are of particular importance to questions of distributive justice and humanization of care. Justice, through impartiality, would demand equal benefits and universal coverage. But if universal coverage of the entire population is not possible, health benefits to the individuals served and health benefits to society generally will be greatest if the poor, children, pregnant women, and women desiring family planning services are provided easy access to services without financial barriers, such as deductibles or coinsurance. Not only must the financial barriers be removed, but outreach programs must be developed in areas where services are currently inadequate. To achieve the greatest health benefits, the needed medical assistance should be provided, and stress should also be placed on measures that promote health and well-being.

Equity requires that priority be given to meeting the needs of those who bear the greatest burden of illness and providing access to those who currently lack it. National health insurance cannot do the job alone. Other programs, such as neighborhood health centers and community mental health centers with easy geographical access and outreach services, should continue to be supported directly. The National Health Service Corps, a federal program employing volunteer health professionals to meet the needs in underserved areas, should be expanded to rural and urban poverty areas. Payment mechanisms, reimbursement policies and the scope of benefits must recognize the need for these outreach services.

In some of the current national health insurance proposals, marked restrictions are placed on outpatient psychiatric services. These restrictions, combined with payment for inpatient psychiatric care, could result in excessive hospitalization of the mentally ill and a serious decline in community mental health services. Thus, the barriers to outpatient care should be removed. It is also important to provide payment for nontraditional health workers such as community health aides who may be able to contribute more to helping patients solve health-related problems than can the highly trained professionals.

Scope of Benefits. Private health insurance in the United States has placed priority on paying for high cost hospital care and the services that physicians provide in the hospital. The result has been needless hospitalization. Medicare and Medicaid slowed this trend somewhat, but unless national health insurance provides adequate coverage for ambulatory care and home care, excessive institutionalization in hospitals and nursing homes will continue. If the national health insurance proposals supported by the American Medical Association and commercial insurance companies are enacted, little would be accomplished to reverse the trend toward excessive hospital care. In contrast to these proposals, a number of others include provision for a comprehensive range of services and definite steps to expand ambulatory care.

The scope of benefits is important in assuring access and equity. There is great interest in providing universal insurance coverage for catastrophic illness because it can be devastating medically, socially, and economically. While providing coverage and equal access to care for people who suffer from illnesses associated with catastrophically high costs, catastrophic insurance could deny many others access to primary medical care and preventive services because available funds will be limited. It is also possible that manpower would be shifted to high technology services if funds are diverted to care of catastrophic illness.

For those who live in areas where needed services are not available, catastrophic illness insurance might have limited value. Patients with end-stage renal disease who are now provided health insurance coverage under Medicare have greater difficulty getting care if they live in rural areas than if they live near a hospital or medical center that provides kidney dialysis and renal transplants.

Catastrophic illness insurance could also contribute to a sharp increase in the price of services, because of increased demand and assured payment. To maximize high quality care in these situations there must be continuing review of the medical necessity of services, their quality, and their effect on people. There must also be some means of containing costs and preventing the proliferation of some services (such as coronary care units) far beyond the needs of the people served.

Quality of Care. Quality control programs and measures designed to improve the quality of care have only recently emerged as significant issues. Insofar as these measures stress the application of complex technology such as X-ray therapy, intensive care units, or automated laboratory facilities, which is often the case, health care can become further depersonalized and dehumanized. In the past, the emphasis on allocating manpower, money, and facilities for such services has tended to diminish the resources available for first-contact primary care and for preventive services. Stress on the technology required can further dehumanize care if the patient is treated as an object or an extension of the machine rather than as an individual. Unfortunately, this has too often been the experience of patients in coronary care and other units where modern technology plays such a vital role.

So far, emphasis in quality control has been placed on the technical aspects of medical care, including the appropriateness of the service provided and the utilization of resources. Congress has mandated that Professional Standards Review Organizations be responsible for this function for Medicare and Medicaid patients. This mechanism for quality control will undoubtedly be extended to whatever program of national health insurance is enacted.

To do an adequate job of peer review, physicians will need more information about the process and outcomes of care than is currently available. One of the tasks of evaluating the appropriateness of a particular service will be to determine its relevance to the caring as well as the curing function of medicine.

Better information and new systems of peer review will not necessarily change behavior and improve the quality of care. The answer will lie in the commitment and the values of health professionals and others who provide medical care. Thus, Brian Abel-Smith commented:

> The health professionals must accept their responsibility for using health resources effectively and efficiently or the immense power we currently give to the health professionals may be challenged and part of it transferred to others. This would, in my view, be the wrong solution.[2]

The Professional Standards Review Organization provides physicians with just such an opportunity and responsibility. A mechanism must also be found for other professionals involved in medical care to review its quality.

Cost Control.   Rapidly rising costs remains one of the major problems in the Medicare and Medicaid programs, and it is one of the major issues that must be dealt with in any program of national health insurance. There are several possible means of cost control:

1. Control of prices (i.e., charges for services).
2. Deductibles and copayments (requiring individual beneficiaries to share the costs at the time services are rendered).
3. Incentive reimbursement schemes, to stimulate payers and payees to find ways of curtailing costs.
4. Limitation of services provided.
5. Control of the availability of health-care resources (e.g., hospital beds, physicians).
6. A global budget for the entire program and special budgets for the various components.

Medicare has emphasized the control of prices for hospital care, surgery, office visits, and other services. Copayments and deductibles have been used as well. Incentive reimbursement schemes have been tried on an experimental basis, but have not had widespread application. In Medicaid the approach has varied from one state to another, and emphasis has been placed on control of prices and limitation on the services provided.

Cost control measures have affected physicians, patients, hospitals and other health-care institutions. Dr. Howard described the reaction of physicians and other providers to many of the restrictions that have been imposed to achieve some measure of cost control:

> Providers of care have complained bitterly about the restrictive hands of third parties such as government agencies, insurance companies, and hospital boards. They feel depersonalized by constrictions on relations with patients, colleagues, and the public; constraints on procedures and regimens deemed necessary for the patient; and the red tape and paper work that accompany third party dealings.[3]

The costs of health care continue to rise more rapidly than most other costs, and more of the increase is due to rising prices without improvements in the quality or quantity of services or increases in the number of people cared for. For these reasons, in any national health insurance program Congress will surely seek ways to constrain this rate of increase. It is likely that Congress will follow the same patterns and approaches used in Medicare and Medicaid, although these appear to have achieved very little in terms of effective control of cost increases.

Each of the methods mentioned would have an impact on the access of patients to care, the scope of benefits provided, or the quality of care provided. One approach that has not been previously attempted is to finance the program publicly and to set a limit on the total amount allocated for medical care. Funds would be distributed to regions on a per capita basis. This approach is similar to the methods used in West Germany where doctors are paid from a local sick fund established by the income of the health insurance system. If services exceed the funds available, physicians receive a reduced fee. This kind of risk sharing has also been proposed for health maintenance organizations.

Public utility regulation of the health-care industry at the state level is receiving increasing attention. Regulatory commissions might control the supply of hospital beds, hospital rates and reimbursement, and specialty services on a community and regional basis. National health insurance legislation may mandate this type of state regulatory commission. It is difficult to assess the potential consequences of such a program because efforts to date have focused on limiting the construction of new hospital beds.

Most of the national health insurance proposals have emphasized deductibles and coinsurance to deter overuse by the patient. These mechanisms, when applied in Canada, did reduce the demand for services by the poor. They had little impact on other groups, and they are no longer used. The principle reason is that the physician, not the patient, is the major determinant of utilization and of medical care costs.

Measures introduced to control rising costs must be carefully considered. They can have serious effects on the individual's right to health care, on access to care, on physician freedom, and the impact of health care on the people served.

Who Should Regulate Medical Care?   The regulation of medical care has focused on the issues of cost and quality control. The federal government, and perhaps the state governments, will be increasingly involved in cost control. The health professions may retain control of the quality efforts and will probably be able to reduce the need for detailed central controls if they concern themselves with issues beyond the care of the individual patient.

Another element in this complex mixture was dicussed by former Health, Education, and Welfare Secretary Elliot Richardson in his 1974 Shattuck Lecture. He stressed the need to diminish the depersonalizing and dehumanizing effects of bureaucratization by limiting the role of the federal government in any national health insurance program.[4] His solution was to provide larger roles for private insurance in underwriting and marketing, and not simply to make them agents of the federal government in the payment of bills. This approach has the strong support of the Ford Administration, the health insurance industry, the hospitals, and the medical profession. In view of this strong political support, it is highly likely that the private insurance companies will play a major role in whatever program of national health insurance is enacted. It is difficult to determine whether this will achieve the desirable objectives described by Mr. Richardson.

A FINAL NOTE.   It is not enough to establish a laudable national health policy or to enact a program of national health insurance. The means to achieve the goals in terms of financing, administration, reimbursement, and controls must be consistent with our concepts of individual freedom, autonomy, and justice.

National health insurance should become a means to increase people's freedom and autonomy. Individuals need to be given more power to control their lives. They need the financial access to medical care that national health insurance can provide, and they need greater knowledge about that care and other factors that may affect their health and well-being.

There are enormous obstacles to creating the means whereby people can share more fully in the decisions that affect their lives, including their health and well-being. The medical profession and the other health professions must share their knowledge and power with individual patients, with groups of consumers, and with the general public. National health insurance can help foster this condition and thus humanize health care, or it can create even greater bureaucratic, financial, and administrative barriers that will have the opposite effect.

The opportunity is clearly present to begin to implement humanization of health care through a program of national health insurance. To achieve this objective will require a careful consideration of the issues, not only within the context of economics and politics, but in the light of a thorough and careful consideration of justice.

NOTES

1. A. R. Jonsen and A. E. Hellegers. "Conceptual Foundations for an Ethics of Medical Care." Delivered at Conference on Human Value Issues in Health Care, Institute of Medicine, November 28-30, 1973.
2. B. Abel-Smith. "Value of Money in Health Services." *Soc Secur Bull*, vol. 37, July 1974, pp. 17-28.
3. Cf. p. "314" of this book.
4. E. L. Richardson. "Shattuck Lecture—The Old Order Changeth, Yielding Place to New." *N Engl J Med*, vol. 291, August 1974, pp. 283-287.

AUTHOR INDEX

SUBJECT INDEX